LIVE LONGER

Revealing Today's Secrets of Longevity & Wellbeing

Dr. MILEHAM HAYES
OAM, MB, BS (Qld), FRCP (Edin), FRCP (Lon).

Live Longer: Revealing Today's Secrets of Longevity & Wellbeing

ISBN: 978-0-9953996-9-3 (paperback)
978-1-7636057-0-1 (eBook)

Disclaimer
The information provided in this book is for general informational purposes only and should not be considered as personal professional advice. The content is based on research and insights that have been available up to the date of publication. Individual health needs and circumstances vary, and it is crucial to consult with qualified medical graduates for personalized advice and recommendations. Any actions taken based on the information provided in this book are at the reader's own risk.

Published in Australia by Dr Mileham Hayes and InHouse Publishing.
www.inhousepublishing.com.au

Printed in Australia by InHouse Print & Design.

InHouse PTY LTD Publishing

National Library of Australia
A catalogue record for this book is available from the National Library of Australia

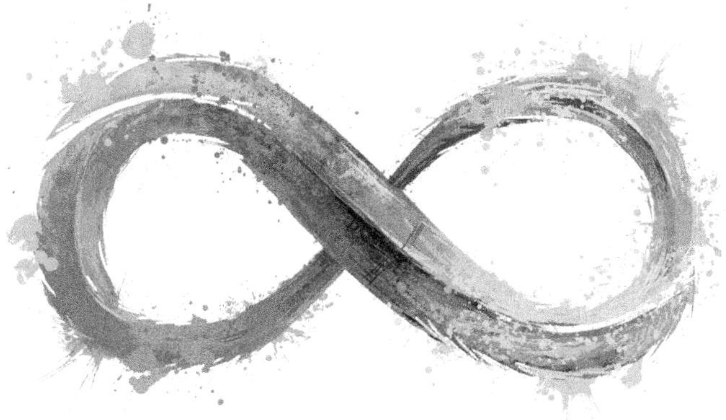

DNA and INFINITY

DNA, or deoxyribonucleic acid, is the hereditary material in humans. It is a molecule that contains the instructions an organism needs to develop, live, and reproduce. It forms a double helix.

The symbol for infinity, "the lazy eight curve", was first used in a geometry treatise in the seventeenth century. It was soon adopted to symbolize infinity and eternity in a variety of contexts.

This basis of life, the DNA double helix, with the infinity's lazy eight has been combined as *Live Longer's* logo.

Purpose and Rationale of Live Longer

Medical progress moves incredibly fast, and it seems we are on the verge of many breakthroughs on innumerable fronts. We may soon be able to modify aging, inoculate against cancer, diagnose potential illnesses with a single blood or urine sample or just retinal changes and exercise by taking a pill.

But not yet, and many will be a long way off.

Live Longer, by contrast, informs you as to what has been proven effective and what you can and should do now.

Man sacrifices his health in order to make money. Then he sacrifices money to recuperate his health. And then he is so anxious about the future that he does not enjoy the present; the result being that he does not live in the present or the future; he lives as if he is never going to die, and then dies having never really lived.

– Dalai Llama.

Author's Note

There are certainly excellent doctors who are older than I and who are still practising… but I claim to be one of the oldest who has specialised in longevity - since 1968, to be precise. Now, I am close to 84, a Superager by the diagnostic criteria, still practising, operating, writing, researching, and even typing this book, I feel I have pragmatically demonstrated "how to live longer" and pass on my experience. I do not endorse or sell any products or commercial entities but disclose what is the best information and advice from the world's best studies which have, obviously, served me well. Very well indeed.

About the Author

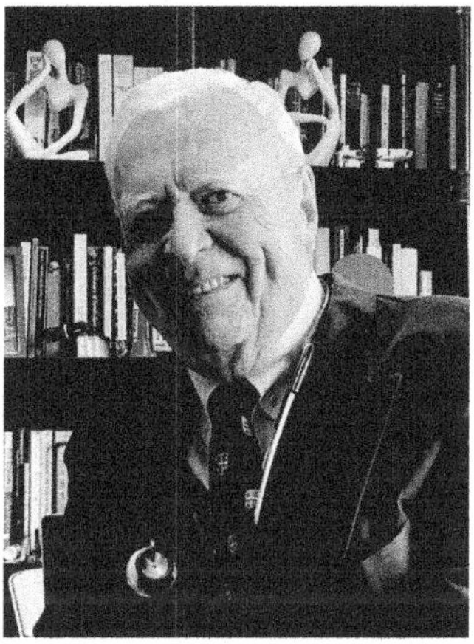

Dr **Mileham Hayes** was appointed to the world's first coronary care unit when heart disease was our greatest killer. It still is, but preventable! This stimulated his research into preventative medicine, and, as he is still working at the age of 83, he wryly notes he has "been there, done that" and is able to offer practical experience and his own evidence as to achieved functional longevity despite a rather full life. That, or as he jokes when people ask him his 'secret', "The Use-by date on his forehead is smeared".

He specialised in Internal Medicine in Edinburgh and London. On returning to Australia, he remained in private practice and has later become interested in melanoma and skin cancers, which cause many preventable deaths.

His early pursuit of preventive medicine put him ahead of the curve (some tests he used 34 years ago are just being recognised as today's preferred best) plus his years of international experience, practising clinical medicine consulting, diagnosing, and treating patients, as well as research, have provided him with a longer view than most as to what makes us healthy and live longer.

He is the author of two critically acclaimed international medical and surgical textbooks as well as health books, including Super-Newtrition. He was an internationally touring jazz musician, volunteered for Vietnam, flew with the CIA, reviewed the best restaurants in the world, writes poetry, played most sports, even playing a Wimbledon, French and USA Champion who kindly let him hit a few balls back. He has farmed, gardened, cooks (invented 'Doctor's Sauce'), loves wine, has five kids, has lived and lives life to the full, and still drives too fast. Not a good role model, and yet…

Contents

Introduction

Longevity is the new hot focus, but you can't live longer if you're dead. What if you could know these worst threats to your health right now and take instant steps to prevent them? *Live Longer* tells you how.

Live Longer has developed an arguably unique '***Predictive Analysis System***' that enables us to do so based on *proven and documented* official government health records, the world's best medical trials and studies, and the authors' over fifty years of clinical medicine.

Understanding Your Health Risks

The illnesses that are going to kill us differ for each decade or so, but also those for a woman and a man are different at the same age. So, if we know what potentially fatal illnesses are most likely to strike us *now*, at our present age, we can take immediate, sophisticated, proven preventive measures.

The Need

Overall, cardiovascular disease-heart attacks are our greatest killer and have been since the author was appointed to the world's first Coronary Care Unit (CCU) when, often at 4 am, he had to go and see the young mother with three kids clinging to her skirt to tell her that her 44-yer-old husband "didn't make it".

These terrible tragedies determined him to pursue the prevention of heart disease and other significant illnesses that kill us prematurely but which are also preventable.

The Epiphany

To do so, he researched official government records and found how some diligent public servants had documented just what illnesses kill or disable us for each decade or so and in order of precedence.

This then allowed for much more focused and targeted, age-specific, prevention tactics. However, it did not seem to be recognised until *Live Longer* developed this Predictive Analysis System.

Common Sense and Priority

This enabled him to prioritize these illnesses and address their prevention in the frequency or 'importance' they occur, which is so obvious, but no one or few seem to have done this. Crazy no!?

Priority One

According to the American Heart Association's 2024 Heart Disease and Stroke Statistics, *heart disease and stroke claimed more lives in the U.S. in 2021 than all forms of cancer and chronic lower respiratory disease combined* and also accounted for approximately 19.91 million global deaths.

This is where to start – preventing heart disease. Then, analyzing what other illnesses prematurely kill us and can be prevented and in what order.

Sensible, yes? (Then why has it not been done until now).

International Experience

This took him to Sydney, Edinburgh (where he walked the same wards that gave rise to Sherlock Holmes, a medical role model), London, San Francisco, Miami, and even Bangkok, where he slowly evolved Predictive Analysis.

Clinical Experience

This book reveals his immense hands-on, clinical, 'coalface' experience, seeing and treating patients daily, and his advice on how to live longer.

Cutting Edge

Live Longer has developed over 50 years by examining and implementing the latest medical advances. For example, the author implemented a heart blood test (ApoB) in 1990, which is only now being recognised as arguably the best test for bad cholesterol; why that's only 34 years for them to catch up—and some are still not there yet.

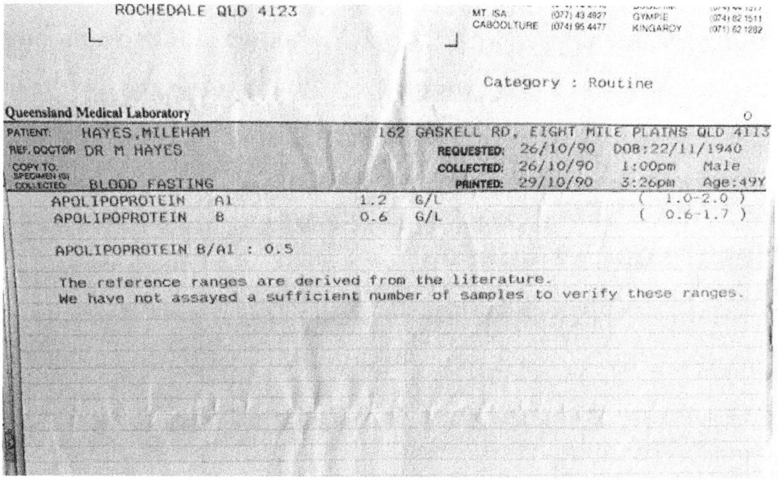
ROCHEDALE QLD 4123

MT ISA (077) 43 4927 GYMPIE (074) 82 1511
CABOOLTURE (074) 95 4477 KINGAROY (071) 62 1282

Category : Routine

Queensland Medical Laboratory

PATIENT: HAYES,MILEHAM 162 GASKELL RD, EIGHT MILE PLAINS QLD 4113
REF. DOCTOR DR M HAYES REQUESTED: 26/10/90 DOB:22/11/1940
COPY TO: COLLECTED: 26/10/90 1:00pm Male
SPECIMEN (S) COLLECTED: BLOOD FASTING PRINTED: 29/10/90 3:26pm Age:49Y

APOLIPOPROTEIN A1	1.2	G/L	(1.0-2.0)
APOLIPOPROTEIN B	0.6	G/L	(0.6-1.7)

APOLIPOPROTEIN B/A1 : 0.5

The reference ranges are derived from the literature.
We have not assayed a sufficient number of samples to verify these ranges.

Ahead of the curve: Dr Hayes did his own ApoB in 1990 but it is only now being recognised as the definitive test for damaging cholesterol…34 years later!

Research and Future Hopes

Today, there is incredible, high-grade research into 'treating' aging by hopefully slowing, stopping, and even reversing it while some people further seek immortality. But, as yet no pill, medicine, or supplement has been *proven* to do so in humans. Not one. None.

The Scammers

As well as the legitimate and brilliant medical research, while we hopefully await their outcome, the scammers, grifters, charlatans, opportunists, mountebanks, snake oil salesmen, frauds, swindlers, quacks, influencers, bloggers, longevity clinics, jade eggs, hydrogen and alkaline water, I.V vitamin drips, coffee enemas, monkey testicle transplants, life coaches, loonies, and con artists have been attracted, like bees to honey to offer the 'promise' of longevity…

Good luck!

Proven Evidence

Live Longer does not offer experimental drugs, supplements or future wishful hopes, with, as yet, unknown downstream side-effects, but rather *proven medical facts* that provide you with the correct medical information you should access to live the longest for your present age and sex.

Healthspan vs Lifespan

In addition, Healthspan has belatedly become as desirable as Lifespan. This, 'Compression of Morbidity', and successful aging (remaining fit, healthy with a good Quality of Life) are also the emphases of this book.

While achieving this for certain populations has been difficult, it is possible by employing this Predictive Analysis System.

Proof Positive

The author speaks from experience: He has achieved the stated objective; he qualifies as a "SuperAger".

Uniquely Just for You

There is a chapter dedicated just for you at your present age and for your sex and then what you should now do.

Finally

There is an Appendix: 'Medical Consultation' which recommends both the 'essential' fundamentals of what tests you should do for your age but also an addendum, of the newer experimental tests, which provides the information for you to take control of your health.

Supplementary update: Biological Age (BA)

The latest emphasis or fad is our Biological Age (BA), which is different to our Chronological Age (CA) and is defined as the age at which our overall physiology or even an individual organ, would be normal or optimal.

The inference is that our heart or other organs may be older than our chronological age, and hence, we die sooner or, if it is younger, we live longer.

BA clocks have been based on DNA methylation and many types of '-omics data', but they have been inaccurate, with different labs providing different answers.

Now, however, it would seem our biological age can be more accurately estimated with second-generation BA clocks that aim to directly predict future mortality from biological parameters. These clocks define true BA as 'Gompertz age', or the age commensurate with an individual's future risk of dying from all intrinsic causes.

In a recent 'Comprehensive Assessment of Long-term Effects of Reducing Intake of Energy (CALERIE)' study of caloric restriction[1] it is claimed, "Unlike existing clinical risk markers,

1 Fong, S., Pabis, K., Latumalea, D. *et al.* 2024, "Principal component-based clinical aging clocks identify signatures of healthy aging and targets for clinical intervention", *Nat Aging*, https://doi.org/10.1038/s43587-024-00646-8

BA clocks can identify individuals likely to remain free from age-dependent dysfunction, morbidity and mortality for years to come. BA clocks can, therefore, provide normative targets for clinical intervention and individual guidance to promote healthy aging" and further that, "Biological age (BA) is the most important risk factor determining individual risk of morbidity and mortality, with true BA of individuals generally different from chronological age (CA)".

It concludes that 2 years of mild caloric restriction significantly reduces biological age. If we can reduce our calorie intake by 12%, the CALERIE study shows that it improves our lifespan and that "Successful aging is more than the absence of specific diseases. Unlike existing clinical risk markers, Biological Age (BA) clocks can (now) identify individuals likely to remain free from age-dependent dysfunction, morbidity and mortality for years to come. BA clocks can, therefore, provide normative targets for clinical intervention and individual guidance to promote healthy aging.

Previous studies aimed for a 25% calorie reduction, which is unsustainable. This 12% reduction, however, may be attainable. That, or we will all need gastric surgery or GLP-1s.

We live in interesting times!

In the interim, *Live Longer* addresses total lifestyle improvements and those illnesses that will prematurely kill us but which we can mostly prevent. Even a young BA is not much use if we are dead from a predictable, avoidable illness.

SECTION A

WHAT IS LONGEVITY?

CHAPTER 1

What is Longevity?

"You'll live to be a hundred if you give up all the things that make you want to."

– Woody Allen

People want to live longer and healthier lives. But how many have thought this through? Is it just another 10 years, 20 years, or more?

And what, exactly, is longevity?

To cut to the chase:

The concept of longevity has been described as the ability *to live a life beyond the species-specific* *average* *age at death.*[2]

The average life expectancy in 2024 in the USA was 79.25 years. In the UK, it was 81.92, and in Australia, it was 84.06.[3]

Living longer than *the average,* however, is *not* living longer or longest, because the average is half-way between the longest and the shortest life expectancies. To live our longest lives, we must, therefore, reach or exceed this upper longest limit and not be dragged down to the average—e.g., if the average age of death is

2 De Benedictis, G. & Franceschi, C. 2006, "The Unusual Genetics of Human Longevity", *Science of Aging Knowledge Environment,* Vol. 10, No. 20.

3 macrotrends.net

80, that would mean it represents both those who lived to 90 and those who died at 70. Hence, the average does *not really* represent longevity, which would actually be living past 90.

Living longer than the average is not what we aspire to today. Today, longevity means *living longer than the upper age of death and not the average.* The longest can only be achieved by not having shortened lifespans dragging the longest one down and the shortest life spans are due to people dying prematurely.

Living longer, or longest, therefore, depends on not dying prematurely.

Definition

Longevity is not dying prematurely.

This may come as a revelation, a contradiction, or a surprise.

Yes, I had to think about it, too.

But a CDC (the American Center for Disease Control) analysis showed that Americans living in rural areas had higher rates of preventable premature mortality from the five leading causes of death than those living in urban areas during the years 2010-2022, and the divide only appears to be growing.[4]

The emphasis here, to me, are the words, ***"preventable premature mortality from the five leading causes of death".***

If then, these five leading causes of death are preventable, to me it is irrefutable logic to attend to these first, if we are to 'live longer'.

However, today, the progress of medical science, combined with the money to back it, longevity objectives are not to prevent

4 Garcia, M. C., Rossen, L. M., Matthews, K. *et al.* 2024, "Preventable premature deaths from the five leading causes of death in nonmetropolitan and metropolitan counties, United States, 2010–2022," *MMWR Surveill Summ 2024*; Vol. 73, No. SS-2, pp. 1-11, https://doi.org/10.15585/mmwr.ss7302a1.

what are prematurely killing us but to hopefully slow, stop, or even reverse aging, as well as adding on years, while some even seek immortality.

But it is difficult to live longer if you are dead.

If your premature death is prevented then these latest developments and research may be approached but, despite some brilliant research, nothing, yet, has been proven.

Preventing your premature death can be incredibly simple. Just checking and controlling your blood pressure is one of, if not '*the*', greatest cause of premature death or disability. It is a simple, painless, often free, check – just a cuff on your arm - yet most of us don't check it! Crazy, no?!

The first World Health Organization (WHO) report dedicated to hypertension indicates that four out of five patients do not receive adequate treatment.[5] Hypertension affects one in three adults worldwide, but nearly half of people with hypertension globally are currently unaware of their condition.

It has been said:

"Longevity is a side-effect of being healthy".[6]

Hold that thought. In fact, it's what this book is all about. At present, our human lifespans are finite. 80 is a reasonable expectation, 90 possible and 122 the record—held by Jeanne Louise Calment, who died on August 4, 1997.[7]

Dmitry Kaminsky, a Moldovan millionaire and longevity investor, then offered a $1 million reward for anyone who lives to 123. But despite the new, incredible longevity industry and the obsessive testing and supplementing of the biohackers, spanners,

---

5 "First WHO report details devastating impact of hypertension and ways to stop it", 19 September 2023, News release, New York.

6 Attributed to Dr. Walter M. Bortz II, a physician, author, and advocate for healthy aging.

7 Wikipedia

transhumanists (see later), and even the 'Immortalists', the reward has not been collected over 27 years later.

A 2023 Norwegian study[8] found that the typical study respondents expressed a desire to live just over 91 years and that quality of life matters just as much as—if not more than—longevity.

In surveys in August 2023 by the 'Say Forever Immortalists' in ten diverse cities such as San Francisco, Haifa, Malmö, Toronto, and São Paulo, respondents only elected their desired lifespan as between 80 and 120, while none elected for longer despite urging by the surveyors.[9]

Therefore, it would seem that 122 is the maximum achievable for humans at present.

Not dying prematurely is the only real working definition until, and if, a new one comes along.

So, I will leave all this current incredible research into mice and animal testing while I get on seeing patients and advising them how they can live longer *now, today*.

I originally wrote this last paragraph as my '*going to see patients who are trying, if not to kill themselves, certainly trying to shorten their lives,*' but my wife admonished me for being 'negative'. But I can say that very many of my patients are, in fact, shortening their lives, and I, or rather modern medicine, can help them live longer and better.

Most developed Western countries set the retirement age around the age of 65; this is also generally considered to mark the transition from middle to old age. Reaching this age is commonly a requirement to become eligible for senior social programs.

8 *Age and Aging*, Vol. 50, No. 6, November 2021, pp. 2012-2018.

9 "Silicon Valley's Quest to Live Forever Has Many Warring Factions", *Bloomberg Longevity Issue*, 19 December 2023.

Old age cannot be universally defined because it is context-sensitive. The United Nations, for example, considers old age to be 60 years or older.[10] But individuals might enter old age at different times, according to their own perceptions as in "75 is the new 65". Researchers at the Humboldt University of Berlin have discovered that we no longer consider ourselves old until we're 74. Middle-aged and older adults believe that old age begins later in life than their peers did decades ago. At age 64, the average participant said old age started at 74.7. At age 74, they said old age started at 76.8. On average, the perceived onset of old age increased by about one year for every four to five years of actual aging.[11]

The World Health Organization (WHO) defines premature death as: Unconditional probability of death between ages 30 and 70 years from cardiovascular diseases, cancer, Diabetes, and chronic respiratory diseases.

As Professor Dole, who lived to 92 and is credited for getting the world to give up smoking in 1949, observed, "Death in old age is inevitable but death before is not."[12]

And that's my message.

The average life expectancy at birth for both sexes combined has been documented above, but there is also a difference in the sexes; women live longer than men. In 2023, women's life expectancy in Australia was 85.16 years, and for men, 81.89; in

---

10 Scherbov, S. & Sanderson, W. 2019, "New Measures of Population Aging", United Nations, archived PDF from the original, retrieved 21 December 2021.

11 Wettstein, M., Park, R., Kornadt, A. E., Wurm, S., Ram, N., & Gerstorf, D. 2024, "Postponing old age: Evidence for historical change toward a later perceived onset of old age", *Psychology and Aging*, online prepublication, https://doi.org/10.1037/pag0000812.

12 Doll, R. 1912, *Journals*, 28 October, royalsocietypublishing.org

the UK, for women it was 83.97 and for men 80.61; while in the USA, for women it was 82.23 and for men 77.27 years.[13]

Other nations, such as Japan, live longer, but I have researched these three (USA, UK, Australia) as being most similar to, and applicable for, most of the developed world.

The common causes of premature deaths in the USA and applicable elsewhere, except for gunshots and fentanyl, are:[14]

- Gunshot wounds: median age at death, 28 years
- Fentanyl: 35 years
- Vehicular crashes: 40 years
- Overdose not otherwise specified (NOS): 46 years.
- Alcoholism: 57 years
- Tobacco addiction: 66 years
- Cirrhosis: 67 years
- Diabetes: 67 years
- Chronic kidney disease: 68 years
- Lung cancer: 71 years
- Cancer not specified: 73 years
- Stroke: 73 years
- Myocardial infarction: 73 years

None of these people lived past 75 years of age despite the longevity 'industry' making dubious and unproven claims. There are the many more causes of premature deaths, all of which *Live Longer* ensures are addressed and part of its essential program of prevention and 'real' longevity.

It's pretty obvious when we think about it.

If we don't know what's going to kill us, how can we prevent it?

13 "Worldometer Life Expectancy of the World Population Life expectancy at birth", data based on the latest United Nations Population Division estimates.

14 Lundberg, G. D. 2023, *Medscape,* 26 June.

But more than half of people in the U.S. (51%) do not know that heart disease is the leading cause of death in the country, according to a recent Harris Poll survey conducted on behalf of the American Heart Association in November 2023. Yet, heart disease has now been the #1 killer for more than a century, according to the 2024 Heart Disease and Stroke Statistics: A Report of U.S. and Global Data From the American Heart Association. The annual update published in *Circulation*, the peer-reviewed, flagship journal of the American Heart Association.[15]

And, to identify the elephant in the room, if you are dead, how then, in goodness name, can you hope to live long, let alone longer or longest?

So, let me run that by you again: more than half the USA, and I would think the same in most Western countries, *don't know what's going to kill them prematurely!*

Yet, 80% to 90% of what prematurely kills them can be prevented.

Even if we did live past 122, of course we would want to be illness free, mobile, financially secure. We would wish for our partner, friends, and dog to still be alive. We would want a nice house or apartment in a good neighbourhood, preferably with a garden (all of which are associated with 'real' longevity), and finally, and most importantly, we would want all our mental facilities intact.

We are being advised and informed by medical doctors, besieged by research articles and the media, inundated by the supplement suppliers, and assaulted by the scam artists touting

15 Martin, S. S., Aday, A. W., Almarzooq, Z. I., *et al.* 2024, "2024 Heart Disease and Stroke Dtatistics: A Report of US and Global Data From the American Heart Association", *Circulation*, Vol. 149, No. 8, https://doi.org/10.1161/CIR.0000000000001209.

miracle mixtures. "All you have to do is take our pill, our special 'scientifically-proven' whiz-bang supplement, our two-week starvation spa. Just send your credit card, subscribe to our newsletter, and live forever!"

This is the actual reality: There are two diets, four to six drugs, and two to three gene mutations which have increased the known usual lifespan of *mice* by some 26% or even 29%[16] and which may well do the same in humans. But, as yet, nothing has been proven for humans, despite the billions being invested.

None, not one, not any, have yet been proven to work... except for in mice, rats, fruit flies, and maybe dogs. These experimental animals, however, share similar growth genes and pathways to humans, which holds significant hope that at least two drugs may work in humans. But in the interim…

Calorie restriction (CR) works. I did have two old friends who were WW2 prisoners of war on the infamous Burma Railway, and one of my physician mentors was on the notorious Sandakan Death March (a series of forced marches in Borneo when only six survived out of 2,434 Allied prisoners of war, which is why he went into medicine). These men were reduced to skeletons—the ultimate calorie restriction—but all lived into their 90s, and I often wondered if they did not provide the human evidence to support CR. But practically, CR is unsustainable (except by reducing intake to 75% for three months as a trial).

This is not to discredit or criticise such legitimate research; one company, after all, has four Nobel Laureates. Some jellyfish and primitive marine animals are immortal. Many animals have cancer-resisting genes, and some don't get heart attacks. We hope to unlock their secrets, but while we wait, *Live Longer* urges

16 Miller, R. "Longevity Supplements – Interventions Testing Program Results", Dr. Richard Miller U-Tube.

caution and provides *proven evidence* of how you can maximise and optimise your health and longevity *immediately*.

Regarding caution, the length of our telomeres (see later) dictates our life span, so it would be reasonable to think that anything that lengthened them would prolong our life. Indeed, but it also promotes the long life of other cells—AKA cancer. So, you can see it is a delicate balance with many potential downstream effects we just don't know about.

One of my coronary care unit colleagues became a professor of epidemiology in San Francisco, then Miami. He was ahead of his time, keen on calcium and the heart and, as such, was "even then" looking at how to prevent heart disease. I visited him frequently in the 70s and 80s to get the inside scoop on the latest research to prevent heart disease. At the time, there was not much we could do other than advise on diet and prescribe drugs, such as fibrates, which had side effects. Statins to lower cholesterol had not been developed yet, so other possible causes such as calcium were being researched.

It was then called preventive medicine (PM), and despite my enthusiasm, in the early 70s, one world authority in London pointed out to me that none of the tests I was researching, such as for cholesterol, were of use. Why? As of then, there were no effective medications or treatments for the diseases these tests could unearth. The first statin, or effective cholesterol-lowering drug, was only introduced in 1987.[17]

In fact, this lack of effective treatment was arguably the stimulus causing preventive medicine to progress with the premature death, in 1945, of President Franklin Delano Roosevelt (FDR), then the most powerful man on Earth. He was widely

---

17 Endo A. 2010, "A historical perspective on the discovery of statins", *Proceedings of the Japan Academy, Series B*, Vol. 86, No. 5, pp. 484-93, https://doi.org/10.2183/pjab.86.484.

considered to be one of the most important figures in the history of the United States, as well as one of the most influential figures of the 20th century.

Today, his premature death would be preventable, He was abysmally incorrectly treated by today's standards. As it was before my time, there were no effective treatments or medications for his increasing blood pressure. I have seen his records, and they were terrifying, tragic, and his death inevitable for his time. He was treated with phenobarbital, a sedative, for goodness' sake! FDR died prematurely of a (preventable) stroke.

Despite this gloomy prospect, I persisted, stimulated by such studies as the famous Framingham Heart Study, and, in fact, I have done my 'bloods', especially cholesterol and triglycerides, every year for 55 years and have lived to see effective treatments for many, many disorders that, as for FDR, would no longer kill people prematurely. In fact, today, FDR would not even get the polio which crippled him.

Preventive medicine (PM) has never reached its promise or potential, but now I have detected a sea change wherein people actually do want to learn how to live longer and healthier. With the development of new investigations and drugs, such as those that lower cholesterol, doctors are addressing such issues. In this time, I have seen PM go from 'not much we can do' to now, when there is a great deal we can do and much more in the pipeline. Preventive medicine has rocketed ahead, and there is a great amount we can do to identify what could kill you prematurely and how we can prevent it. But you have to get the right information and be aware of the forces against you.

I hasten to say these 'forces' are not the sinister forces of evil but are often only responding to public demands, as is evident with the fast-food industry.

For one example, our affluent lifestyle now provides cheap, delicious artificial foods we can't metabolise. These foods don't provide the essential nutrients we need. But these large corporations have the money and advertising budgets to kill any legitimate voice in the wilderness—such as this.

Even still, as you will see, there are many other 'forces' after your health dollar.

I inherited the shrewd observations of my father, who graduated in medicine before there were x-rays, antibiotics, modern anaesthetics, MRIs, and such. Though he lived to use all these (he was one of the first doctors in the world to use penicillin as a major at the biggest WW2 hospital), he also knew the benefit of fresh air, fresh food, and exercise. He did give up smoking in 1947, two years before the rest of the world was persuaded to do so by Sir Robert Dole.

I was also intrigued by populations who reputedly lived longer than most. These were later identified by Dan Buettner as 'The Blue Zones'. What was, or is, their secret? *Live Longer* examines this, too.

Unfortunately, as will be seen, observations or associations do not confirm or prove causation, and this is the big bugbear for longevity studies. The classic was when Caesar drained Rome's Pontine Marshes, as it was thought it was the fog which caused malaria. It worked! No fog, no malaria! Ah yes, but this was association and not the real mosquito parasite cause.

The main problem with diet and health studies, unless they are to test new drugs, is that there is no way to harness 10,000 people, divide them in two, and strictly monitor their different diets or habits to see which group lives longer (Framingham and North Karelia may be the exceptions).

Nevertheless, some observations and associations are pretty obviously beneficial.

John Rowe and Robert Kahn (1987) conceptualized the successful aging model, advocating views of "better than average" aging as a combination of three components: avoiding disease and disability, maintaining high cognitive and physical function, and keeping engagement with life.[18]

Their model solidified a major turning point in gerontology (the scientific study of old age, the process of aging, and the particular problems of old people) and offered views of elders as able, valuable societal members who benefited from engaging lives. Many of the studies that followed required that individuals have great physical health and good memory and cognitive performance, but they rarely paired both cognitive performance and physical performance together.

Successful Aging Concepts

Successful aging includes longevity but also requires optimising cognitive physical, social, spiritual, emotional, and economic parameters, while considering quality of life (QOL) and the capacity to cope with change. There's not much use living past 122 years, with no friends, no money, no wits, no 'nuthin'.

Factors people defined as necessary for successful aging included:[19]

1. Health
2. Psychological factors
3. Social roles and activities
4. Finances
5. Social relationships
6. Neighbourhood

---

18 Rowe, J. W. & Kahn, R. L. 1997, "Successful Aging", *The Gerontologist*, Vol. 37, No. 4, pp. 433-440, https://doi.org/10.1093/geront/37.4.433.

19 Bowling, A. & Dieppe, P. 2005, "What is successful aging and who should define it?", *BMJ*, Vol. 331, No. 7531, pp. 1548-1551, https://doi.org/10.1136/bmj.331.7531.1548.

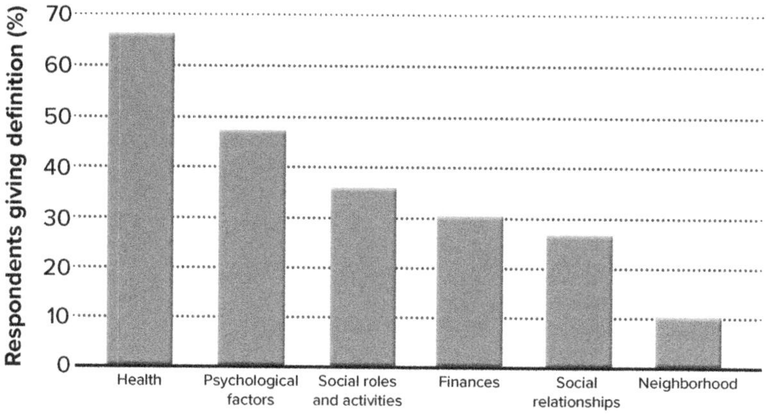

Figure 1: Most common definitions of successful ageing given by 854 people aged ≥50 in Britain.

As the graph shows, our health is number one, by a long way, and I guess the psychological factors could also be amalgamated, making health, by far and away, even more our greatest concern.

What to Address First

While we are slurping our super-supplements at the gym, what are the real percentages of health issues adults found most important for the U.S. as of 2019 and 2023?[20]

To inject common sense, don't you think we should address these concerns first—in the order they are most likely to affect us and the order in which we can prevent them? Rather than test for some non-agreed biomarkers and take some unproven supplements, shouldn't we take verifiable action?

Eternal Youth

The wish for eternal youth is as old as humanity—just check-out the Greek myths. The difference today is the incredible advances

20 Vankar, P. 2023, "Most important health issues facing the U.S. according to U.S. adults", *Statistica*, 1 June.

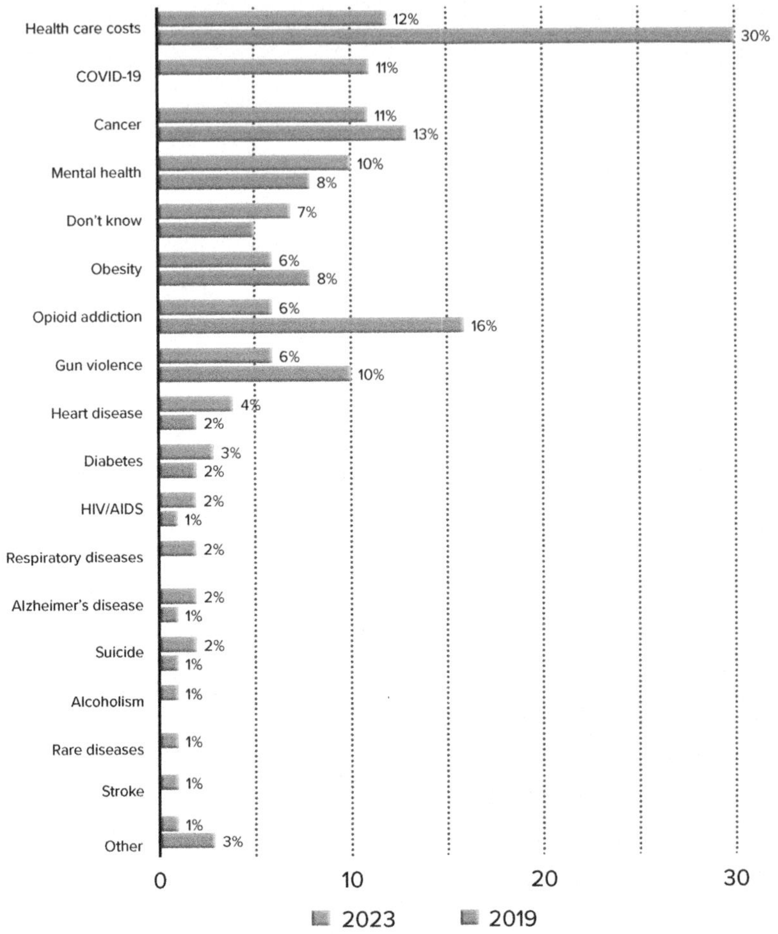

Figure 2: Most important health issues facing U.S. adults in 2019 and 2023.

in medicine and science, and the money to back them, have made the allure of eternal youth feel closer than ever.

Today, many of the richest people on the planet believe aging can be slowed, stopped, cured, and even reversed. These people are investing billions. The global longevity and anti-senescence therapy market was valued at $25.1 billion in 2020 and is projected to reach $44.2 billion by 2030, growing at a CAGR of 6.1% from 2021 to 2030.[21]

21 Allied Market Research, March 2022.

But Are We Living Too Long?

UK data shows, on average, women are ill for the last 19 years of life, while for men, it's around 16 years.[22]

Are we going to live longer as cancer-cardiac cripples with addled minds, alone in a nursing home, eating splodge denuded of all nutrition?

Even then, there are six conditions patients regard as worse than death and four more that were rated as "somewhat better than death" (?!)—these are listed later.

One prominent doctor who was an advisor to President Obama, doesn't want to live past 75 or will, at least, refuse treatment for serious illnesses after that time—we will talk about him later.

To live longer thus means being healthy rather than simply being alive. This introduces the concepts of lifespan vs healthspan and compression of morbidity.

So, is there a way to live longer, and well, and healthy... and happy?

Staying Healthy

While sometimes unavoidable, it is very preferable for you to avoid the hospital and illnesses (the whole purpose of this book). While modern medicine has made incredible progress, there are still many missed and mis-diagnoses, leading to patient deaths or disabilities as per the Johns Hopkins Armstrong Institute Center for Diagnostic Excellence, which found in a new analysis of national data that across all clinical settings, including hospital and clinic-based care, an estimated 795,000 Americans die or are permanently disabled by diagnostic error each year.[23]

---

22 https://www.kingsfund.org.uk

23 Newman-Toker, D. E., Nassery, N., Schaffer, A. C., *et al.* 2024, "Burden of serious harms from diagnostic error in the USA", *BMJ Quality & Safety*, Vol. 33, pp. 109-120.

These figures can be extrapolated to all first world countries, which means you could have a more than 10% chance of being mucked up. But this has also been reviewed elsewhere wrt medications (see later – Ch. 2 Prescribed Drugs).

In other research I did, I found medications were the sixth greatest cause of premature deaths.

Avoiding Premature Death

If you do really want to live longer, this is how to go about it and why I developed *Live Longer*.

This must now be our number one priority. And again, to be logical, we should seek the illness that mostly kills us and then investigate how to prevent it.

The above list (the illnesses we fear most in 2023), is however, *not* what is going to kill *you* this year.

To actually find out, the *Live Longer* program has been created from accessing new official data so you can find out what specific illness or activity is most likely to kill *you*, *this year, for your age and sex.*

Hence, you can now take *immediate preventive measures* and maximize your chances to live longer and well and happy.

An article in the *New York Times* in 2023,[24] "Suddenly, It Looks Like We're in a Golden Age for Medicine", pointed out how "we may be on the cusp of an era of astonishing innovation—the limits of which aren't even clear yet," and expands on the exciting potential developments.

But these 'astonishing innovations' are sometime in the future, if ever (but I do think some are inevitable).

Age, it has been observed, remains the biggest threat to our health. It was, in fact, listed, in its own right for the first time, by the World Health Organization in 2018, as a condition in

24 *New York Times*, 23 June 2023.

its International Classification of Diseases.[25] As a result, we are being bombarded by pills, the latest favourites are metformin and rapamycin (addressed in detail later), potions, supplements, dubious 'treatments', wellness centres, stem cells, plasma transfusions (parabiosis), and even the macabre act of freezing your detached head.

The 10th Aging Research and Drug Discovery (ARDD) conference, a five-day non-profit event organized by the University of Copenhagen was held in September 2023, while the first Longevity Med Summit was in Cascais Portugal, in May 2023.

Longevity clinics are popping up like mushrooms in New York, London, and Melbourne. I assume the same is true for the rest of the developed world.

However, a recent study found "three approaches with a reputation for slowing aging processes have proven largely ineffective".[26]

One of them is *intermittent fasting*, in which the calories consumed are reduced. Number two targets a central node of cell metabolism (mTOR), which is also the target of the supposed "anti-aging drug" *rapamycin*. Number three, in turn, interferes with the release of *growth hormone*. Similar treatments are also used by humans, although their efficacy with regard to aging has not been sufficiently proven.[27]

Regarding diet, humans are opportunistic omnivores, and a little meat is beneficial, but 'the world's best diet' is at the end of the book (it's vegan-friendly, too).

---

25 The WHO has formally recognized aging as a disease in its latest version of the International Classification of Diseases (ICD-11),14 February 2022.

26 Xie, K., Fuchs, H., Scifo, E. *et al.* 2022, "Deep phenotyping and lifetime trajectories reveal limited effects of longevity regulators on the aging process in C57BL/6J mice", *Nature Communications*, Vol. 13, No. 6830, https://doi.org/10.1038/s41467-022-34515-y

27 *Ibid.*

As for exercise, while it is arguably the best investment we can make for our health, we should 'go gently', avoiding long-term damage and consequences. All the world champion athletes I know have had hip replacements. They ran miles and miles and hours and hours every day, and the wear and tear on their hip joints must have been incredible. But, in 2013, a Norwegian group found their data suggested that a single bout of four minutes of AIT (Aerobic Interval Training) performed three times per week may be a time-efficient strategy to improve VO_2max and reduce blood pressure and fasting glucose levels in previously inactive but otherwise healthy middle-aged individuals.[28]

And so it is that *Live Longer* certainly explores all that is new but does not push the unknown boundaries and concentrates on what is known, what has been proven, and what can actually be achieved.

And a hell of a lot can be done, elegantly and simply, to ensure we live longer.

While there have been no major new breakthroughs, relatively young individuals are eagerly submitting themselves to extreme regimes in unproven hope. One 46-year-old man, Bryan Johnson, as detailed later, is spending $2 million a year trying to live longer (he found his son's plasma transfusions have not helped) and boasts he is the most tested man in the world, which I do not doubt.[29]

---

28 Tjønna, A. E., Leinan, I. M., Bartnes, A. T., *et al.* 2013, "Low- and high-volume of intensive endurance training significantly improves maximal oxygen uptake after 10-weeks of training in healthy men", *PLoS One*, 29 May, https://doi.org/10.1371/journal.pone.0065382.

29 "The Man Who Thinks He Can Live Forever", 2023, *Time Magazine*, https://time.com, 20 September.

Unproven Hopes

I have pursued and researched the actual evidence as to what can make us live longer. The new promised pills, supplements, and innovations *may* be developed... but not yet. Nothing is proven.

While medicine often moves at a dazzling pace, the human body is incredibly complex. We have just witnessed the 100-year anniversary of the discovery of insulin, yet in these 100 years, there have been no real advances in treating diabetes 1. All that has happened is that the insulin is purer, the blood glucose reading is more elegant, and the delivery systems are more sophisticated. But in 100 years, no actual significant advance has been made.

Delaying aging treatments will undoubtedly occur, but one would think that curing diabetes is a lot simpler than 'treating' or delaying aging.

What, then, if anything, is actually ***proven*** to let us live longer? What are the latest advances? Can we live longer, and if so, how is it possible? Is it practical? And is it worth it? Or are we, in fact, living too long? *Live Longer* provides evidence-based and proven ways to optimize our health and longevity now. Its exclusive Predictive Analysis Program helps you avoid the illnesses that kill us prematurely and how to adopt the best lifestyle to remain healthy as long as possible.

It has worked for me despite my being a bad patient.

Here, I must add that I wished I had known all this when I was younger in that I would have adopted a Mediterranean Diet and EVOO a lot sooner instead of the heavy red meat diet I was brought up on, even creating my meat sauce based on cream! And I would have eaten a great deal more fruit and vegetables, which is why I say I was a bad patient. That, and too many late nights and long hours. Be that as it may, the fundamentals as espoused here in *Live Longer*, nevertheless, have obviously kicked in to protect me such that I am still with it, working and apparently qualifying to be a 'SuperAger'. So, it's not too late for you too.

It's not much use if you can complete a triathlon, eat a plant-based diet, earn a $million – only to die prematurely.

CHAPTER 2

Factors Affecting Our Health and Longevity

"If I had known I was going to live so long,
I'd have taken better care of myself."

– Billy Noonan

Sometimes attributed to Eubie Blake who wrote
'Memories of You' and died aged 96.

Do You Want to Live 12 Years Longer Starting Today? Yes, *Today*!

A study in the prestigious medical journal *Circulation*[30] revealed how 'simple' lifestyle behaviour modifications can extend our lives by more than a decade.

Researchers found that people who, at age 50, were practicing ***five healthy habits*** added between 12 and 14 years to their lives.

30 Li, Y., Pan, A., Wang, D. D. *et al.* 2018, "Impact of Healthy Lifestyle Factors on Life Expectancies in the US Population", *Circulation*, Vol. 138, No. 4, pp. 345-355, https://doi.org/10.1161/CIRCULATIONAHA.117.032047.

These habits are:

1. exercising regularly
2. eating healthy
3. not smoking
4. maintaining healthy weight
5. not drinking excessive alcohol

These recommended healthy habits may seem too simple, too pathetic when we want to take a super-supplement, consume metformin or rapamycin, run an ultra-marathon, do powerlifting, and get a life coach. But apart from the exercise, none of these can or will offer you a decade more of life at the moment.

Don't disparage the five healthy habits.

It has been found that, to achieve such lifestyle changes, we must enforce small, acceptable changes or mini steps. But, if you smoke, I urge you to quit cold turkey, without vaping.

But apparently, we have other, more immediate, concerns than living longer.

Health Concerns for 2023: *The Forbes Health/ One Poll survey*[31]

- Improved mental health (45%)
- Improved fitness (39%)
- Lose weight (37%)
- Improved diet (33%)
- Improved finances (30%)

As part of addressing our immediate concerns, longevity clinics have erupted, offering ETK—Every Test Known. These include our biological age, whole body MRIs, life coaches, psych

31 Forbes Health/One Poll survey of 1,005 U.S. adults conducted 18-22 November 2022.

Table 1: The Forbes Health/One Poll survey.

Which health concerns are you worried about?	**USA**	**Canada**	**Australia**
The risk of someone I care about falling ill with a serious illness	38.1%	45.7%	49.2
The risk of someone I care about being diagnosed with cancer	39.4%	44.1%	48.5%
The risk of being diagnosed with cancer	41.6%	44.4%	48.1%
The risk of falling ill with some other serious disease	37.5%	41.3%	42.1%
The risk of significant physical injury to someone I care about	37.8%	34.4%	38.7%
Long waiting lists for surgical/medical appointments	14.3%	36.2%	36.9%
My stress levels impacting my health	29.8%	34.3%	36.8%
The risk of significant physical injury to myself	35.2%	31.7%	34.5%
Not being able to afford the healthcare I need	22.8%	23.9%	32.6%
None of the above	18.8%	12.3%	12.8%

support, pampering, antioxidants, supplements, vitamins, jade eggs, alkaline spiritual water, influencers, spanners, loonies, and anything other than these five ostensibly simple, but medically proven, pieces of advice.

The five healthy habits listed at the outset, even though they will increase our lives by more than anything else, are now seen as too simple, too easy, too pathetic.

But they are not.

The research into extending, pausing or reversing aging is dazzling, exciting, incredible, and of high quality, with billions invested and new discoveries made almost every day. It would seem interference, manipulation, and alteration of our genes and metabolic or aging pathways is extremely promising and inevitable, but given the incredible complexities, they are a long way off. And, sad to say, there are absolutely no new breakthroughs for humans at present.

> ***Live Longer*, therefore, addresses what is known, safe, and proven to maximise our human longevity *now*.**

When I studied for what were considered the world's toughest exams (for the Royal College of Physicians in Edinburgh and London), the competition was intense, with selected doctors from all around the globe and then an exam every year for three years with a 10% pass rate. I went to bed at 4 am, but the Hong Kong doctors' lights in the room opposite were always still on.

And so, I developed a plan. I allocated my study time in direct proportion to the number of pages apportioned to each disease in my two major textbooks (both American, Cecil and Loeb and Harrison). I then duplicated my study time accordingly in proportion; if cardiovascular disease took 40% of their books, I gave it 40% of my study time. If another disease took 10% of its contents, I gave it 10% of my time, as I figured Drs. Cecil, Loeb, Harrison, and their illustrious contributors were no fools.

I didn't spend much time at all on the fish that swam up the male urethra in Thailand, the toxicity of the Ackee plant in Jamaica, or the nutritional value of the mushroom (all of which I was later examined on!).

But my plan worked. My examiners were no fools, either, and it has stood me and my patients in good stead. Over 50 years ago, I prioritized the importance of our illnesses, determining which were the most relevant i.e., which were going to kill us and in what order and in what order and then how to prevent them.

This is my proven path to living longer by researching the illnesses and prioritizing them in the order that affects us most. But, in addition, I consider what can be prevented and how by researching what occurs at your present age (as it's pretty obvious what is most likely to kill a 30-year-old man is different from that for a 65-year-old woman).

I would add that I did have a great doctor friend in Bangkok, but I only swam in the pool at the British Club, and my sister practised in Jamaica where her husband had the leading article in the New England Medical Journal—The Seablue Histiocyte—before moving to Albany and Seattle, and I do recommend mushrooms for their vitamin D, fiber, and as a good source of ergothioneine, which is linked to lower triglyceride levels and may help prevent the formation of arterial plaque. But this is trivia, whereas *Live Longer* concentrates on the big issues that will do more than anything else to help us live longer.

Being appointed to the world's first coronary care unit was, undoubtedly, the stimulus for my passion for preventing illnesses. Heart attacks and cardiovascular disease were our greatest killers, and I saw, even then, that this could, and *should*, be prevented.

Then, as noted, much more complete official government records became available, which provided prioritized lists *specific to our present ages*.

The next step was to provide what essential investigations and tests to get (those proven as to best diagnose these illnesses) and to advise what can be done to prevent them.

This onslaught of new tests has been a challenge. Which, if any, should I list? Which should I ignore? I agonized over this, and my solution is to also list the names of the doctors and researchers who list their new recommendations for you to access their websites or YouTube lectures to accept or reject. I detail them later.

What Affects Our Longevity?

Established Criteria

1. Genetics
2. Age
3. Nutrition—the food we eat
4. Weight
5. Hygiene—mainly a clean water supply
6. Environment—where we live and air pollution
7. Medical markers—especially weight, blood pressure, lipids, blood, and biochemical profile
8. Exercise
9. Mental status—personality, lack of stress, happiness, Alzheimer's
10. Skin
11. High-risk behaviors

New Criteria- Live Longer

1. Illnesses specific to age and sex

Established Criteria

1. Genetics

We can't alter our genetics (at present), but many inherited, genetic or chronic problems such as Diabetes 1, Coeliac Disease, and other autoimmune illnesses can be dramatically ameliorated today with the advances in medicine.

2. Age

Age is the greatest risk factor for our health.

Atrial fibrillation, where the heart beats rapidly, is now an age-related epidemic, along with osteoarthritis, reduced eyesight, and poorer dentition. While these conditions may be obvious, less obvious ones, such as reduced hearing, can be part of increased social isolation, which contributes to premature demise.

One of the great tragedies I encounter almost daily is patients who simply have never addressed these inevitable age changes and are bewildered and devastated when illness strikes, or their spouse dies. To live past 75, you should plan your old age now. And not just you; think about what your spouse will do if you depart. The key to this, after coping with the grief, is social integration and mobilization—friends, clubs, and hobbies are absolutely essential. If you are under 50, this may seem all too far away. It is tragic when those in their 70s and older just won't face it and plan accordingly. Then, the survivor often becomes a recluse with an ever-accelerating downward spiral as to their own personal care and health.

3. Nutrition—the food we eat

A global survey concluded that, "Poor diet is consistently responsible for more disease and death than physical inactivity, smoking and alcohol combined."[32]

Higher diet quality scores have been consistently associated with a lower risk of mortality. All-cause mortality was reportedly reduced by 11–42%, cardiovascular disease mortality by 17–60%, and cancer mortality by 11–40% in individuals within the highest category of scores of diet quality compared to individuals within the lowest category.[33] Fresh fruit and vegetables may

32 "Global Burden of Diseases, Injuries, and Risk Factors Study 2013", *The Lancet*, 22 July 2014.

33 Jackson, J. K., MacDonald-Wicks, L. K., McEvoy, M. A. *et al.* 2020, "Better diet quality scores are associated with a lower risk of hypertension and non-fatal CVD in middle-aged Australian women over 15 years of follow-up", *Public Health Nutrition*, Vol. 23, No. 5, pp. 882-893, https://doi.org/10.1017/S1368980019002842.

initially cost more than processed junk, but as you can see, they pay off in the long-term.

Recently, I examined a not overweight gas station attendant who, like most of us today, is working longer harder and feels "too tired" to cook when he gets home at night. Instead, he fills up on the processed food at his Servo—sausage rolls, with their high saturated fat pastry and dubious contents, were his nominated favourite. He may not be overweight now, but our modern lifestyle and access to prepared processed, cheap, and delicious food does not augur well for his future.

When I ran through my advice, he agreed it was good and he liked it... but would never do it. The processed food was simply too easy and convenient. At least he was a realist and not blaming anyone else.

You will have to make an effort, which is why this book is for the motivated individual. The government is not going to home-deliver healthy food to you, do your exercise, or organize the other proven preventive health measures you need.

I have written a book I titled *Super-Newtrition* (being revised) that was initially stimulated by the famous studies of Ancel Keys who promoted the Mediterranean Diet, the North Karelia Project (see later), and a study by Professor De Logeril in 1994, in the fine food capital of the world, Lyon (yes, I dined at Paul Bocuse's Restaurant twice, and he kindly signed my menu, now on our dining room wall).

de Logeril swapped half his post-heart-attack patients to an essentially Mediterranean diet, and they lived while the others who ate as before didn't do so well.[34] It became my benchmark

---

34 de Lorgeril, M., Renaud, S., Mamelle, N. *et al.* 1994, "Mediterranean alpha-linolenic acid-rich diet in secondary prevention of coronary heart disease", *Lancet,* Vol. 343, No. 8911, pp. 1454-1459, https://doi.org/10.1016/s0140-6736(94)92580-1; erratum in *Lancet,* 1995, Vol. 345, No. 8951, p. 738.

model, I adopted it, and all my patients were given handouts based on it. That was 30 years ago. Since then, I have done a great deal of research to tweak, and based on the reports, improve this diet, which resulted in my *Super-Newtrition* book (as outlined at the end of this book).

But they asked for more and more information, and I became intrigued with what foods were beneficial and why. We all know about vitamins, but there are only 13, whereas I found there are in excess of 5,000 micronutrients which do seem to confer benefits.

4. Weight

Losing weight is the hardest thing we can do in an affluent society with delicious junk food, researched and developed to make you want more, advertised and available in excess 24 hours a day, seven days a week, and home delivered. Most, in fact all, fad diets don't work long-term. Long-term sustenance of lost weight is challenging, and weight regain is typical. In a meta-analysis of 29 long-term weight loss studies, more than half of the lost weight was regained within two years, and by five years more than 80% of lost weight was regained. Indeed, previous failed attempts at achieving durable weight loss may have contributed to the recent decrease in the percentage of people with obesity who are trying to lose weight and many now believe that weight loss is a futile endeavour.[35] Some think only 5% to 10% lose weight long term.

The New Weight Control Drugs

The development of the glucagon-like peptide-1 (GLP-1) receptor agonists would seem to promise significant weight loss for those who cannot otherwise reduce their intake (like the 95%

35 Hall, K. D. & Kahan, S. 2018, "Maintenance of Lost Weight and Long-Term Management of Obesity", *Medical Clinics of North America*, Vol. 102, No. 1, pp. 183-197, https://doi.org/10.1016/j.mcna.2017.08.012.

of us). With the injected drug, tirzepatide, approved in the U.S. in May 2022 to treat Diabetes and sold as Mounjaro, nearly 29% of those taking the drug lost at least a quarter of their body weight, compared with just over 1% of those taking a placebo, which is higher than the results for semaglutide (Wegovy/Ozempic) and similar to the results seen with bariatric surgery.[36] It's early days, but here's hoping not only do they lose the weight but also improve their heart risk profiles. After that, there is Gastric Banding or Sleeves, and the patients in my practice are very happy with the results.

The 'Obesity Paradox', i.e., a positive relationship between obesity and mortality, is a fable: for each five-unit increase in BMI above 25 kg/m2, the corresponding increases in risk were 49% for cardiovascular mortality, 38% for respiratory disease mortality, and 19% for cancer mortality. The hazards of excess body weight were greater in younger than in older people and in men than in women.[37]

Note: As I wrote years ago, BMI is not a good measure as detailed in the exercise chapter.

The Waist-Hip Ratio (WHR)

WHR is better than the BMI but has some inherent problems—mainly in that a young person may have a BMI of 24 with a waist of 80cm and hips of 100cm, giving a WHR of 0.80. But then they put on weight over the next decade, and their waist is now 100cm and their hips are 125cm, so their BMI is 35 and they are obese, but their WHR is still only 0.80.

---

36 Lin, F., Yu, B., Ling, B. *et al.* 2023, "Weight loss efficiency and safety of tirzepatide: A Systematic review", *PLoS One*, Vol. 18, No. 5, https://doi.org/10.1371/journal.pone.0285197.

37 Global BMI Mortality Collaboration, 2016, "Body-mass index and all-cause mortality: individual-participant-data meta-analysis of 239 prospective studies in four continents", *Lancet*, Vol. 388, No. 10046, pp. 776-86, https://doi.org/10.1016/S0140-6736(16)30175-1.

Waist Circumference (WC)

Just the waist circumference is good. The 'recommended' measurements are: for men, a waist circumference below 94cm (37in) is 'low risk', 94–102cm (37-40in) is 'high risk', and more than 102cm (40in) is 'very high'. For women, below 80cm (31.5in) is low risk, 80–88cm (31.5-34.6in) is high risk, and more than 88cm (34.6in) is very high.

But these are not specific enough, as they infer a person of six feet should have the same waist size as a five-footer. My gut (pun intended) recommendations for tall people are:

- Men: < 104cm ~ 41inches
- Women: < 90cm—certainly < 95cm (35.5 - 37.5")

Waist measurements over the above figures reflect a direct correlation with the deposition of (injurious) intra-abdominal/ visceral fat.

Slight reductions result in improvements in several cardiovascular risk factors.

A recent study[38] reports that women over the age of 60 who maintained a stable weight were more likely to experience what the authors referred to as exceptional longevity (living to the age of 90 or older). For the study, weight stability was considered as not altering more than 5% from baseline weight.

5. *Hygiene*

Forgive me, but I do rant on here a bit. This is because I was brought up in a household wherein my father had graduated in medicine before antibiotics, and so basic hygiene was the routine.

---

38 Shadyab, A. H., Manson, J. E., Allison, M. A. *et al.* 2023, "Association of Later-Life Weight Changes With Survival to Ages 90, 95, and 100: The Women's Health Initiative", *The Journals of Gerontology: Series A*, Vol. 78, No. 12, pp. 2264-2273, https://doi.org/10.1093/gerona/glad177.

Today, however, this routine has lapsed, as we think antibiotics will fix us when hygiene may well have prevented us from becoming ill.

Hygiene is mainly the province of public health/ government authorities and requires a clean water supply, a good sewerage system, and cleanliness in food processing plants and restaurants. However, recent epidemics such as Ebola and bird flu demonstrated the need for personal improvements. The introduction of antibiotics has made us all blasé. We now feel disdain for illnesses that struck terror into the population prior to the introduction of antibiotics in the mid-1930s; now, we don't wash our hands (even doctors), and we cough and sneeze over all and sundry, thus spreading the flu and respiratory infections. There are, however, many everyday behaviours that can better protect us.

COVID-19, however, has made us more aware. Such viruses are airborne and can drift and infiltrate everywhere, contaminating surfaces and our hands. When I first started practising in 1969 (yes, electricity had been invented), I had a discrete fan between the patient and me to blow their germs away from me, and I still do!

I also use alcohol-based hand wash between every patient and nitrile gloves for examinations, as a courtesy to them and a protectant for both of us.

We cannot live our lives in a sterile bubble, and it is thought that exposure to germs stimulates our 'natural resistance', or our immune system. That said, I am appalled at the general lack of knowledge and, therefore, practice of basic hygiene, which must invariably lead to more infections, illnesses, and reduced longevity. A recent survey of 2,200 UK residents found almost one in ten people wash their towels twice a year only. Five per cent of men admitted to washing them just once a year compared to 1 % of women. The study found that 11 per cent of respondents weren't concerned at all by bacteria or hygiene issues, despite the NHS' advice that towels can spread germs if not washed frequently.[39] Fomites are objects or materials that are likely to carry infection, such as clothes, utensils, and furniture. Germs breed in and on such fomites. As such, Doctors' ties were banned in UK hospitals.

My father banned tea towels as being 'filthy'. He was right, and we stacked and air-dried our washing up. Today's dishwashers and paper towels have replaced most tea towels.

The men who don't wash their towels, of course, are the minority extreme, but they do reflect how some elements of society are almost totally ignorant of basic hygiene. Sadly, this also extends to nutrition, exercise, and most basic, healthy lifestyles.

As an aside, some 20 years ago, I approached the top politician who governed the state I live in to urge that nutrition and sun-smart awareness be introduced into our schools. She had been a teacher and surrounded herself with 'advisors' who were also teachers and who, I got the distinct message, only saw this as 'more work for them'. It went nowhere. Later, an old friend who was the top state public servant laughed, assuring me how naive I had been, saying, 'The politician will only do what benefits them and if they can claim ownership and credit'.

COVID-19 woke us up or should have, regarding the airborne and fomite transmission of germs, but even so, I have patients who don't cover their mouths when they sneeze or cough—and sometimes straight at me—whose fingernails and hands and whole demeanour and clothes are dirty. Even people who are 'dressed up to the nines' when stripped off have fungal infections under their unkempt toenails and such. The conclusion I draw is that if they can't address this, then what is the rest of their hygiene like? Not good, I guarantee.

39 *Daily Mail,* 5 January 2024

Another colleague eschewed baths as 'lying in one's perianal excretions', and his observation is hard to refute.

Hidden cameras found doctors in UK hospitals were not washing their hands frequently enough, and I would think the same is true elsewhere.

As said, I now wear nitrile gloves to examine patients and use an alcohol-based hand rub between every patient contact. Even at home, pump containers are scattered strategically all around our house. Still, I use the back of my hand to depress the pump and my knuckle for the toilet cistern. If I have to use a public toilet, I wait until someone else opens the door so I don't have to touch the knob(s). And a recent UK survey (*London Telegraph,* 30 April 2024) of three Lanarkshire Hospitals in Scotland found men's lavatory door handles had eight times the germs of the women's and unisex were the dirtiest of all.

An English doctor in Bangkok taught me the best analogy for germ transmission. He used to tell his patients to imagine their hands were covered in a red dye representing germs. If they went to wash their hands, the dye would first be transferred onto the bathroom doorknob, then the tap knob, then even the soap. While their hands may have then been washed, they then pick the germs up again, turning off the tap and transferring them to contaminate the hand towel. This is why operating theatres have elbow taps and elbow press alcohol-based hand-wash—and even then, two minutes of systematic, ritual washing is the minimum.

Obviously, doctors should be aware of all this, but in my experience, the most meticulous are those with the more potentially serious infections, such as cardiac or orthopaedic surgeons.

Wound infections (in patients) should not exceed 2%, and I can't remember the last one I had, whereas at a clinic where I worked, one doctor had so many I had to leave as that clinic wouldn't address this obvious problem.

As noted, these hygiene procedures should be a basic, unthinking ritual and routine. Shower every day, inspect your nails, groin, skin, and brush your teeth, especially gum/gingival margins, twice a day. Very few patients have to strip off to their underwear as mine do and, as such, I am appalled as to many smartly dressed who have badly looked after feet. It's kinda my criteria now (as to how well people are looking after themselves – the "Heel Sign".)

Spring cleaning should not wait until spring. My wife and I are dismayed at the lack of basic housekeeping, and any new staff we employ must be shown how to do it.

As I said, this may sound precious and pedantic, but it served my father's family, and now my family, better than most.

The Aggregation of Marginal Gains

The British Cycling Team had never won a major event in some 100 years until their new coach, Dave Brailsford, coined this phrase and, in 2003, set about addressing what most of us neglect. As well as caring for the minute gear and equipment changes, he hired a surgeon to teach his team how to wash their hands properly; he selected the best pillow and mattress for each rider and painted the inside of the team truck white to spot dust.

These, and hundreds of other, small improvements added up to a significant increase in their performance.

Within five years of implementing this strategy, the British Cycling Team won 60 percent of the gold medals at the 2008 Olympic Games in Beijing and seven world records at the 2012 Olympic Games in London. They also won the Tour de France five times between 2012 and 2017.

I cite this as the need to address the basics of our lifestyle and health practices that we dismiss while we frantically search for unproven supplements, diets, biomarkers, fads, and self-help podcasts when practising basic hygiene—a clean home, fresh air, basic tests such as blood pressure, ApoB, eating a variety of basic fresh produce, minimisation of intake of known 'toxins' such as pollution, stress, smoking, drugs (including prescription), alcohol, and high-risk behaviours—has been proven to help us.

These habits are not as groovy as having your serum-uranium and kryptonite biomarker taken by your new laboratory and health coach podcaster, who will then sell you the unproven supplements that differ for each laboratory or guru, but they have been *proven* to enhance health and longevity.

Sadly, the conmen, mountebanks, supplement scientists, et al. have all the keywords, PR, and guff to make hygiene sound too simplistic. On their path to immortality, they sell you more tests, more supplements, and more courses—but getting you to wash your hands and avoid people coughing and sneezing at you just isn't groovy or profitable.

So often, we overestimate the importance of making big, drastic changes, while underestimating the impact of small, daily tweaks.

6. Environment—where we live

Western societies with 24-hour availability of junk food have seen the development of the "Diseases of Affluence", viz: heart disease, strokes, hypertension, peripheral vascular disease, hyperlipidaemia and obesity, with the resulting downstream conditions of Diabetes type 2, depression, certain forms of cancer, auto immune disease, arthritis, asthma, alcoholism, and possibly a range of other psychiatric illnesses.

Polluted air is linked to 1.6 million deaths a year in China;[40] Air pollution has now been found to cause up to 30%

40 Rohde, R. A. & Muller, R. A. 2015, "Air Pollution in China: Mapping of Concentrations and Sources", *PLOS ONE*, Vol. 10, No. 8, https://doi.org/10.1371/journal.pone.0135749.

of strokes.[41] The pollution from car fumes, especially diesel, in cities is well known. Sitting in traffic immediately behind the car in front's exhaust is the worst—so close all vents. A screen of trees can prevent the exhaust from intruding into our homes.

No matter where we live, there are some 80,000(+) untested chemicals, invented since WW2, in our water and food containers, and we all now contain microplastics.[42]

7. Medical markers

Weight, blood pressure, blood glucose, lipids, and blood and biochemical profiles are fundamental. Hand-in-hand with these are the newer investigations and tests that can better identify conditions early so preventive measures can be instituted.

One example is coronary artery calcium screening. I was an early advocate of this and watched as the medical journals endlessly debated its worth—which, of course, should be done. In the end, it was found useful and is now widely used as a screening test. My enthusiasm arose when I was screening an eye surgeon whose every other parameter, including both his routine and stress ECG/EKGs, were normal, but he had chest pains; and, while it was not yet an approved test, I found his coronary calcium was very high. He nearly retired then and there. That was 2002. He was still operating 18 years later.

Many more tests are being offered today, but many are frankly useless, while others are dubious, but they have responded to the anxiety COVID has wrought.

---

41 Chen, G., Wang, A., Li, S. *et al.* 2019, "Long-Term Exposure to Air Pollution and Survival After Ischemic Stroke", *Stroke*, Vol. 50, No. 3, pp. 563-570, https://doi.org/10.1161/STROKEAHA.118.023264.

42 Lloyd-Smith, M. & Sheffield-Brotherton, B. 2008, "Children's environmental health: intergenerational equity in action – a civil society perspective," *Annals of the New York Academy of Science*, Vol, 1140, pp. 190-200, https://doi.org/10.1196/annals.1454.051.

Today, the buzzword is 'biomarkers.' It is beloved by longevity spammers, but there are often no agreed-upon standards or selections for many. *Live Longer* concentrates on the tests, investigations, and biomarkers that have been proven to provide essential data and for which something can be done if they are abnormal.

8. Exercise

Exercise is the best health investment—see the dedicated chapter within this book. But, as noted, a free VO_2max app is available on smartphones or watches to track your oxygen absorption and motivate you to improve.

9. Mental status

For normal emotions, albeit extreme ones like grief over the death of one's partner, which we once coped with via emotional support and time, we now expect some pill to alleviate or even cure our feelings. Our vulnerability is exploited by ruthless Big Pharma (drug companies) such that "depression" is considered an epidemic, and their profits sit at record levels. In 2008, the NEJM published an article that reviewed over 70 major studies of antidepressants. Thirty-eight showed positive results, and most of these were published. Of the remaining 36 showing negative results, 22 were buried, and 11 were published while giving a positive slant; only three were published accurately.[43]

While there is no doubt that these psychiatric disorders exist, what I am suggesting is that drug therapy is not always

---

43 Turner, E. H., Matthews, A. M., Linardatos, E. *et al.* 2008, "Selective publication of antidepressant trials and its influence on apparent efficacy", *New England Journal of Medicine*, Vol. 358, No. 3, pp. 252-60, https://doi.org/10.1056/NEJMsa065779.

needed. Review of one's lifestyle and coping strategies, along with cognitive behavioral therapy, may be the first priority.

Dementia and Alzheimer's are covered later.

10. Skin

The Sun Belt (across the southern United States) and Australia are witnessing an epidemic of melanoma and skin cancers. It used to be that 'melanoma was the only disease the rich got more than the poor' (because they had holidays, and then on the 'advice' of Coco Chanel). But now, increased holidays for all where we bake in the sun, don't wear sunglasses, and refuse to cover up have resulted in an epidemic of skin cancer and melanoma. However, *some* daily sun exposure is important to produce vitamin D.

The worst behaviour for fair-skinned people, is "binge-burning"—getting severe exposure and burning.

11. High-risk behaviours

These are not obviously dangerous escapades like base jumping or mountaineering but *everyday habits and lifestyles* which account for over 50% of health problems. High-risk behaviours are lifestyle actions that increase medical problems.

Table 2: High-risk behaviors that increase medical problems.

High-risk behavior	Quick fix
Tobacco—cigarette smoking	Support. No vaping.
Nutrition: processed, junk foods, lack of fruit/vegetables	Immediately cease. Adopt Newtrition foods (see end).
Exercise patterns—inactivity	Try HIIT 4 minutes, alt. Days.
High blood pressure	Check. Lose weight. No salt or sugar.
Drinking habits—alcohol harm	Reduce to 1 to 2 glasses per day.
Weight—overweight	GLP-1 Agonists (Wegovy, Mournjurno).
High LDL	Get checked. Newtrition Diet. Statins.

Driving style	Independent opinion: don't speed.
Hobbies—high risk	Base jumping, Mt. Everest, seriously?
Occupations—high risk	Outdoors, machinery, quad bikes.
Unsafe sex	HIV kills. STDs are on the increase.
Illicit drugs	Are you serious? Just don't do them.
UVR—ultraviolet—sun damage	Cover up.
Not being vaccinated	Vaccinate for everything.
Hygiene—poor	Hygiene—immaculate.
Environmental pollution	Trees. Shut windows to traffic.
Head trauma from sport	Tennis, anyone?

As a physician, I fully realize some medications are necessary. My attitude is to minimize them in general and also to use the minimum effective dose. The tragic truth, however, is that it is easier to take a pill than to run (or even walk) around the block, so the bulk (pun intended) of us prefer to take pills.

Vaccination

See chapter 'Flu, COVID-19, Chest Infections'

Prescribed Drugs

One statistic has been understandably, but disturbingly, missing. That is the problems caused by prescribed drugs or medical errors. It has been listed at number six, but some authorities have felt it may be as high as fourth. Now, medical errors have been alleged as being the third leading cause of hospital death.[44]

It is not, as revealed by the BBC program "More or Less" on 8th June 2024 and available for a year (on Google) and analyzed by Professor Mary Dixon-Woods, Director of the Healthcare Improvement Studies Institute at Cambridge University.

44 Makary, M. A. & Daniel, M. 2016, "Medical error-the third leading cause of death in the US", *BMJ*, Vol. 353, https://doi.org/10.1136/bmj.i2139.

This false allegation was a comment article that, in essence, reported on conditions that potentially contributed to rather than caused deaths. The authors only consulted four very small studies, none of which were to investigate medical errors, and used "very flawed methods to reach their conclusions."

However, high-quality studies, done at Yale University in 2020, found the rate was 3%, not 30%.[45]

The latest and more accurate estimate in 2022 comes from Johns Hopkins Armstrong Institute Center for Diagnostic Excellence who have estimated 795,000 Americans die or are permanently disabled by diagnostic error each year.[46]

More Elderly Using Dangerous Drug Combinations

One in six older adults now regularly use potentially deadly combinations of prescription and over-the-counter medications and dietary supplements—a twofold increase over a five-year period. While it is not known how many older adults in the United States die of drug interactions, the risk seems to be growing and public awareness is lacking.[47]

If you are taking any medications, see what can be reduced or stopped. Recently, it has been found that:

---

45 Rodwin, B. A., Bilan, V. P., Merchant, N. B. *et al.* 2020, "Rate of Preventable Mortality in Hospitalized Patients: A Systematic Review and Meta-analysis", *Journal of General Internal Medicine*, 2020 Vol. 35, No. 7, pp. 2099-2106, https://doi.org/10.1007/s11606-019-05592-5.

46 Newman-Toker, D. E., Nassery, N., Schaffer, A. C., *et al.* 2024, "Burden of serious harms from diagnostic error in the USA", *BMJ Quality & Safety*, Vol. 33, pp. 109-120.

47 Qato, D. M., Wilder, J., Schumm, L. P. *et al.* 2016, "Changes in Prescription and Over-the-Counter Medication and Dietary Supplement Use Among Older Adults in the United States, 2005 vs 2011", *JAMA Internal Medicine*, Vol. 176, No. 4, pp. 473-482, https://doi.org/10.1001/jamainternmed.2015.8581

- Many statins are now not needed, as the heart risk calculators were wrong. But they are beneficial if needed.
- Aspirin is not recommended for primary cardiovascular prevention and can cause gut bleeds.
- NSAIDS cause bleeding and heart attacks.

As a young medical registrar, my first action on admitting a patient was to "cease all medications". At the time of admission, I well remember many patients taking over 15 different drugs—and one (which I think represents a personal record) was on some 33 different drugs. Most of these patients, when later discharged, feeling much better, were only taking the three or four essential drugs actually needed.

Obviously, the patients' doctors are not trying to poison their patients, and, too often, the patient is reluctant to complain of side effects. Frequently, when a patient is seeing different doctors, a new drug is added but an old one is not ceased. However, all drugs have side effects, so it behoves the patient to *balance their greater benefit against any downside.* Many people have idiosyncratic responses to even the most common drugs. So, don't ignore side effects; note any new problems that occur after you start any new medication, and *get your whole medication regime reviewed at least annually.* Make a specific appointment just for this and nothing else.

Older patients are being prescribed numerous "invisible" anticholinergic drugs that interfere with our nervous systems and put them at risk of side effects such as cognitive impairment. While drugs for urinary incontinence and tricyclic antidepressants are traditionally recognized for their high-level anticholinergic risks, most of the anticholinergic burden for elderly patients comes from the unwitting prescribing of low-level anticholinergic drugs.

The top 8 anticholinergic drugs to be aware of:[48]

1. Warfarin
2. Oxycodone
3. Furosemide
4. Prednisolone
5. Prochlorperazine
6. Digoxin
7. Fentanyl
8. Morphine

Overall

I am not advocating that we cocoon ourselves in cotton wool, but I am advocating that we are fully made aware of the dangers so we can minimize the risks. How tragic it is to read how kids were killed on a quad bike because they perceived it as a fun vehicle, and no one told them otherwise.

Had I known such risks, would I have changed my habits? You bet! I played (too) many years of rugby when hard knocks were never admitted to, but I gave up my skateboard (in my 50s) when I read how a champion international athlete my age had fallen off his and broken his hip. My friend's squash racquet opened my eyebrow, but my eye at least remained intact. I now know how to hold in and control a champagne cork after I witnessed one actually hitting someone in the eye. When the angle grinder kicked back, I couldn't believe how sudden, violent, and dangerous it was and having owned three quad bikes, I only wish the man who sold us the first one had warned us of the

48 Fountain, J., Griffiths, P., Farrell, M. *et al.* 1998, "Diversion tactics: How a sample of drug misusers in treatment obtained surplus drugs to sell on the illicit market", *International Journal of Drug Policy*, No. 9, Vol. 3, pp. 159-167, https://doi.org/10.1016/S0955-3959(98)00013-9.

inherent design dangers (they tip over very easily if turned too sharply).

No one over 60 should climb a ladder, let alone stand on a chair, to reach or fix something. My mother rang me to say my elderly father "couldn't get up". He had been standing on a chair, putting up kitchen curtains, and he wouldn't believe my "spot diagnosis" of a fractured neck of his femur (thigh bone). The injured person lies in a characteristic position, so the spot diagnosis can be made immediately. Like most formerly active men, he didn't know when not to pursue activities that may not have been dangerous when younger.

One surgeon I knew slipped off his ladder cleaning out the gutters of his roof and ended up as a vegetable in a nursing home. Do I get up on chairs to get the special condiments from the high cupboard shelf? Well, yes, but I am very aware of the risks and make sure it is a solid wooden chair and that I have support. I now also slide my hand down the staircase rails. My excuse is that I do know the dangers, unlike most men, and I am super careful. This gets back to not wrapping ourselves in cotton wool.

We can continue most of our previous activities if we know the dangers and how to avoid them.

A little-known issue that most young people don't think about until it's too late is hearing impairment, which is often preventable but condemns the sufferer to a great deal of social isolation in their old age. The rock concerts, the boom boxes, the surround-sound high-volume car speakers, and the earphones are all harbingers of deafness. Deafness is one of the worst causes of social isolation, loneliness, and early death.[49]

49 Shukla, A., Harper, M., Pedersen, E. *et al.* 2020, "Hearing Loss, Loneliness, and Social Isolation: A Systematic Review", *Otolaryngolgy–Head and Neck Surgery*, Vol. 162, No. 5, pp. 622-633, https://doi.org/10.1177/0194599820910377.

With Global Warming heat exhaustion and heat strokes are becoming more prevalent. Avoid the middle of the day. Stay in the shade and hydrated.

Finally, always wear a smart-watch or carry a phone that triggers a fall warning as to where you are. Better still avoid being alone.

Small, Pleasant, Acceptable Changes: Micro Steps

Any necessary improvements have been shown to be best applied by small, pleasant, acceptable, evidence-based changes, substituting good for bad. One such example for nutrition is using olive oil (and extra virgin at that) instead of butter.

CHAPTER 3

How to Live Longer

"The secret of longevity... Is to keep breathing!"

– Sophie Tucker

Lifespan vs Healthspan

Premature Deaths

Is there a way to live longer but maximise health and enjoyment? Have the latest medical advances provided better evidence to live longer, healthier, and happier?

Yes!

This information has been available for some time but, until now, has not been functionally utilised.

Compression of Morbidity:

Living Healthier Longer vs Sicker Longer

Are we living too long as we encounter more and more illnesses and disabilities?

The concept of the healthspan has evolved with the aim to "live longer, healthier" or the "life in our years". This is affected by the *Compression of Morbidity*, with fewer ill years and longer healthy years. With a good healthspan, old age is to be enjoyed, not endured.

Increase Healthspan, not Lifespan, or Make Them the Same

In 1980, Dr. James F. Fries, a Stanford University physician who studied chronic disease and aging, proposed that a "compression of morbidity" would enable most people to remain healthy until a certain age, perhaps 85, before they die naturally or after only a brief illness.[50]

While diverse strategies—from caloric restriction to genetic manipulation—have proven to extend life span in model organisms in the lab, these animals are not necessarily enjoying longer periods of health. Increasing lifespan also increases the acceleration of the age-dependent mortality rate of the population.

The "future ideal" is *Compression of Morbidity*—living healthier, longer (with a good quality of life) by preventing age-related disease and physical decline. While minor progress is being made to try and reverse aging, this goal will be years away. What can be done immediately, however, is the predicting and preventing or minimizing of these disorders and illnesses.

Laboratory researchers, such as Intervention Testing Program's Prof Richard Miller, have found their mice have both extended their lifespans and healthspans, and this, of course, would be the ultimate objective. But for us humans, the data says otherwise.

---

50 Swartz, A. 2008, "James Fries: Healthy Aging Pioneer", *American Journal of Public Health*, Vol. 98, No. 7, pp. 1163-1166, https://doi.org/10.2105/AJPH.2008.135731.

Compressing Mortality

Such that Healthspan = Lifespan

Think about two points on a typical human lifespan, with the first point representing the time at which a person becomes chronically ill or disabled and the second point representing the time at which that person dies. Today, the time between those two points is about 20 years or so years. During the early portion of those years, chronic disease or disability is minor, but it increases nearer to the end of life. The idea behind compression of morbidity is to squeeze or compress the time between the onset of chronic illness or disability and the time in which a person dies.

As this graph shows, the average lifespan now is some 80 years, with the years from age 63 and on encumbered with increasing illnesses and disabilities.

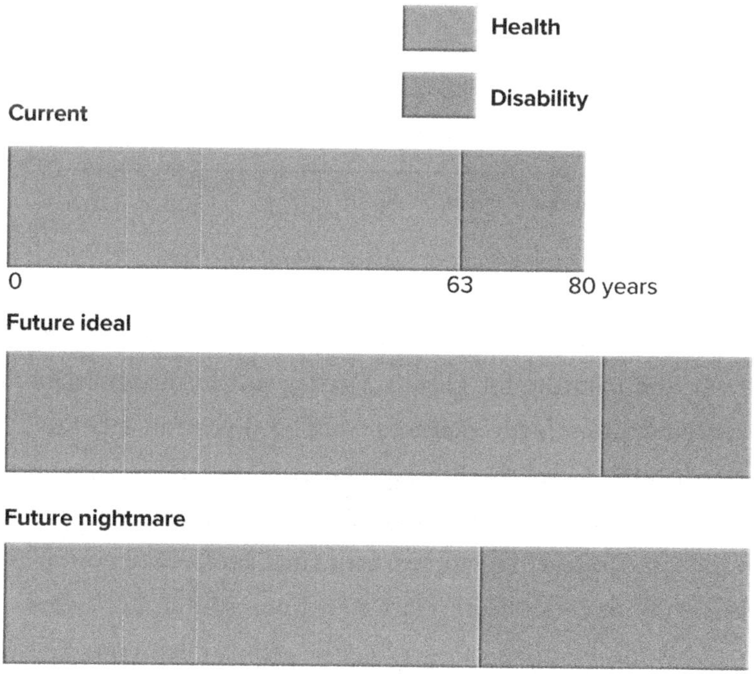

Figure 3: Compression of morbidity.

As can be seen from this later graph below, we spend some 12.7 or more years unwell before we die. The obvious aspiration for us all, and the aim of this book, is that we not only live longer but do so while being healthy.

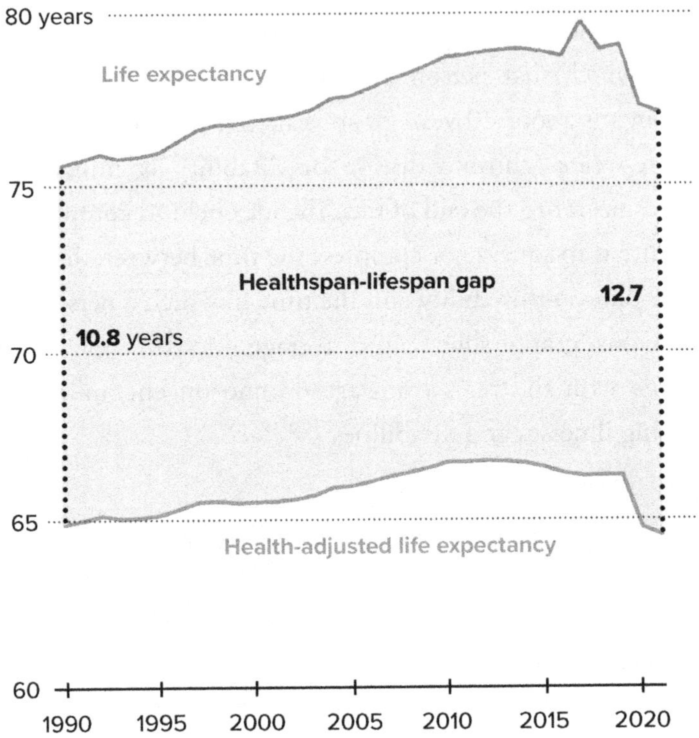

Figure 4: Healthspan-lifespan gap (*Source: Institute for Health Metrics and Evaluation).*

In the Institute for Health Metrics and Evaluation data, life expectancy from birth increased from 75.6 years in 1990 to 77.1 years in 2021. Healthy life expectancy, a measure of how many years we can expect to enjoy good health, fell from 64.8 to 64.4 in the same period. The average estimated gap between our overall years and our good-health years grew from 10.8 to 12.7 years.

Our Health Span can get as close as possible to our Lifespan by specifically identifying these fatal or debilitating illnesses that plague our later years and then how to avoid and minimize (compress) them.

Can Compression of Morbidity Be Achieved?

While most people struggle with an ever-increasing burden of disease and disability as they age, it has been found that those who live exceptionally long lives have the additional benefit of shorter periods of illness—sometimes just weeks or months—before death. These findings suggest that discoveries made in one group of centenarians can be generalized to diverse populations. And they contradict the notion that the older people get, the sicker they become (and the greater the cost of taking care of them).

That said, Dr Dhruv Khullar pointed out in the New Yorker (April 15, 2024), "Fries died of end-stage dementia in 2021, at the age of eighty-three, and his broader prediction never seemed to come true. If anything, longer lives now appear to include more difficult years. The "compression of morbidity may be as illusory as immortality," two demographers, Eileen Crimmins and Hiram Beltrán-Sánchez, wrote in 2010. According to the World Health Organization, the average American can expect just one healthy birthday after the age of sixty-five".

However, elsewhere, I point out the dichotomy in American health, which, to me, explains this paradox and does not negate the pursuit or, indeed, the attainment of, compression of mortality. As I am writing this, typing it myself, at the age of eighty-three, I can only suggest it can be done!

Quality of Life

In addition, our quality of life must be addressed. Being healthy but living in poverty is not to be recommended.

Avoid the Nursing Home!

Although people are now living longer, they are not necessarily healthier than before. Many people are indeed "dying longer"—being kept alive without much quality of life, in many cases. Their healthspan does not match up with their lifespan. Nearly a quarter (23%) of the overall global burden of death and illness is in people aged over 60, and much of this burden is attributable to long-term illness caused by diseases such as cancer, chronic respiratory diseases, heart disease, musculoskeletal diseases (such as arthritis and osteoporosis), mental and neurological disorders. This long-term burden of illness and diminished wellbeing affects patients, their families, health systems, and economies, and is forecast to accelerate. For example, the latest estimates indicate that the number of people with dementia is expected to rise from 44 million now to 135 million by 2050.[51]

At present, despite the billions being spent to reverse aging, we all still age. In doing so, we incur some presently unavoidable changes, such as our hair whitening, our eyesight reducing, and the loss of muscle (sarcopenia). Many of these changes can be disguised or minimized. Elderly women look quite smart with hair dyed to look natural; laser surgery can make spectacles a thing of the past; regular exercise minimizes muscle loss.

Even so, we are not the same healthy bouncing ball we were at 11 years old; inevitably, we will incur some impost. The aim at present, and a key point to this book, is to minimize any such imposts and live longer, being "HAFFI": healthy, alert, fit, functional, and independent.

---

51 Prince, M. J., Wu, F., Guo, Y. *et al.* 2015, "The burden of disease in older people and implications for health policy and practice", *Lancet,* Vol. 385, No. 9967, pp. 549-562, https://doi.org/10.1016/S0140-6736(14)61347-7.

Premature Deaths

The most obvious way to live longer is not to die prematurely

Yet, most of us do!

Surely, it is blatantly obvious (and therefore missed), that we should *prevent* what we know can kill or disable us. First things first. But the history of preventive medicine is remarkably short. In fact, it has all happened, essentially, in my lifetime.

Men vs. Women

It has long been observed that women live longer than men, but the reasons why have not been clear. Humans are the only species in which one sex is known to have a survival advantage, and this sex difference in longevity may be one of the most robust features of human biology. The Human Mortality Database has complete lifespan tables for men and women from 38 countries that go back as far as 1751 for Sweden and 1816 for France; and for all 38 countries for every year in the database, female life expectancy at birth exceeds male life expectancy.[52] The Gerontology Research Group data for the oldest of the old show that women make up 90% of the supercentenarians, those who live to 110 years of age or longer.[53]

The birth cohorts have been studied from the mid-1800s to the early 1900s for Iceland. This small, genetically homogenous country—which was beset by catastrophes such as famine, flooding, volcanic eruptions, and disease epidemics—provides a particularly vivid example of female survival. Over that time, life

52 The Human Mortality Database (HMD)

53 Perls, T. T. 2017, "Male Centenarians: How and Why Are They Different from Their Female Counterparts?", *Journal of the American Geriatrics Society*, Vol. 65, No. 9, pp. 1904-1906, https://doi.org/10.1111/jgs.14978.

expectancy at birth fell to as low as 21 years during catastrophes and rose to as high as 69 years during good times. Yet in every year, regardless of food availability or pestilence, women at the beginning of life and near its end survived better than men.

A 2015 study found that vulnerability to heart disease is the biggest culprit behind a surge in higher death rates for men vs. women during the twentieth century.[54] Women are reaping the longevity benefits at a much faster rate, with a massive but uneven decrease in mortality. This uneven impact of cardiovascular illness-related deaths on men, especially during middle age and early older age, raises the question of whether men and women face different heart disease risks due to inherent biological risks and/or protective factors at different points in their lives.[55]

Play the Percentages and Odds

It is not only heart attacks which can now be prevented, but most of the top 10 (or even 20) fatal or debilitating illnesses specific to your age. Now, by reviewing the lists of the causes of death and disabilities, the top 10 illnesses can be analyzed. Now, there can be far fewer young widows or widowers. Knowing the odds against us allows us to best respond to even up those odds.

The high-risk behaviors responsible for an estimated 50% or more of our premature demise or disabilities include some quite surprising behaviors we often take for granted. By knowing these risk factors along with the prevalence, incidence, and specific-age-related illnesses, we can reduce the odds.

---

54 Beltrán-Sánchez, H., Finch, C. E. & Crimmins, E. M. 2015 "Twentieth century surge of excess adult male mortality", *Proceedings of the National Academy of Sciences*, Vol. 112, No. 29, https://doi.org/10.1073/pnas.1421942112.

55 Woodward, M. 2019, "Cardiovascular Disease and the Female Disadvantage", *International Journal of Environmental Research and Public Health*, Vol. 16, No. 7, https://doi.org/10.3390/ijerph16071165.

We understand that reducing the odds against us offers us the greatest chance of success when it comes to sports and games. We know that "backing the long shot" is just that; it does not offer the best odds. Having played tennis against Wimbledon, the US, and French Champions, who kindly let me occasionally hit the ball back, I quickly learned how much, even against an inept opponent like myself, they play the percentage game and thereby reduce the odds. They know which shot has the greatest chance of success. The center of the net is some six inches lower than the outside net on the singles lines, so where do they hit most shots? Across the center. It is lower; it offers a greater percentage for success. Knowing the odds, they do not make high-risk shots. The same principle applies to world championship poker or any other competitive venture.

To win at health, we also have to know the odds and play the percentages. What are the odds of a heart attack at your age? What are the odds of depression? If one illness occurs 70% more than others at your age, you can improve your chances by knowing how to avoid it. Most people, including my doctor colleagues, don't know the exact odds that would improve their patients' health (nor their own with such a specific analysis).

When it comes to health, we seemingly blunder on, following disproven rituals such as the "annual check-up or physical", which is tantamount to blindly playing cards without knowing the rules or going for a backhand down the line, which only has a 15% chance compared with a forehand across the middle of the net at 90% success. What are the odds (the rate of occurrence) for a 40-year-old woman to get breast cancer? Are they more or less than her odds of having a heart attack or suffering from depression, suicide, and Diabetes? If the chances are greater, would it not make sense to concentrate on this instead of the 360-to-1 option? Yet many of us do the latter because we don't know the age-rates and order in which illnesses occur.

At best, we buy vitamins and supplements (very bad odds), follow some fad diet (bad odds), exercise incorrectly (well, at least it's exercise, but there are now better methods), and get an annual check-up from our doctor, which all health authorities now recognize as being not very effective[56] (not good odds but at least it may pick up something). Then, out of the blue, to our complete surprise because we are so super-fit and health-nutty, we get struck down with an illness which, had we known what to look out for, we may well have prevented.

Or, at worst, we eat the wrong foods, don't exercise, don't get checked and get heart disease, high blood pressure, have a disabling stroke, get Diabetes, have to gobble down 17 drugs a day in a nursing home while wearing diapers, and die 20 years before we should.

This need not be.

The point here is that we must address being healthy if we are to live longer, whereas most of us just go on not facing facts, not thinking about our future health, and not actively doing something about it. Knowing what to do and being proactive is the main thrust of this book.

---

56 Gold, J. 2015, "Ritual Not Science, Keeps the Annual Physical Alive", *Medscape*, 6 April.

SECTION B

WHAT CAN KILL US THIS YEAR & IN WHAT ORDER & WHAT CAN BE PREVENTED

CHAPTER 4

Overview: What Kills or Disables Us Prematurely and Recent Changes

"Like one that on a lonesome road doth walk in fear & dread,
And having once looked round walks on and no more turns his head,
Because he knows a frightful fiend doth close behind him tread."

– Samuel Taylor Coleridge

As of May 2, 2023, the outbreak of the coronavirus disease (COVID-19) had spread to almost every country in the world, and more than 6.86 million people had died after contracting the respiratory virus. Over 1.16 million of these deaths occurred in the United States.[57]

57 "Number of novel coronavirus (COVID-19) deaths worldwide as of May 2, 2023, by country and territor", *Statista.*

The number of deaths from COVID-19 surpassed that of the 1918 flu pandemic. According to data from the CDC, about 675,000 people died from the flu pandemic in the US between the early spring of 1918 and 1919.[58]

The following tables are not age-specific but summarise the whole spectrum of illnesses. The changes from 2003 to 2022 are particularly interesting, as are the ravages of Covid.

The following table shows 'The Burden of Disease'. What has changed?

The following table is an overall picture of the top 25 illnesses that not only kill us but can disable us and the changes since 2003. These figures are applicable, in the main, to all first world countries with only minor modifications, if any.

Heart Disease is still our greatest killer, and cancer number two if colon, lung, breast, and prostate are amalgamated.

There has been a dramatic *fall in strokes*, probably because of better blood pressure control, but an impressive *rise in dementia* (Alzheimer's Disease). Is this because of better awareness and diagnosis?

Poisoning has plummeted, but I am not sure if these figures have included erstwhile friends of the Kremlin.

Suicide has risen, and so has atrial fibrillation—these sadly at opposite ends of the age spectrum (in that suicide is more common in the younger age groups).

Hearing loss and alcohol disorders have dropped, but I don't think they are linked, whereas chronic liver disease has increased, and alcohol did play a part there—so what has changed?

Asthma has increased (pollution?) while lung cancer plummeted—in direct proportion to the cessation of smoking—

58 *Perspectives in Health*, 2003, Vol. 8, No. 3.

but I await with trepidation for its inevitable return unless vaping can be outlawed.

Bowel cancer has also dropped even though it is increasing in 30-year-olds, and we don't know why.

Breast cancer and osteoarthritis have gratifyingly fallen, along with eating disorders and dental caries.

The rest, out of some 25 major health conditions, viz: heart disease, back pain, anxiety, COPD, type 2 Diabetes, rheumatoid arthritis, and alcohol disorders, have remained much the same, but COVID has not been included.

'The Burden of Disease' and changes since 2003

The overall causes of death, while interesting, do not give us the information needed for your age but are provided here for your interest.

Covid came out of left field and caught us all unaware, some more than others, and we must learn how to protect ourselves. The below graph shows the effect of vaccination: Blue vs Red. Personal hygiene is essential; hand washing (alcohol based), social distancing, avoiding peoples' coughs and sneezes, and masks are fundamental.

COVID altered the order of what was our greatest killers, now assuming fourth place, but our greatest killers are still heart disease, cancer and unintentional injuries (accidents), and we must focus on preventing these and as many causes of premature death as we can.

Causes of Premature Death by Age and Sex (USA, UK, Australia)

In addition to national laws, which can make one entity more dominant in another country (e.g., gun laws), various statistical

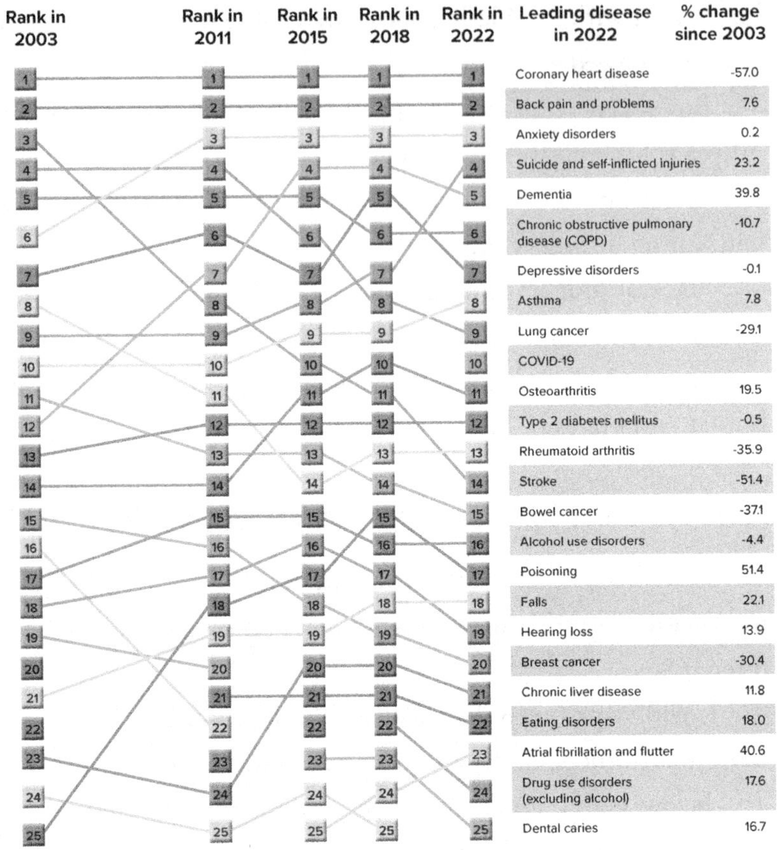

Figure 5: The Burden of Disease (*Source: AIHW: Australian Burden of Disease Study 2022, 13 December*).

authorities in the same country may have different recording criteria or methodology, and so these lists may vary in a minor way, not only from country to country but also in the same country where there is more than one recognized authority.

These lists should be used as an overall guide. By comparing one country with another, the figures most applicable to one's own community or socio-economic status can be best identified.

Death after the age of 80 years is the ambition, and I then do not consider it as "premature".

These have not changed much since 2002, which allows us to focus on the main health issues which are historically affecting us.

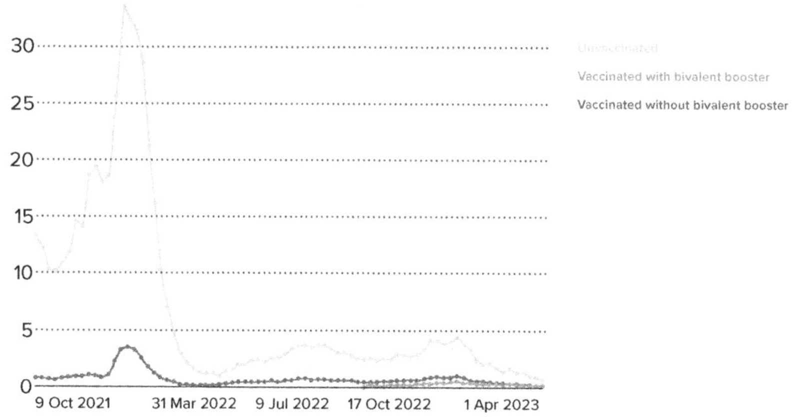

Figure 6: COVID-19 weekly death rate by vaccination status in the United States, all ages. Death rates are calculated as the number of deaths in each group, divided by the total number of people in this group. This is given per 100,000 people. The mortality rate for the 'All ages' group is age-standardized to account for the different vaccination rates of older and younger people (*Source: Centers for Disease Control and Prevention, Vaccine Breakthrough/ Surveillance and Analytics Team*).

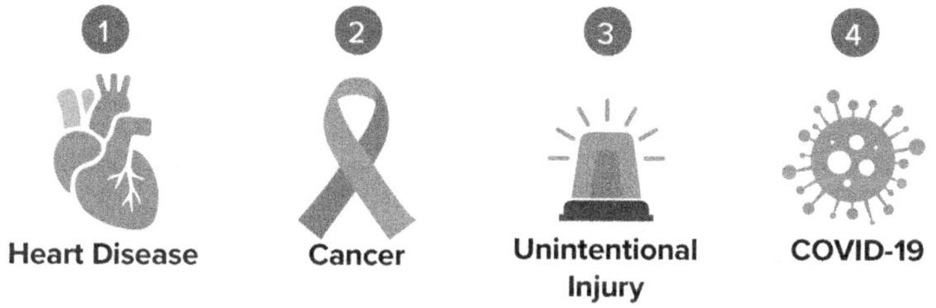

Figure 7: Leading causes of death in 2022 among US residents.

But the risks and deaths due to medications are not usually registered.

The Treatment, Not Error, Is Biggest Risk to Elderly[59]

The greatest threat to older patients' safety in primary care is the risk posed by treatment itself, not treatment error or negligence,

59 *Annuals of Family Medicine*, Vol. 13, No. 5.

Table 3: Top 10 causes of death in the USA (CDC/National Center for Health Statistics; last reviewed 18 January 2023), UK (Office for Nations statistics, Census 2021) and Australia (13 Doctor certified deaths by cause AIH).

	USA 2021	UK 2022	Australia 2023
1	Heart disease	Heart disease	Cancer
2	Cancer	Malignant neoplasms of trachea, bronchus, and lung	Dementia/AD
	Covid	Dementia and Alzheimer's (AD)	Heart (IHD)
3	Unintentional injuries	Colorectal cancer	Respiratory disease
4	Stroke and Cerebrovascular diseases	Cerebrovascular diseases	Other Cardiac conditions
5	Ch low respiratory diseases	Breast cancer/ Pancreatic cancer	Cerebrovascular diseases
		COVID	COVID
6	Alzheimer's disease	Prostate cancer	Diabetes
7	Diabetes mellitus	Emphysema COPD	Colon, sigmoid, rectum cancer
8	Influenza and pneumonia	Injuries	Blood, lymph cancer (leukemia)
9	Kidney disease	Oesophageal cancer	
10	Suicide	Brain cancer	

according to an analysis of no-fault claims data from New Zealand. Medication injuries were the main source (34%) of all treatment injuries among the elderly, and within that category, antibiotics were, by far, the biggest culprit (51%). Next highest among injury sources were nonsteroidal anti-inflammatory drugs (9%) and angiotensin-converting enzyme inhibitors (9%). Antibiotics also topped the list for causes of serious or sentinel injuries for patients aged 65 years and older. Antibiotics caused 39% of such injuries in that age group, followed by warfarin (14%) and steroids (7%). The serious/sentinel category was defined as having "the potential to result in" or "has resulted in" "unanticipated death or major permanent loss of function".

Most medication injuries overall were allergic and idiosyncratic reactions, without a suggestion of error (1295; 91% of medication injuries and 34% of all injuries), according to the study. The elderly are particularly susceptible to antibiotic injury, the author notes, because they often take multiple medications, leaving them vulnerable to drug interactions. Even when medications can be reconciled, it does not take into account everything a patient is taking over the counter.

Infirmities and Disabilities

While we may survive these serious illnesses, we are then often left with a permanent disability, making life miserable and often shortening it. But, in addition, there are behaviours which can easily be avoided but, if not, lead to disabilities, which we may dismiss as minor when young but which, when old, are major. Hearing loss is a good example. These people are effectively socially isolated.

When we are young, high-risk and even low-risk (but cumulative), behaviours are often treated as a "rite of passage" or relegated to be addressed when older. Drinking and now, binge drinking are epidemic. Smoking has gratifyingly been recognized as 'not cool', but a stupid, injurious affectation and drug of addiction… until vaping came along.

Cars pull up beside me with speakers that would do Carnegie Hall justice with some young man with a baseball cap on backwards gyrating to the beat, which seems to lift his car off the ground while ensuring his accelerated hearing loss. Meanwhile, in my rear-vision mirror, some 18-year-old or so girl is tailgating me until she cuts me off with the one-finger salute and absolutely no idea how to control a skid. And both of these people are drinking a cola and eating pizza or some processed food and are overweight. The only exercise they get is from their thumbs texting. They have little or no idea of nutrition or hygiene, and getting a tan is most desirable to them.

I have no answer to these behaviors, other than alerting those readers under 40 years of age or their parents or anyone (!) to these avoidable disorders, let alone fatal illnesses.

Of course, I was perfect and never indulged in such practices... pig's bottom. I often say the only reason I'm alive is that when I arrived at the Pearly Gates (or was it the other place), the "Use-By Date" on my forehead was blurred and they sent me back.

But a friend of mine, a Rock' n Roll Drummer who, of course, has a hearing loss, told me how he wished someone had told him to wear earplugs and warned him of the dangers of loud noises. But I don't think he would have listened (bad pun).

Forecast Bigger Increases in Lifespan in Affluent vs Disadvantaged Areas

A UK study forecasting how life expectancy will change in England and Wales has predicted that people living in the longest-living areas in 2012 are expected to live seven or eight years longer than those in disadvantaged parts.[60] By 2030, the gap is projected to grow to more than eight years. Even within London, inequality between districts is stark, with residents of Kensington and Chelsea living five to six years longer than those in Barking

60 Bennett, J. E., Li, G., Foreman, K. *et al.* 2015, "The future of life expectancy and life expectancy inequalities in England and Wales: Bayesian spatiotemporal forecasting", *The Lancet,* Vol. 386, No. 9989, pp. 163-170, https://doi.org/10.1016/S0140-6736(15)60296-3.

and Dagenham or Tower Hamlets (suburbs of London).[61] Studies have shown the same suburban longevity inequality exists in Glasgow.[62]

61 *Ibid.*

62 Marmot, M. 2015, *The Health Gap*, Bloomsbury.

CHAPTER 5

What's Going to Kill *You* This Year

"Health is not valued till sickness comes."

– Thomas Fuller

The Live Longer Predictive Analysis System

The Live Longer Predictive Analysis System is arguably unique in that it accesses official government data, only relatively recently available, that identifies which illnesses are most likely to affect us for our sex and present age, followed by providing the best tests, investigations, and medical advice to prevent them.

Screening

A recent study concluded that screening is overused for some diseases and that it is possibly perceived as more effective and cost-effective than it is. However, the study *did advise* that "the role of screening should be considered on a disease-specific basis,"[63] which is exactly what the Live Longer Predictive Analysis system does.

63 Saquib, N., Saquib, J. & Ioannidis, J. P. A. 2015, "Does screening for disease save lives in asymptomatic adults? Systematic review of meta-analyses and randomized trials", *International Journal of Epidemiology*, Vol. 44, No. 1, pp. 264-277.

Many illnesses are not preventable, but most are, or are eminently treatable if diagnosed early. But we must be aware of what they are and when they are most likely to "attack" us. If we have this information, if we know when and where the enemy is, we are at least and at last in a position to fight back. Yet, every day, we blunder in making dangerous health mistakes, which accumulate to shorten our lives or to cause us to become housebound or nursing home invalids.

Analyse, Predict, Prevent

It was only in the late part of the last century, in the 1970s in my experience, that death certificates were expanded to include details of comorbidities (what other illness the deceased were suffering from). Before that, just the main, terminal illness was recorded, while other illnesses or disabilities were mostly ignored.

These far more detailed, massive Official Government National Death and Disability Data Records of the USA, UK, and Australia not only showed the 'Cause of Death' but also any co-existing illnesses (comorbidities) which contributed to death or disabled the person.

As a hypothetical example, no longer was a woman's cause of death listed only as a 'Road Traffic Accident' but now included her Alzheimer's disease, which caused her to wander off from the nursing home, her blood pressure-hypertension, Diabetes, obesity, and arthritis, which slowed her down and blurred her vision so she didn't see the big truck that hit her.

Analysis of these lists and tables allows for prediction and, thus, prevention. While they have been available for some time, they have not apparently been accessed or utilised to improve our health.

However, they now provide the complete information as to what kills or disables each sex for each decade. This then allows precise predictive analysis to identify and so *prevent* those illnesses most likely to affect you, now and in the future.

This great leap forward in medical records and statistics has allowed for officially recorded decade-by-decade statistics regarding:

- Causes of Premature Deaths
- Causes of Non-Fatal Burdens of Disease (NFBD)
- Most Prevalent Health Conditions
- Most Common Reason for Attending a Doctor

By combining the lists of causes of death with those of illness burden, a more complete picture of our health emerges—in fact, the most complete invaluable picture of our health possible. Not all countries have such in-depth statistics, but for Western countries, these figures provide a similar complete picture.

The Big "40"

Further, the statistics show the incredible, sudden, usually unrecognized, deteriorations at age 40 as detailed in a later chapter:

1. Cardiovascular disease
2. Blood pressure
3. Cholesterol
4. Diabetes
5. Cancer
6. Lung disease
7. Rheumatoid arthritis
8. Osteoporosis and Osteoarthritis
9. Eyesight
10. Weight

All of the ten above "suddenly" get worse at around age 40.

But this onslaught is not really sudden. It is, of course, not the first puff of a cigarette that causes the lung cancer or the one sunburn that causes the melanoma, but rather the repeated exposure to these irritant carcinogens. In the same way, it is not the one bad meal that causes the cardiovascular disease, hyperlipidemia, obesity, and Diabetes but rather the long-term, chronic abuse of our bodies by high-risk habits and behaviors from that peak health age of 11 (if not before, even in the womb).

Like lung cancer or a melanoma, which may seem "sudden", they all are, in fact, just the end result of long-term abuse.

The good news, however, is that it's never too late to reverse or improve much of this damage.

If you know what's most likely to kill or disable you this year, you can best avoid it.

If you don't know, you are not going to live longer.

All you now have to do is look up the chapter for your age, and then the world's best data provides you the answer—those evidenced illnesses or activities, prioritized and listed in order, for you to now avoid.

CHAPTER 6

Age-sex Specific Analysis

"To look at something as though we had never seen it before requires great courage."

– Henri Matisse (1869-1954)

"No one is so old that he does not think he could live another year."

– Cicero (106 BC- 43 BC)

How to Use This Section:

- Look up the chapter for your age and sex,
- Find what is most likely to kill or disable you this year, then
- Take the provided avoiding action.

The Graphs: Don't be put off—they save you reading!

Leading Causes of Death by Age, 2019–2021

Table 4: Leading Causes of Death by Age, 2019–2021 (*Source: AIHW: Australian Burden of Disease Study 2022, 13 Decmber 2022*).

Age group (years)	Rank 1st	2nd	3rd	4th	5th
Under 1	Perinatal and congenital conditions	Other ill-defined causes	Sudden infant death syndrome	Selected metabolic disorders	Accidental threats to breathing
1–14	Land transport accidents	Perinatal and congenital conditions	Brain cancer	Other ill-defined causes	Suicide
15–24	Suicide	Land transport accidents	Accidental poisoning	Other ill-defined causes	Assault
25–44	Suicide	Accidental poisoning	Land transport accidents	Coronary heart disease	Other ill-defined causes
45–64	Coronary heart disease	Lung cancer	Suicide	Colorectal cancer	Liver disease
65–74	Lung cancer	Coronary heart disease	Chronic obstructive pulmonary disease	Colorectal cancer	Cerebrovascular disease
75–84	Coronary heart disease	Dementia, inluding Alzheimer's disease	Lung cancer	Cerebrovascular disease	Chronic obstructive pulmonary disease
85–94	Dementia, inluding Alzheimer's disease	Coronary heart disease	Cerebrovascular disease	Chronic obstructive pulmonary disease	Diabetes
95+	Dementia, inluding Alzheimer's disease	Coronary heart disease	Cerebrovascular disease	Heart failure	Influenza and pneumonia

Specific Analysis: Each decade has its own, more detailed chapter, for both men and women.

These figures are applicable, in general, to all developed nations. Exceptions are easily identified. For example, in the USA, for the 24-44 age group, gunshot wounds and fentanyl head the list.

Introduction

In 2023, life is more stressful now than in the 1990s, especially for the middle-aged, those aged 45 to 64, new research from Penn State University has found. But then, it seems stress decreased with age. For example, 25-year-olds reported stressors on nearly 50% of days, while 70-year-olds reported stressors on only 30% of days. In addition to the decrease in the number of daily stressors reported, the study found that as people age, they are less emotionally reactive to daily stressors when they do happen.[64]

According to a recent study, our happiness, averaged across the 187 country estimates for peoples' age, found happiness steadily increased through our 50s and 60s.

National, Ethnic, and Social Differences

There are significant national differences. While high-risk behavior in young males is universal, the United States adds a greater dimension to this, with Fentanyl and homicide featuring.

There are also socioeconomic class differences. I stand to be corrected, but I would think homicide is more prevalent in deprived areas than the affluent or educated suburbs.

The figures for suicide are alarming and probably shadow depression, which is not an official cause of death.

Terminology

Terminology also differs. Ischemic Heart Disease (IHD), Coronary Artery Disease (CAD), and Coronary Heart Disease (CHD) are synonymous.

---

64 Almeida, D. M., Rush, J., Mogle, J. *et al.* 2023, "Longitudinal change in daily stress across 20 years of adulthood: Results from the national study of daily experiences", *Developmental Psychology*, Vol. 59, No. 3, pp. 515-523, https://doi.org/10.1037/dev0001469.

What the United States calls a "stroke", other countries may call cerebrovascular disease. Emphysema, asthma, and bronchitis can be covered by Chronic Obstructive Pulmonary Disease (COPD).

Changes Over Time

Some statistics have altered slightly since I first researched them for my books. This is to be expected, as prevention has improved. For example, decreased male smoking has seen lung cancer drop from second to third.

The overwhelming fact remains that cardiovascular disease remains the leading cause of death and burden for both sexes. If it doesn't kill you prematurely, it will turn you into a dependent invalid more so than any other illness.

The USA's Disadvantage[65]

The United States suffers from a health disadvantage in that the US population experiences poorer health than populations in other countries, and the disadvantage has grown over time. One component of this phenomenon is the US life expectancy disadvantage: survival in the developed world has increased over the past century, but growth in US life expectancy has not kept pace with that of other industrialized countries. The gap with other countries widened dramatically after 2010, when life expectancy plateaued in the United States but continued increasing elsewhere.

During the COVID-19 pandemic, when the United States experienced more COVID-19 deaths than any other country and was among the highest per capita death rates, US life expectancy

65 *American Journal of Public Health (AJPH)*

decreased by 2.1 years between 2019 and 2021, the largest decrease in a century. The US life expectancy disadvantage began decades ago but exactly when remains unclear. Studies typically date the onset to the 1980s or 1990s, raising intriguing research questions about events in history that might explain this timing.

Age-Specific Analysis

These graphs and tables represent the illnesses, in order, which are most likely to disable us at our present age. Being disabled is usually the result of a serious condition that may have killed us but didn't, thus causing a permanent disability. While most countries identify the causes of death for each age group, few identify the illnesses or conditions that disable us.

Unfortunately, these graphs are not made any more but are included as they still provide the best visual comparisons and information.

As to the Following Graphs:

The immediately following is an example graph (more age/sex specific graphs follow). Combined graphs are provided at the end of each age group.

All You Need to Know is That:

- Light bar = Disability = Chronic illness
- Dark bar = Premature death by the same illness

Years lost to disabilities, as per the graph below, are always greater than from premature deaths. Hence, as will be seen, many people are living longer, escaping death, but in chronic ill-health or with disabilities. The objective is to 'compress' these so that healthspan and lifespan are as close to the same as possible.

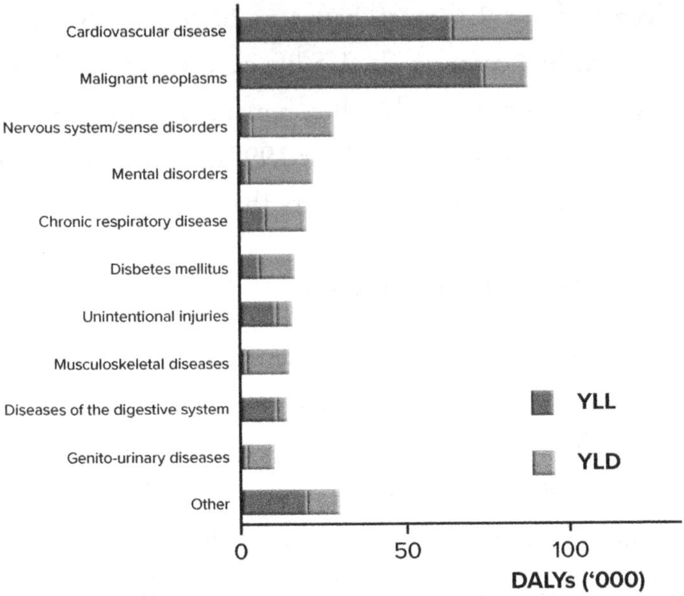

Figure 8: Example graph.

Explanation Combination Graph

Don't be put off with the statistician-speak of "YLD, YLL, and DALYS".

The DALY is the *total years of healthy life lost.*

How to Use These Graphs and Lists

Each chapter is dedicated to a decade for both men and women.

Each is stand-alone, complete in itself, so you don't have to refer back and forth. This may seem repetitious if, out of interest, you read them sequentially, but it is necessary to provide a quick refresher without having to recap.

The illnesses that affect us 'progressively' alter but with overlaps. Again, it was an editorial decision to make these entire rather than referring you to other pages.

In the same way the graphs are explained (light and dark bars, YLL, YLD, etc.), these concepts are explained each time. Again, to save you referring elsewhere.

In other words, select the chapter for your age, and that should tell you the whole story.

You may wish, in fact it is advisable, to read the next chapter to see what the future may bring (and how to avoid it).

Causes of Death by Age and Sex

Male and female are in separated sections. Identify the chapter appropriate to you for your age.

We should all live to be over 80 years of age. If this is not achieved, there are some illnesses or accidents that cause our premature demise. If these age specific illnesses are identified, avoidance or preventive measures can be instituted for each age group below 80 years. Males accounted for 62% of premature deaths. One in two premature deaths were considered potentially avoidable.[66]

Many of the illnesses and conditions (like blood pressure, high cholesterol, and early cancers) have no symptoms. Prioritizing them allows for specific focus, with the appropriate investigations and preventive measures, rather than the previous generalized, one-size-fits-all recommendations will allow you to know exactly what to focus on.

Hence, when you examine the tables, if you are a 45- to 54-year-old female, you are most likely to die from breast cancer in the United States and United Kingdom, but from coronary artery disease (CAD) if Australian.

The overall data (for all ages combined) is included for interest only; it highlights that heart or cardiovascular disease is the overall number-one killer for essentially all first world nations.

66 *Premature mortality in Australia 1997–2012,* https://www.aihw.gov.au/reports/life-expectancy-deaths/premature-mortality-in-australia-1997-2012/contents/summary

Emergency Signs and Prevention

The other essential is recognizing any acute and potentially serious symptoms and signs if and when they occur. Early medical attention results in the best outcomes. When I ran the coronary care unit, the greatest delay in patients being admitted occurred because they "didn't want to bother anyone". The average delay, from memory, was some four to six hours before they called the ambulance, and in those days the ambulance response time was slower. Today, however, while people may still "not want to bother anyone," most are either in denial or don't recognize their symptoms as being potentially serious.

The Following are Emergency Signs:

If you experience any of these, get checked out *immediately:*

1. Chest pain like indigestion that won't go away. This is a heart attack until proven otherwise.
2. FAST: Face—drooping; Arms—weakness; Speech—slurred, difficult; Time—urgent.
3. Momentary loss of vision. This may be a Transient Ischaemic Attack warning of a stroke.
4. Chronic cough, especially in smokers.
5. Change in bowel habit.
6. Unexplained loss of weight or tiredness.
7. Nocturia (having to get up to void at night).
8. Intermenstrual bleeding.

A Note:

I recommend **The Three Ps**

1. Project
2. Purpose
3. Participate (socialise)

for people who are retired, as they often find themselves somewhat lost, but it has been pointed out it is good advice for all ages.

And a Further Note

As to the sources for all the following causes of death the official Government Data is quoted viz:[67]

Overall, Cardiovascular disease is our greatest killer

Little wonder as the human heart pumps about 2,000 gallons (7,571 liters) of blood and beats around 100,000 times each and every day. Extra fat makes your circulatory system work overtime. Every pound (0.45kg) of (extra) fat contains 5 miles (8km) of blood vessels, ('The lean live longest'). Any elevated blood pressure then forces our hearts to work even harder. It is essential to regularly check your BP and lipids.

67 *CDC/National Center for Health Statistics*, Office for National Statistics (ONS), released 15 December 2023, ONS website; Statistical bulletin, "Deaths registered in England and Wales 2022"; Australian Institute Health and Welfare (AIHW) National Mortality Database.

CHAPTER 7

Men Under 24 Years

"The Difficult Years"

Table 5:

USA Males 20-24	**UK Males 5 - 19 yrs**	**Australia 15-24**
Unintentional injuries 42.7%	Transport Accidents (Land)	Suicide
Suicide 18.8%	Suicide	Land Transport Accidents
Homicide 16.8%	Homicide	Accidental Poisoning
Cancer 4.2%	Lymphoid Cancer	Assault
Heart Disease 3.0%	Congenital Defects	Event of Undetermined Intent
Birth Defects 0.8%	Cerebral Palsy / Paralytic Syndromes	
Diabetes 0.6%	Brain Cancer	
Flu & Pneumonia 0.5%	Accidental Poisoning	
Ch Lower Respiratory D	Accidental Threats to Breathing	
Stroke 0.5%	Emphysema / Bronchitis	

Although we know that high-risk behavior is common in young men and leads to injuries and deaths, the data on "fun activities" is not well known.

A study of youth and adolescents, 5–19 years of age, who were treated in US emergency departments (EDs) found that over a 19-year period, there were an average of 176 visits a day for skateboarding-related injuries.[68]

Quad bikes are the greatest cause of injury and deaths on farms.[69]

Diving into shallow water, drugs, alcohol, and driving too fast are perhaps better known.

Many of these are a matter of "boys being boys" or an inevitable rite of passage as testosterone surges. Some "primitive" tribes controlled this by initiation ceremonies, but these are high risk years for youths testing their boundaries.

What to Do

As can be seen in the next age group, "Drugs, Booze, and Testosterone" are also manifesting here. It is a too-often deadly combination as youths' experiment.

Parental control can give way to guidance and advice, but this age group consider themselves "bullet proof", and only the death of a close friend may alert them to modify their high-risk behaviors.

Sport has been a traditional outlet to attenuate the aggression that testosterone brings, but the electronic age has witnessed less and less sport being played.

Suicide figures prominently, and any signs of withdrawal, depression, or "problems" must be acted on urgently. But, again, this depends on parental competence and dedication which decreases in poorer families.

---

68 Epidemiology of skateboarding-related injuries sustained by children and adolescents 5-19 years of age and treated in US emergency departments: 1990 through 2008. *Injury Epidemiology*, 2016; 3 (1) DOI: 10.1186/s40621-016-0075-6

69 accc.gov.au 19 August 2020

Homicide would seem inexorably linked to permissive laws.

In the USA, fentanyl and guns dominate deaths, but now the drug xylazine, better known as "tranq", a powerful horse and cattle sedative used to enhance the effects of heroin, cocaine, and fentanyl is taking over.[70]

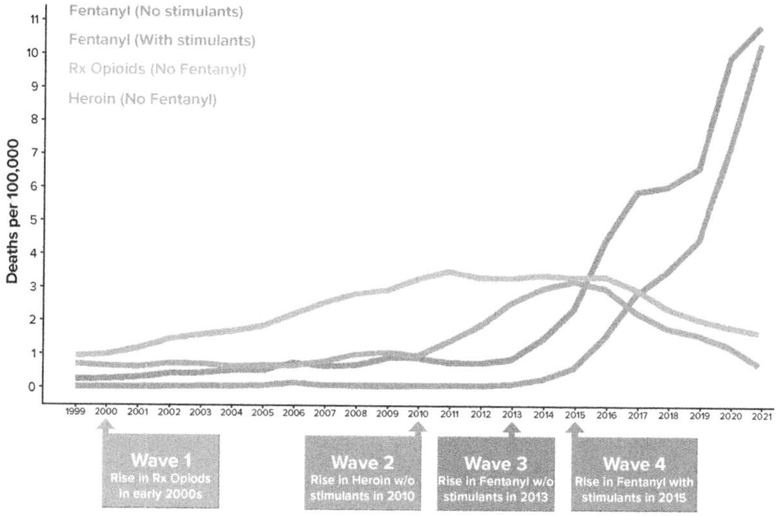

Figure 9: A simplified schema of the four waves of the US overdose mortality crisis. Waves 1 and 2 include deaths involving commonly prescribed opioids, and heroin, respectively, but excluding fentanyl co-involved deaths. Wave 3 and Wave 4 show fentanyl deaths not involving, and involving, stimulants respectively as distinct trends *(Source: Friedman, J. & Shover, C. L. 2023, "Charting the fourth wave: Geographic, temporal, race/ethnicity and demographic trends in polysubstance fentanyl overdose deaths in the United States, 2010–2021",* Addiction, *Vol. 118, No. 12, pp. 2477-2485 https://doi.org/10.1111/add.16318).*

70 Friedman, J. & Shover, C. L. 2023, "Charting the fourth wave: Geographic, temporal, race/ethnicity and demographic trends in polysubstance fentanyl overdose deaths in the United States, 2010–2021", *Addiction*, Vol. 118, No. 12, pp. 2477-2485 https://doi.org/10.1111/add.16318.

CHAPTER 8

Men 25–34–44 Years

More Drugs, Booze, and Testosterone

Drugs, Booze and Testosterone

Drugs, booze, and testosterone account for 70% of all deaths and disabilities in this age group, which is where to focus.

Causes of Deaths

As a group, the greatest cause of disabilities in this 25–44-year-old age group for men is mental disorders, which in turn are mainly due to substance abuse—alcohol and illicit drugs (38%) with fentanyl and 'tranq' (xylazine) taking over. Then, depression (27%) causing disability rather than premature deaths.[71] In fact, deaths in this first group have the lowest ratio to disabilities in the top six causes. Knowing that drugs, substance abuse, and

71 *Substance Abuse and Mental Health Services Administration*, 2022, "Key substance use and mental health indicators in the United States: Results from the 2021 National Survey on Drug Use and Health", Center for Behavioral Health Statistics and Quality, Substance Abuse and Mental Health Services Administration, https://www.samhsa.gov/data/report/2021-nsduh-annual-national-report.

Table 6:

	USA 25 - 34 yrs	**UK 20 - 34 yrs**	**Australia 25 - 44**
1	RTA (Road Traffic Accidents), Guns, Drugs	Suicide	Suicide
2	Homicide	Accidental Poisoning	Accidents
3	Suicide	RTA	Cancer
4	Poisoning	Homicide	Cardiovascular Disease
5	Other Injuries	Liver Disease	Infections / Parasitic Diseases
6	Drownings	Epilepsy	Mental Disorders
7	Endocrine Disorders	Heart Disease	Others
8	Congenital Abnormalities	Brain Cancer	Nervous System Disorders
9	Inflammatory/Heart	Lymphoid Cancer	Digestive System disorders
10	Leukemia	Cerebrovascular Disease	Chronic Respiratory Disease

Table 7:

	Evidenced prevalence (in order)	**Symptoms and preventive measures**
1	CVS	Shortness of breath on effort, chest pain. Screen. Better nutrition.
2	Infections	Cause. Overseas travel, prophylaxis.
3	Chronic Respiratory Diseases	Asthma/emphysema. Cease smoking. Treat aggressively.
4	Musculoskeletal Diseases—Back Pain	Back pain starts at 20. Lifting advice. No strong man show-off. Bend knees.
5	Nervous System Multiple Sclerosis	No preventive measures as yet.
6	Digestive System	Heartburn: Lose weight, stop smoking, reduce booze, avoid PPIs. Investigate any others.

depression cause so many problems may facilitate an earlier diagnosis. Today, it would seem naïve not to suspect substance abuse, which may also be a contributor to depression. Getting on

Table 8:

	Evidenced prevalence	Preventive measures
1	Drugs & Booze – 38% Depression	Suspect all males in this age group as substance abusers. Warn and advise. Watch for depression—suicide.
2	Homicide (USA/UK)	Access to guns is the problem.
3	RTA/Accidents – 15%	Fast cars, testosterone, and booze. Again, advice and counselling. Motor bikes are very dangerous: 5% of vehicles but 25% of MVAs.
4	Suicide – 12%	Heightened awareness that this age group is at risk. Early diagnosis, support, advice + antidepressants.
5	Cancer	Not as common as above but, smoking and processed foods promote. Alert for change of bowel habit, change in behaviour, smoker's cough.

the front foot and aggressively treating rather than suspecting depression is also arguably warranted.

In the United States, with easy access to firearms, homicide is high on the list.

Unintentional injuries are second and *contribute more to death than disabilities* (as do the next five causes). As above, they account for 15.5%, of which almost half are from road traffic accidents (RTA). This group represents the testosterone-fueled, high-risk behaviour group—smoking, drinking, "never thinking of tomorrow," experimenting, showing off, driving too fast. The best prevention is to start early with advice, warnings, defensive driving courses, and even a visit to the spinal injuries unit if the message isn't getting through.

Intentional injuries come third, making up some 12% of the total. Breaking down such injuries, 85% are due to suicide or self-inflicted injuries.

However, the largest *single* cause of disease and injury burden in this age group is suicide and self-inflicted injuries, at 10.3%; then depression (7.4%), road traffic accidents (6.6%), alcohol dependence/misuse (5.8%), HIV/AIDS (4.5%).

The message here is to get on the front foot and proactively assume depression and seek support, intervention, and treatment to prevent suicide or attempted suicide. This, I feel, cannot be over-emphasized.

Age-specific Tests

Now is the time to get your whole baseline tests, as per the appendix.

Cancer, or malignant neoplasms, are next, with brain cancers more common than most of us think; these are invariably fatal. Again, early diagnosis offers the best hope. Watch for any change of behaviour. These changes may be subtle but should not be ignored. Headaches are not often a symptom but, again, should not be ignored, while paralysis or altered movement is an advanced sign. Cancer of the colon (CAC) is another we don't really associate with young men, but there are some famous young widows whose husbands died from CAC. Unexplained loss of weight, change of bowel habit, passing mucus, slime or blood, and undue fatigue are signs.

Cardiovascular disease usually manifests later. Report any undue fatigue, and shortness of breath on exertion must be investigated. While the annual physical has been found a pretty useless ritual, getting one each decade in your 20s and 30s would seem warranted to listen for heart murmurs, ECG/EKG abnormalities, and lipids. In this age group, congenital abnormalities are more to be found than those caused by poor diet.

Infectious and parasitic diseases are usually communicable diseases spread by bacteria or viruses by airborne droplets, insects, and contaminated food; or, they are sexually transmitted. Everyone should be vaccinated against as many illnesses as possible. After that, continue to take care of personal hygiene.

Chronic respiratory disease is invariably the result of smoking, either active or passive, tobacco or marijuana and, as such, is preventable. Asthma is also an underestimated chronic illness where research reveals sufferers under-treat themselves. Neglecting regular prevention medication and only seeking immediate emergency relief leads to unnecessary hospitalizations and even deaths. Again, a very preventable illness.

Musculoskeletal diseases in these statistics don't cause death. They include osteo and rheumatoid arthritis, chronic back pain, and even gout, all of which are popularly considered as occurring in the older populace. Back pain increases dramatically at age 20 years (to 54), unlike the arthritides, which increase later at 40 years. There can be no doubt that these conditions can be a severe problem, ever since, as the medical observation goes, "man became the only animal with enough arrogance to walk upright on his hind legs." Often, a cause cannot be found, and this has led to abuse of the welfare system and a complicated psychiatric roundabout of "pain" gets reward. Much can be prevented by strong core muscles (para-spinal and abdominal), being fit, reducing abdominal fat, and avoiding unnatural postures, especially while lifting (bend the knees). Back surgery has improved by leaps and bounds.

Nervous system disorders at this age are usually epilepsy or multiple sclerosis. Unfortunately, there are no prevention methods except for avoiding traumas that cause epilepsy.

Digestive system diseases run the spectrum from indigestion to cancer (covered above) and include ulcers, irritable bowel syndrome, Crohn's disease, ulcerative colitis, and piles.

Looking ahead, there is a dramatic change after 45, when heart disease and cancer raise their ugly heads. This fact should alert all to cease smoking and eat the ***Newtrition Diet*** (see end). The most obvious, and therefore frequently the most overlooked deduction, is that heart disease and cancer *don't* suddenly start at 45. If males do manage to live through their high-risk behavior years, avoiding unintentional or intentional injuries, they have, however, not avoided causing the pathology that will kill or burden them. So, as well as addressing these high-risk behaviors by being alert to possible depression and potential suicide, we should also be looking at what prevents the diseases that manifest after 45.

You will also see that mental illness and suicide dramatically decrease with age. It would be more than cynical to suggest that this is because all the fragile males have already topped themselves. Rather, it is the accepted medical wisdom that if we can get them through these high-risk years, their mental state stabilizes to normal, so it's worth being aware and making the effort.

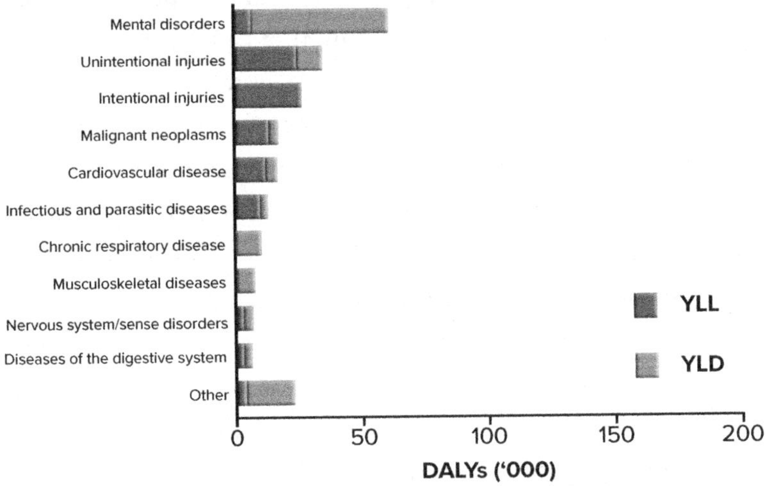

Figure 10: Leading causes of burden of disease and injury in men aged 25-44 years. YLD = Years Lost Due to Disability = Non-fatal burden of illness, i.e., chronic illnesses. YLL = Years of Life Lost due to premature death by the same illness. DALY = YLL + YLD = Total Burden (*Source: Australian Burden of Disease and Injury Study*).

CHAPTER 9

Men 35-64

The Male Menopause, Heart Attacks, and Cancer

Life is more stressful now than in the 1990s, especially for the middle-aged, those aged 45 to 64, research in 2023 from Penn State University has found.[72]

Overall

The drugs, booze, smoking, junk food, and obesity have now caught up, and cardiovascular disease and cancer affect over half of these men. Look ahead at what illnesses are most likely when over 65. These are what you must now try to prevent, as well as getting early diagnosis of any current ailments (CVD increases significantly at 65 but cancer does not).

72 Penn State, 2020, "Middle age may be much more stressful now than in the '90s", *ScienceDaily*, 7 May, www.sciencedaily.com/releases/2020/05/200507094745.htm.

Table 9: Causes of Male Deaths

	USA 35 - 44 years	UK 35 - 49	Australia 45 - 64
1	Suicide	Suicide	CVD
2	Poisoning	Heart Disease	Cancer
3	CAD	Liver Disease	Accidents
4	RTA	Accidental Poisoning	Digestive D
5	Homicide	CVD	Ch Lung D
6	Liver Disease	Lung Cancer	Diabetes Mellites
7	Hypertension	RTA	Nervous Syst
8	Diabetes Mellitus	CAC	Mental
9	CVA	Lymphoid Cancer	Genito-urinary
10	CAC	Brain Cancer	Musculoskeletal

Causes of Premature Deaths and Disabilities, in Order, 45-64

1. Cardiovascular disease (CVA)
2. Malignant neoplasms (cancer)
3. Nervous system disorders
4. Mental disorders (disability far greater than deaths)
5. Chronic respiratory diseases
6. Diabetes mellitus
7. Unintentional injuries
8. Musculoskeletal diseases (100% disabilities)
9. Digestive system diseases
10. Genito-urinary diseases
11. Other

Disabling conditions most affecting 45–64-year-old males:

1. Ischemic heart disease 17%
2. Lung cancer 7%
3. Nervous system 7%

4. Mental disorders 6%
5. COPD (Chronic Obstructive Pulmonary Disease) 5%
6. Diabetes 5%
7. Hearing Loss 5%

Causes of disease and injury burden: Men aged 45–64

1. Cardiovascular disease 26%
2. Ischemic heart disease 64%
3. Strokes 17%
4. Cancer 25%
5. Lung 26%
6. Colorectal 16%

What to do:

Get help if depressed or if having any suicidal thoughts.

At 35 or 40, it is time to get a base-line level for all medical tests as per, but especially: blood pressure, lipids (cholesterol), blood glucose, liver function tests, and CT scan chest/angiogram done.

Immediately stop smoking.

Adopt the Mediterranean diet of ***Newtrition Foods.***

Consider low-dose aspirin twice a week to help prevent stomach and colon cancer (but needs 10 years and side effects and serious bleeding events are becoming more and more recorded).

Get fit.

Report wheeze, difficulty breathing, chronic cough, and bloody phlegm to your doctor.

Get a hearing test if any difficulties.

Suicide

It is a surprise that suicide is the number one killer for men aged 35 to 50 years in the USA and England/Wales. One can only conjecture as to the causes—unfulfilled ambitions, failed love, business failure, the male menopause—but psychiatry for too long has gotten bogged down as to etiology (cause) and not got on with treatment. It is rather like asking someone bleeding to death from a leg wound 'how it happened' rather than staunching the loss and applying a tourniquet.

A little-known fact is that it is not known how anti-depressants work and that the only reliable anti-depressant over the last 25 years is called a placebo.

All are at risk, and the best help is support from all sources—family, health workers, friends, social groups. Any talk of suicide, even a seeming joke, is a red-flag emergency.

Cardiovascular disease

Ischemic heart disease means the blood supply to the heart is compromised by cholesterol plaques and narrowing of the coronary (heart) arteries. This usually first manifests as heart pain on exertion (angina) and must be treated and monitored. Any chest pain, undue fatigue, or shortness of breath on exertion must be investigated. It would be advisable to get your blood pressure checked, have your doctor listen for heart murmurs, request a lipids panel (LDL/ApoB), and have an ECG and/or EKG done when you are 35, then repeat each of these tests every five to10 years.

Cancer. This age group, between 35 and 64, is where cancer is most likely, and early diagnosis affords the best chances of cure or survival. Be aware of the early symptoms and signs. Report any cough, loss of weight, altered bowel habit, passing or coughing up of blood or mucus.

Cancer of the colon (CAC): unexplained fatigue, loss of weight, change of bowel habit, and passing mucus, slime, or blood are symptoms and signs. Get a blood test, and if slightly anaemic, get a colonoscopy. Faecal blood tests may pick up some problems, but a colonoscopy is the gold standard. People who took an aspirin tablet (325 or 81 mg) at least twice a week (usually for headache or muscle pain) had a lower incidence of gastrointestinal tract cancers, especially colorectal cancers. Again, aspirin is being recorded as causing increasing serious bleeding events. I would only consider using it if there was a strong family history.

Lung cancer and Chronic Obstructive Pulmonary Disease (COPD) are invariably due to smoking tobacco or marijuana and are preventable. But be alert to any past workplace contaminants such as asbestos, which may be as "innocent" as wrapping/lagging on factory or ships' pipes. If you are a smoker, you must get regular chest x-rays. If you have a cough that hangs on, also get a chest x-ray. Better still, stop smoking.

Skin Cancer and Melanoma, like all cancers, "take off" after the age of 40 and increase. This is due to excessive ultraviolet radiation—sun exposure. Like lung cancer, it is not the one packet of cigarettes but the regular exposure to the carcinogens (smoke or sun) over some 20 years that initiates the mutation of the DNA in our cells to become cancers. The best feature of skin cancer is that it can be seen and, therefore, most can be diagnosed early enough to effect a cure. Get checked annually.

Aspirin for Preventing CVD and Colorectal Cancer-But, with Reservations.[73] In 2016, the United States Preventive Services Taskforce (USPSTF) recommended initiating low-dose aspirin use for the primary prevention of CVD and CRC in

73 US Preventive Services Task Force, 2022, "Aspirin Use to Prevent Cardiovascular Disease: US Preventive Services Task Force Recommendation Statement", *JAMA*, Vol. 327, No. 16, pp. 1577-1584, https://doi.org/10.1001/jama.2022.4983. PMID: 35471505.

adults aged 50 to 59 years who have a 10% or greater 10-year CVD risk, are not at increased risk for bleeding, have a life expectancy of at least 10 years, and are willing to take low-dose aspirin daily for at least 10 years. However, the decision to initiate low-dose aspirin use in adults aged 60 to 69 years who have a 10% or greater 10-year CVD risk should be an individual one. The USPSTF previously found that the evidence was insufficient to assess the balance of benefits and harms of initiating aspirin use for the primary prevention of CVD and CRC in adults younger than 50 years or adults 70 years or older.

It does not prevent primary CVD but does carry significant risks of brain and GIT bleeds.

Seniors who took low dose aspirin[74] daily for primary prevention had no reduction in the risk for first strokes in a large, randomized trial that followed them for about 5 years.

But those who took aspirin at 100 mg/d, compared with placebo, did show a significant 38% jump in risk for intracranial (IC) bleeding. Rates for ischemic stroke[75] and for hemorrhagic stroke[76] were similar between the aspirin and control groups.

Low dose aspirin, however, is recommended for secondary prevention, i.e., for patients at risk of having a heart attack in people who have heart disease. It is also used to reduce the risk of stroke in people who have previously had a stroke or "mini stroke" (transient ischemic attack) due to a blood clot (and not a haemorrhage).

Among such individuals with a self-reported history of cardiovascular disease, aspirin use for secondary prevention was 40.3% in the pooled sample and ranged from 16.6% in

---

74 Medscape aspirin (Rx, OTC), 2023

75 Medscape Ischemic Stroke, updated 14 Jul 14y 2022

76 Medscape Hemorrhagic Stroke, updated 22 April 2019

low-income countries to 65.0% in high-income countries, which authorities suggest is suboptimal use.[77]

In other words, if you have heart disease or had a TIA, you should be on it.

Aspirin works by stopping platelets from clumping together and forming blood clots that can cause a heart attack or stroke.

Nervous system disorders at this age are multiple sclerosis or more rare degenerative disorders, for which there are no prevention or treatments except for specialized rehab centres. Report any unexplained limb weakness, incoordination, vision disturbances, altered sensations, or headaches.

Mental problems, usually anxiety or depression, should be addressed with cognitive behavioral therapy.

The "Male Menopause" or Mid-Life Crisis

Female Menopause is when the ovaries shut down and hormones cut off. Humans are only one of a few animals that undergo menopause. The others are Cetaceans, marine mammals, It is dramatic and often very symptomatic and debilitating.

By contrast, the male hormones continue on, only slightly lessening with time. However, the 'Male Menopause', or mid-life crisis, would seem a real entity. It is best explained where and when the man feels he is losing his youthful vitality, hasn't achieved his dreams, and seeks to recreate it with a sports car, a trophy mistress, and even by seeking longevity treatments.

While this may be an object of derision, it has been pointed out that monogamy is unnatural to most species and humans. By living much longer, we have not been "prepared" by evolution

77 Yoo, S. G. K., Chung, G. S., Bahendeka, S. K. *et al.* 2023, "Aspirin for Secondary Prevention of Cardiovascular Disease in 51 Low-, Middle-, and High-Income Countries", *JAMA*, Vol. 330, No. 8, pp. 715-724, https://doi.org/10.1001/jama.2023.12905

for the long monogamous relationships that our new longevity provides. It is a subject too complex to deal with here, but an equitable divorce is better than a poisonous marriage, the ultimate objective being the welfare and prosperity of all concerned.

I have also noted that this current obsession by longevity entrepreneurs seems to be dominated by mid-aged men. My interest, however, began in the world's first coronary care unit when I was 27 and when I witnessed people dying too young from preventable heart attacks. You can't live longer if you're dead. First things first.

Asthma and emphysema are also very "underestimated" chronic illnesses where research shows sufferers under-treat themselves, especially as to regular prevention medication rather than immediate emergency relief leading to unnecessary hospitalizations and even deaths. Again, a very preventable illness.

Diabetes 2 we associate with being fat, but there are many skinny diabetics. Get a blood glucose test.

Musculoskeletal diseases in these statistics don't cause death. They include osteo and rheumatoid arthritis, chronic back pain and even gout.

Back pain increases dramatically at age 20 years to 54, unlike the arthritides, which increase later at 40 years. There can be no doubt that it can be a severe problem ever since "man became the only animal with enough arrogance to walk upright on his hind legs." Often, a cause cannot be found, and this has led to abuse of the welfare system and a complicated psychiatric roundabout of "pain" gets reward." Much can be prevented by strong core muscles (para-spinal and abdominal), being fit, reducing abdominal fat, and avoiding unnatural postures, especially while lifting. Getting a diagnosis allows for the most appropriate treatment.

Physiotherapy, weight loss, and having fit muscles, while maintaining flexibility and movement, are all important while using the minimum of analgesics. NSAIDS used as anti-inflammatories, while effective, cause heart attacks, and I try to avoid them. There is a pecking order as to cardio toxicity, with Naproxen being the least toxic.

If musculoskeletal issues persist, an MRI is mandatory for a diagnosis.

Digestive system diseases run the spectrum from indigestion to cancer (covered above) to ulcers, irritable bowel syndrome, Crohn's Disease, ulcerative colitis, and piles. Weight loss and tiredness are often the early symptoms, and the passing of blood or mucus is an early sign.

Genito-urinary issues usually mean "prostate trouble" or benign prostate hypertrophy (BPH) where the prostate enlarges, then pushes into the bladder or urethra causing difficult or frequent urination and nocturia—having to get up at night to void.

There are drugs available, but one type causes feminizing side effects and reduced libido or performance. An interesting alternative may be one of the erection enhancers—Tadalafil (Cialis)—which, in smaller doses, relaxes the bladder's small muscle wall and relieves the nocturia. Bladder and kidney cancers are not unknown—report passing any pink-blood urine.

The usual treatment for BPH was a TURP—Trans Urethral Resection of the Prostate, which is a rather brutal "re-bore' of the penis. Now, radiology departments offer Prostate Artery Embolization (PAE) with less risk, less pain, and less recovery time than traditional surgery. They also offer water vapor thermal therapy (WVTT).

Water vapor thermal therapy (WVTT) involves using a special steam-creating device to reduce the size of the prostate. The hot steam travels through a tube in the urethra and damages excess prostate tissue. Over time, the body reabsorbs this tissue. After multiple sessions, the prostate should decrease in size and put less pressure on the urethra.

Outcome and success rates

Some evidence suggests that WVTT is effective. According to a 2020 review, WVTT may improve symptoms in people with moderate to severe symptoms of an enlarged prostate.[78] Adverse effects are usually temporary and relatively unserious. However, further research is necessary to evaluate this treatment.

Prostatic urethral lift

Prostatic urethral lift (UroLift) uses implants to hold the prostate back and reduce pressure on the urethra. Doctors begin the UroLift procedure by inserting a device into the urethra. This device can hook tiny stainless-steel implants onto the prostate. Once these implants are secure, they move the prostate away from the urethra. The latest survey found it more effective than WVTT.

Outcome and success rates

Research suggests that UroLift may be an effective treatment for an enlarged prostate. According to a 2021 analysis of real-world UroLift procedure outcomes in hospitals across England, the complication rate tends to be relatively low. Within two years of undergoing UroLift treatment, only 11.9% of people required further retreatment for an enlarged prostate.[79]

---

78 Miller, L. E., Chughtai, B., McVary, K. *et al.* 2020, "Water vapor thermal therapy for lower urinary tract symptoms secondary to benign prostatic hyperplasia: Systematic review and meta-analysis", *Medicine*, Vol. 99, No. 30, https://doi.org/10.1097/MD.0000000000021365.

79 Page, T., Veeratterapillay, R., Keltie, K. *et al.* 2021, "Prostatic urethral lift (UroLift): a real-world analysis of outcomes using hospital episodes statistics", *BMC Urology*, Vol. 21, No. 55, https://doi.org/10.1186/s12894-021-00824-5.

Prostate artery embolization

Prostate artery embolization (PAE) aims to restrict blood flow to the prostate, causing it to shrink.

During the procedure, a medical professional enters a thin tube into an artery in the groin or wrist. Using imaging technology, they guide the tube into the prostate arteries and inject tiny round particles that help restrict blood flow.

Outcome and success rates

Results on the effectiveness of PAE are unclear.

Some research suggests that symptoms of enlarged prostate recur in 23% of cases post-PAE. Additionally, the complication rate for PAE is around 32.9%, although 99% of these are minor. However, the same analysis suggests it can significantly reduce symptoms.[80]

Other

Hearing loss negatively affects your life. It is important you become aware as to any reduction in your hearing. While there are different types, most are caused by loud noise (amplified music, machinery). Reduce exposure. Use earmuffs. Turn the TV and radio down.

80 Naidu, S. G., Narayanan, H., Saini, G. *et al.* 2021, "Prostate artery embolization—review of indications, patient selection, techniques and results", *Journal of Clinical Medicine*, Vol. 10, No. 21, https://doi.org/10.3390/jcm10215139

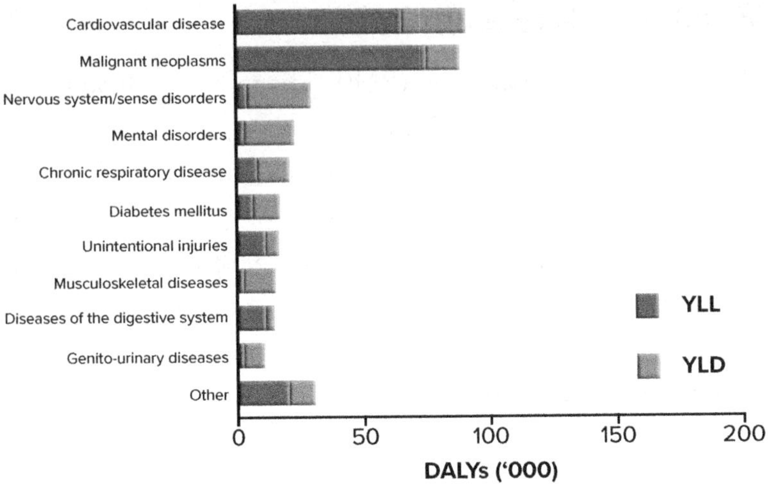

Figure 11: Leading causes of burden of disease and injury in men aged 45-64 years. YLD = Years Lost Due to Disability = Non-fatal burden of illness, i.e., chronic illnesses. YLL = Years of Life Lost due to premature death by the same illness. DALY = YLL + YLD = Total Burden (*Source: Australian Burden of Disease and Injury Study*).

CHAPTER 10

Men 65 years and over

No Mental Issues, More Fatal Heart Attacks & Cancer

Table 10: Causes of Deaths and, for Australia, Disabilities.

	USA 65 years+	**UK 65+**	**Australia 65+**
1	CAD	IHD	CVD
2	Lung Disease	Cancer, Lung & Trachea	Cancer
3	Diabetes	Lower Respiratory D	Nervous Syst
4	Stroke	CVD	Ch Lung D
5	Homicide	Ca Prostate	Genito-urinary
6	Cancer Colon		Diabetes melitus
7	Hypertension		Digestive D
8	Cancer Pancreas		Musculoskeletal
9	Liver Cancer		Accidents
10			Endocrine/Metabolic

Thankfully, the black 'Slough of Despond' has been crossed, and suicide is no longer high on the list. Both the previous major problems of heart disease and cancer have increased in this age group, and both of these now cause significantly more deaths than disability.

Cardiovascular disease has increased from 26% to 36% (i.e., more than a third), which makes it priority number one.

Cancer has only increased by some 2%, but it is still one of the major problems.

I am continually amazed at old people who groan as they undress and have to be helped onto the examination table and complain "It's awful getting old, doctor." They are slow, bent, dull and look old, but when I check their age, they are up to 10 years younger than I am! Most of them, in fact, add and admonish me, "Wait till you're my age!" They have no debilitating illnesses, but their whole attitude is wrong.

Someone recently said, "75 is the new 60", and due to improved nutrition, public health measures, and modern medicine, this is indeed the case. So, being "65 and over" does not condemn you to the retirement village—rather, it is a call to increase your pursuit of health and vitality. Be an optimist. There are a lot of people worse off.

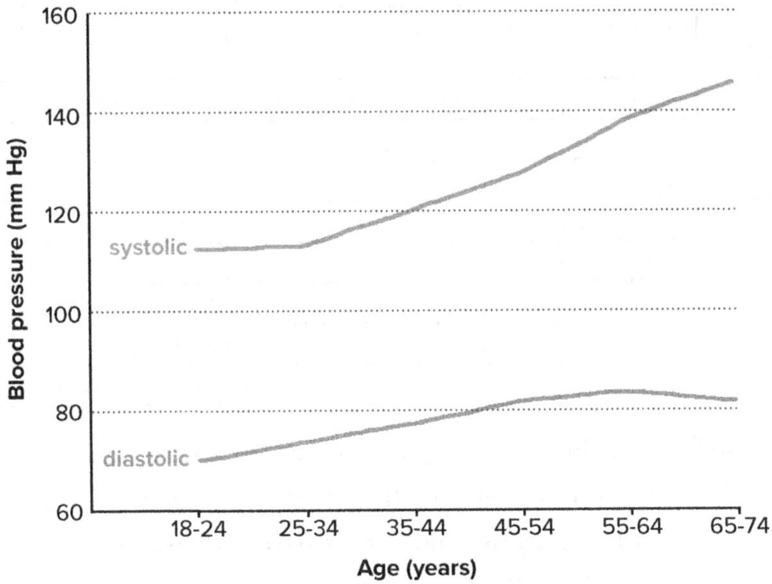

Figure 12: Relation between age and blood pressure (*Source: van Katwijk, C. & Peeters, L. L. 1998, "Clinical aspects of pregnancy after the age of 35 years: A review of the literature",* Human Reproduction Update, *Vol. 4, No. 2, pp. 185-94, https://doi.org/10.1093/humupd/4.2.185*).

When I had whining, introspective patients in hospital with not much wrong but who pestered me out of proportion to their ailment, I had them moved beside someone terminally ill. When that patient died, the change in the hypochondriacs was always startling.

One of my "treatments" for bad sleep, if and only if it is suitable after I have assessed the patient—usually a stressed businessperson who keeps mulling over their work—is to recommend the patient listen to the news. After the suicide bombings, refugee drownings, and the ghastly tsunami of bad news upon bad news, the penny drops, and they realize they don't have such horrors to contend with. Their anxiety over what was keeping them awake is not as great as these life-and-death struggles; with this new-found objectivity, they can go to sleep. But more, this newfound objectivity can and should be applied to every-day living. Carpe diem.

We all have to die, despite Silicon Valley's efforts, but the whole essence of this book is to live it up as long as you can. Don't become a premature invalid. At 65 and over, there is the distinct danger of people winding down because that is how they think society is geared. Well, read *The New York Times* obituaries and see just how many were rock and rollin' into their 90s.

Cardiovascular Disease

Cardiovascular disease is mostly IHD (60%).

This is where to place greatest priority. The best advice has been already documented above.

What to do:

Don't smoke.

Report any chest pain, shortness of breath, and ankle swelling.

Get BP, LDL, and BG checked.

Get an ECG/EKG or a Kardia—or a smart watch—to exclude silent atrial fibrillation, which isa major cause of strokes and now an epidemic for those over 60 years.

Learn to feel your own pulse, and if thready and irregular, get another ECG/EKG. AF can strike at any time and causes an irregular pulse.

An abdominal ultrasound is now recommended to exclude an aortic aneurysm.

Adopt *Newtrition Diet.*

Exercise and weight programs (lose weight, cope with stress, challenge the brain).

Cancer

Lung cancer accounts for 26% of cancers, so get a low dose CT scan or x-ray of chest.

Prostate 19%.

Colorectal cancer (CRC) 14%.

Skin

Get checked annually

What to do:

Report any urgency, frequency of urination, or nocturia (having to get up at nights to void). There were no satisfactory tests for cancer of the prostate, and in any event, it is often so slow growing that men die from something else. It is alleged that every male over 90 has cancer of the prostate. But now, a specific prostate MRI gives higher diagnostic results.

Report any alteration of bowel habit, passage of blood, mucus, or unexplained loss of weight.

Consider having a colonoscopy. Cancer of the colon is curable if resected early enough.

Nervous System Disorders

Alzheimer's/Dementia may begin at this age. Be alert to signs and symptoms (see specific later chapter).

It is now more important than ever to accept new challenges and force the brain along. Adopt the *Newtrition Diet.*

The Rest

There is now greater urgency not to ignore what you may consider "minor" symptoms. It is the proactive patient who achieves the best results for their health.

Stay fit, slim, and active with plenty of new mental challenges.

Finally, see the Appendix for detailed age-specific tests and investigations.

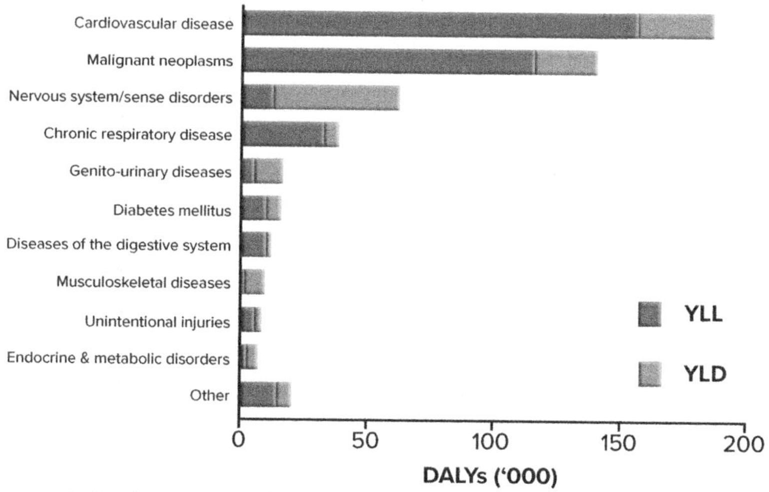

Figure 13: Leading causes of burden of disease and injury in men aged 65 years and over. YLD = Years Lost Due to Disability = Non-fatal burden of illness, i.e., chronic illnesses. YLL = Years of Life Lost due to premature death by the same illness. DALY = YLL + YLD = Total Burden (*Source: Australian Burden of Disease and Injury Study*).

CHAPTER 11

Women

Women's Greatest Concerns (UK)

1. Heart disease
2. Breast cancer
3. Osteoporosis
4. Depression
5. Autoimmune diseases

Table 11: Leading causes of burden of disease and injury. Note, these are conditions which make someone an invalid or disabled and may or may not include the cause of death (*Source: Australian Burden of Disease Study 2022, 13 December 2022*).

25 - 44 years		45 - 64 years		65 years and over	
Condition	**% of Total**	**Condition**	**% of Total**	**Condition**	**% of Total**
Depression	12.1	Breast Cancer	10.0	Ischemic Heart Disease	20.3
Anxiety	6.2	Osteoarthritis	6.6	Stroke	10.7
Breast Cancer	4.9	Ischemic Heart Disease	6.5	Alzheimer's/ Dementia	8.9
Genito-urinary Diseases	4.2	Diabetes Mellitus	5.6	Ch Obstructive Pulmonary D	4.0
Asthma	3.5	Depression	5.2	Breast Cancer	3.6

CHAPTER 12

Young Women

Road Accidents and Suicides

Table 12: (*Source: CDC/National Center for Health Statistics, Mortality in the United States, 2021, 17 January 2024; Office for National Statistics (ONS), released 15 December 2023, ONS website, statistical bulletin, Deaths registered in England and Wales, 2022*).

USA Females 15 – 24	**England and Wales 5 - 19**
RTA	RTA
Suicide	Suicide
Poisonings	Homicide
Homicide	Lymphoid Cancer
Endocrine Disorders	Congenital Defects
Other Injuries	Cerebral Palsy
Congenital Anomalies	Brain Cancer
Maternal Conditions	Accidental Poisoning
Leukemia	Accidental Breathing Threats
Influenza and Pneumonia	Emphysema / Bronchitis

The England and Wales figures are from age 5 years, so more infantile conditions occur.

For the 15 to 24 years old age group, road accidents predominate. Suicide is second, and this is where most emphasis needs to be placed.

Counselling youths not to drink and drive and to wear seat belts cannot be over emphasized or repeated enough.

Suicide watch is all important. Note any mood changes, withdrawal, sadness, volatility, or frank depression. If these signs are observed, immediate attention and intensive observation and support are required.

CHAPTER 13

Women 25-44

Depression, Anxiety, & Cancer

Table 13: Causes of female deaths (*Source: AIHW National Mortality Database*).

	USA 25 - 34	England & Wales 20-34	Australia 25 - 44
1	Unintentional Injuries	Poisoning	Suicide
2	Cancer	Accidental Poisoning	Accidental Poisoning
3	Suicide	RTA	RTA
4	Heart Disease	Breast Ca	CAD

Disabilities

As noted, causes of premature death are not always in the same order as causes of premature disabilities.

In this age group, depression and anxiety far outstrip any cause of deaths, where cancer claims most victims.

Causes of Premature Deaths and Disabilities in Order 25 - 44yrs

1. Mental Disorders (disability far greater than deaths)
2. Malignant Neoplasms (cancer)
3. Chronic Respiratory Diseases
4. Genito-urinary Diseases (100% disability—not fatal)
5. Musculoskeletal Diseases (100% disabilities—not fatal)
6. Unintentional Injuries
7. Cardiovascular Disease
8. Intentional Injuries
9. Digestive System Diseases
10. Nervous System Disorders

Disability Problems for this Age Group (25-44 years) Are:

1. Mental Illnesses

Depression 38%
Anxiety 33%

As a group, the greatest cause of disabilities in this 25–44-year-old age group for women is dominated by mental disorders, which in turn are mainly due to depression (38%) and anxiety (33%), causing disability rather than premature deaths.

While deaths, according to this data set, are relatively few, it is to be noted that for "8. Intentional Injuries", by which we can only assume suicide, deaths are 100% and surely the result of a mental illness, be it acute or chronic depression.

Drugs or illicit substances do not seem to play as much a role as with young men, but the liberation of women may make this an impression rather than an actual fact. After all, women are smoking and drinking alcohol more, which usually shadows drug and substance abuse.

The explosion of hormones, now or earlier, provides a roller coaster ride for many young women with unrealized and confused ambitions. Marrying your childhood sweetheart and having kids before the age of 20 is no longer the preferred career move. But what is? A world perceived to be male-dominated and offering less career satisfaction might frustrate, confuse, and depress the more ambitious. Coping with the workplace and accepting responsibility can engender anxiety in those promoted beyond their experience or competence. A turbulent home life only exacerbates the problem(s).

Most seem to settle in their 30s, but the "Big 4-0" would seem to make women sit up, look around and wonder if there isn't more to life.

While unpleasant, most of these mental disorders respond to treatment and do not account for many deaths.

2. Cancer

Cancer accounts for 13% of the disabilities in this age group, of which breast cancer predominates at 37% and is one of the greatest causes of death. Early diagnosis is essential.

What to do:

Mammograms, examinations, and pap smears should be done. The time intervals differ from country to country and are often updated—check with your local authority.

Genetic counselling is encouraged if there is a family history.

3. Chronic Respiratory Disease

Chronic respiratory disease is invariably the result of smoking, either active or passive, tobacco or marijuana and, as such, is preventable. Asthma is also an underestimated chronic illness where research reveals sufferers under-treat themselves. Neglecting regular prevention medication and only seeking immediate emergency relief leads to unnecessary hospitalizations and even deaths. Again, a very preventable illness.

4. Genito-Urinary Disease

Sexually transmitted diseases (STDs) are likely and increasing in the sexually active with multiple partners. Intercourse, childbirth, and the anatomy where the opening of the urethra is so close to the vagina and anus make women much more susceptible to urinary tract infections. It is essential that these be completely cleared each time, or there is the chance of chronic infection, which can then ascend to the kidney—a far greater problem. The gold standard is to get a mid-stream urine specimen to identify the germ, prescribe the best antibiotic, and then repeat the test after the course of antibiotics to make sure the urine is now sterile.

Childbirth can also distort the anatomy, making infections more easily acquired, as well as causing the uterus to displace.

Regular checks are mandatory—see Appendix.

5. Musculoskeletal

Musculoskeletal disorders don't often cause death and include osteo and rheumatoid arthritis and chronic back pain. Back pain increases dramatically at age 20 years to 54, unlike the arthritides, which increase later at 40 years. There can be no doubt that it can be a severe problem. Often, a cause cannot be found. Much can be prevented by strong core muscles (para-spinal and abdominal), being fit, reducing abdominal fat, and avoiding unnatural postures, especially while lifting. Getting a diagnosis allows for the most appropriate treatment.

Physiotherapy, weight loss, and having fit muscles while maintaining flexibility and movement are all important while using the minimum of analgesics. NSAIDS used as anti-inflammatories, while effective, cause heart attacks, and I try to avoid them. There is a pecking order as to cardio toxicity, with Naproxen being the least toxic.

6. *Cardiovascular Disease (CVD)*

CVD, surprisingly, manifests later in women or is under-diagnosed. Any undue fatigue, shortness of breath on exertion, or chest pain must be investigated. Get BP checked regularly and have an ECG/EKG if asymptomatic when you hit 40. Get your LDL/ApoB and Lp(a), if not previously done at 30, as a baseline record.

7. *Digestive Tract Disorders*

Digestive system diseases run the spectrum from indigestion and cancer (covered above) to ulcers, irritable bowel syndrome, Crohn's Disease, ulcerative colitis, and piles. Weight loss and tiredness are often the early symptoms, while the passing of blood or mucus is an early sign. Recurrent abdominal pain, swelling, or diarrhea must be investigated.

8. *Nervous System Disorders*

At this age, these are Multiple Sclerosis or rare degenerative disorders for which there are no preventions or treatments except for specialized rehab centers.

The following graphs are to show the proportions as to different causes of premature deaths (UK) and then the most helpful combining causes of both premature deaths and disabilities.

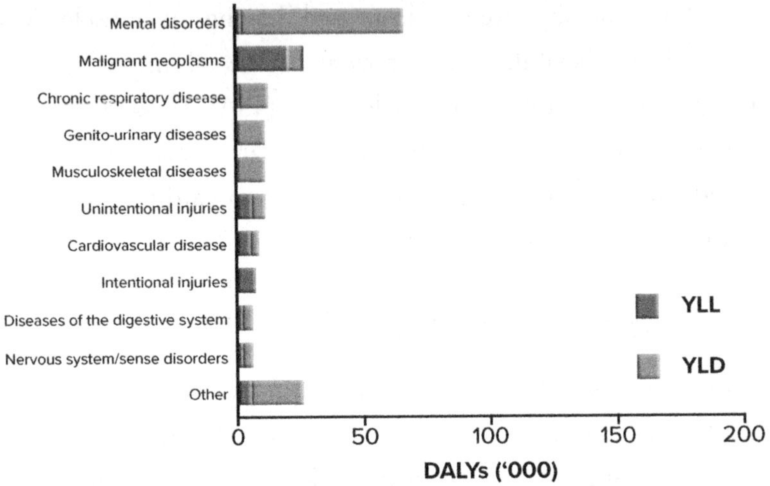

Figure 14: Leading causes of burden of disease and injury in women aged 25-44 years. YLD = Years Lost Due to Disability = Non-fatal burden of illness, i.e., chronic illnesses. YLL = Years of Life Lost due to premature death by the same illness. DALY = YLL + YLD = Total Burden (*Source: Australian Burden of Disease and Injury Study*).

CHAPTER 14

Women Aged 45–64 Years

Cancer (breast, lung, colon) and Heart

Table 14: Causes of premature deaths.

	USA 45 - 54	**England & Wales 35-49**	**Australia 45 - 64**
1	Cancer (Breast, Lung, CRC)	Breast Ca	CAD
2	Heart Disease	Liver D	Lung Ca
3	Unintentional Injuries	Accidental Poisoning	Breast Ca
4	Ch Liver D	Suicide	Suicide
5	Ch Lower Respiratory D	IHD	CRC

Australia Causes of Premature Deaths and Disabilities

1. Malignant Neoplasms (cancer) 13%
2. Cardiovascular Disease 5.7%
3. Mental Disorders (disability far greater than deaths)
4. Musculoskeletal Diseases (100% disabilities- not fatal)
5. Nervous System Disorders
6. Chronic Respiratory Diseases
7. Diabetes Mellitus
8. Unintentional Injuries
9. Digestive System Diseases
10. Oral Health

This is quite a difference from the younger previous group, wherein the dominant mental issues of depression and anxiety and intentional injuries have been displaced by cancer and heart disease. Surprisingly, there no genito-urinary issues. presumably addressed in the earlier sexually active and child-bearing age group. The respiratory diseases are mostly due to smoking, then asthma, but Diabetes Mellitus (Type 1—insulin dependent) makes its first appearance. Oral health makes its first and only appearance. Time to get your teeth fixed—pity about the lack of fluoride as a kid.

Problems for age 45–64 Women:

This is the most dangerous age for breast cancer, but other cancers occur as well, while heart disease and strokes impact health.

Cancer

Breast cancer 30%
Lung 14%
Colorectal 13%.

Cardiovascular Disease 14%

IHD 47%
Strokes 29%

Mental Disorders

Depression 51%.
Anxiety 33%

Osteoarthritis 7%

Diabetes 6%

The cancer and cardiovascular disease are more often fatal, whereas the others more often result in non-fatal burdens.

What to do:

Menopause

Menopausal symptoms vary from mild to severe. Not much helps except Hormone Replacement Therapy (HRT), which has received bad reports, but these have now been found to be the subject of misinformation. HRT can be helpful and is recommended if symptomatic.

Breast Cancer

One in eight women will develop cancer of the breast.

Regular examinations by your doctor are necessary.

Learn to self-examine—you have more time than anyone else.

Regular mammograms are recommended. Mammograms are arguably the best screen test, but some one in six cancers are missed.

Have regular pap smears.

Lung Cancer

Don't smoke.

Get a low dose chest CT scan/MRI if coughing blood/losing weight.

Lung cancer and COPD are invariably due to smoking tobacco or marijuana and are preventable. But be alert to any past workplace contaminants such as asbestos, which may be as "innocent" as insulation/lagging on factory or ships' pipes or on old roofs and walls.

Colorectal Cancer

Have a colonoscopy if any passage of blood or mucus.

Cardiovascular Disease

Ischemic heart disease means the blood supply to the heart is compromised by cholesterol plaques and narrowing of the coronary (heart) arteries. This, usually, first manifests as heart pain on exertion (angina) and must be treated and monitored.

Report any chest pain or heart flutters—get an ECG/EKG and possibly CT angiography –see Appendix.

Also see note regarding aspirin in relevant men's age group.

Strokes

Make sure you are on a low-dose pill.

Skin Cancer and Melanoma

Like all cancers, they "take off" after the age of 40 and increase. This is due to excessive ultraviolet radiation—sun exposure. Like lung cancer, it is not the one packet of cigarettes but the regular exposure to the carcinogens (smoke or sun) over some 20 years that initiates the mutation of the DNA in our cells to become cancers. The best feature of skin cancer is that it can be seen, and therefore, most can be diagnosed early enough to effect a cure. Get checked annually.

Mental Issues

Treat depression/anxiety. Cognitive behavioral therapy may be preferable to drugs.

By now, suicide seems to not be the potential threat it is with younger women, so support is what is needed.

The average age for menopause is 53, and this comes as a psychological as well as hormonal insult. Here, the estrogen is abruptly cut off. It is a violent hormonal change with no male equivalent but, obviously, can herald many mixed emotions.

Osteoarthritis

My best analogy is that OA is "rust" in the joints. It can run the gamut from inconsequential to being completely debilitating.

Report any finger joint lumps and hand, knee, or hip pain or stiffness.

Keeping mobile (like moving and using a rusty hinge) is all-important.

Diabetes

Get a Random Blood Glucose test.

As noted elsewhere, Diabetes 2 is usually associated with being overweight, but I have some very slim and fit diabetics in my practice, and some with no family history.

The first line of treatment is to adopt the *Newtrition Diet*.

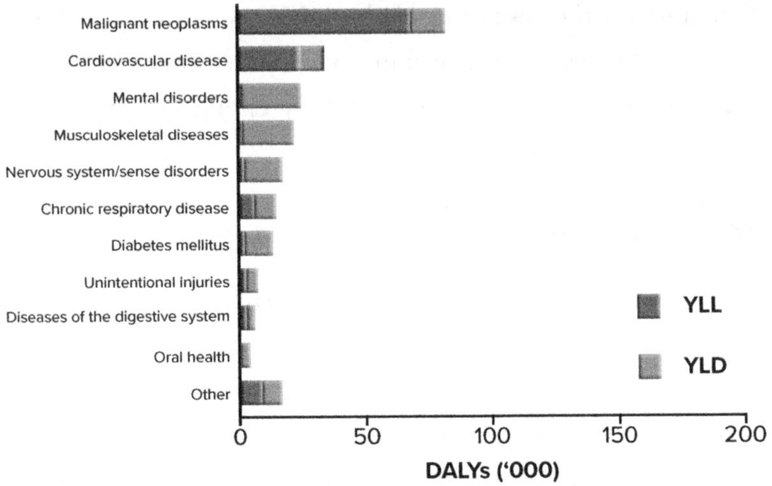

Figure 15: Leading causes of burden of disease and injury in women aged 45-64 years. YLD = Years Lost Due to Disability = Non-fatal burden of illness, i.e., chronic illnesses. YLL = Years of Life Lost due to premature death by the same illness. DALY = YLL + YLD = Total Burden (*Source: Australian Burden of Disease and Injury Study*).

CHAPTER 15

Women 65 Years and Over

Be Still My (Irregularly) Beating Heart[81]

Table 15:

	USA 65 - 74	**England & Wales 65-79**	**Australia 65 - 74**
1	Cancer	Lung and Trachea Ca	Lung Ca
2	Heart Disease	Ch Lower Respiratory D	CAD
3	Ch Lower Respiratory D	IHD	COPD
4	Stroke	Dementia & Alzheimer's	CVD
5	Diabetes	CVD	CRC

81 Apparently the earliest citation for the term 'be still my beating heart' comes from William Mountfort's Zelmane from 1705.

Causes of Premature Deaths and Disabilities in Order

1. Cardiovascular Disease
2. Malignant Neoplasms (cancer)
3. Nervous System Disorders
4. Chronic Respiratory Diseases
5. Musculoskeletal Diseases (100% disabilities—not fatal)
6. Diabetes Mellitus
7. Digestive System Diseases
8. Unintentional Injuries
9. Genito-urinary Diseases
10. Acute Respiratory Diseases

Cardiovascular problems now take over from cancer as the greatest cause of disabilities.

The early signs of dementia and Alzheimer's manifest; eyesight and hearing start to deteriorate. Heart attacks and strokes present most problems: control of blood pressure and any heart arrhythmias must be checked and controlled. Mental disorders have disappeared, and teeth have been fixed. Eyesight and hearing problems manifest.

The early signs of dementia and Alzheimer's manifest, and nervous system disorders, rare in the younger, such as Parkinson's Disease manifest with increasingly small handwriting, frozen expression, shuffling and "pill rolling" tremors.

As noted in the men's section but repeated here, you are now "old", but as with the age-old saying, "You are only as old as you feel"; in other words, you can still have "joie de vivre"—the joy of life.

I am continually amazed at these old people who groan as they undress and have to be helped onto the examination table and complain, "It's awful getting old, doctor." They are slow, bent, dull, and look old, but when I check their age, they are up to 10 years younger than I am! Most of them, in fact, admonish me, "Wait till you're my age!" They have no debilitating illnesses, but their whole attitude is wrong.

Someone recently said, "75 is the new 65", and due to improved nutrition, public health measures and modern medicine, this is indeed the case. So, being "65 and over" does not condemn you to the retirement village but, rather, is a call to increase your pursuit of health and vitality. Be an optimist. There are a lot of people worse off.

When I had whining introspective patients in hospital with not much wrong but who pestered me out of proportion to their ailment, I had them moved close to someone terminally ill, and when that patient died, the change in the hypochondriacs was always startling.

We all have to die, but the whole essence of this book is to live it up and stay healthy as long as you can. Don't become a premature invalid or prematurely old because of a bad mental attitude. At 65 and over, there is the distinct danger of people winding down because that is how they think society is geared. Well, read the *New York Times* obituaries and see just how many were rock and rollin' into their 90s.

The Main Health Problems in Older Women Are:

Cardiovascular 37.2%

IHD is the main cardiovascular problem at 54.4%, then stroke at 28.8%.

Cancer 20.8%

Colorectal Cancer 16.4%

Breast 15.1%

Lung 15.1%.

Nervous System Disorders 17.9%

Of which Alzheimer's/dementia make up 49.7%.

Hearing and Vision Loss 32.1%

Parkinson's 12.2%

Acute Respiratory Infections

What to do:

An ECG/EKG is now mandatory to rule out silent atrial fibrillation and reduce strokes.

Get a CT angiogram if any cardiovascular symptoms appear.

CAC: Colon cancer has now overtaken breast cancer, so report any change of bowel habit, undue/unexplained fatigue or anemia, and chronic diarrhea; consider a colonoscopy.

Continue mammograms and breast examinations.

Report any ongoing coughs.

Get a low dose chest CT if there is past history of smoking.

Staying fit with mental challenges is all-important. Alzheimer's and Parkinson's, while inevitable, can be remarkably delayed by doing so. Even ballroom dancing and bridge helps.

Get eyes and hearing checked.

Report any tremors, shuffling, or smaller writing.

Get any chest infections treated aggressively and promptly. Review the results and repeat annually.

Get skin checked more regularly if damaged and living in a sunbelt zone.

Many of these deaths and disabilities may seem sudden, like a heart attack or a stroke; but in truth, most have been brewing and incubating for decades. If we are at our healthiest at age 11, then by 40 years, our tests reveal a sudden spurt of bad results. Most of these, we don't notice. Our raised blood pressure and blood lipids are asymptomatic; we may be a little thirstier and void more from Diabetes, but the joint pains are usually mild and just starting, and any symptoms of cancer are not usually flagrant—perhaps a little tiredness, usually passed off. And so, most usually from self-inflicted abuse of high-risk behaviours, we have spent three decades, from 10 to 40 years of age, accumulating damage. The only outside sign is obesity, and the only one we notice is pushing the paper farther away to read.

The Three Ps

As previously discussed, it is essential you get a:

1. Project
2. Purpose
3. Participate - socialise

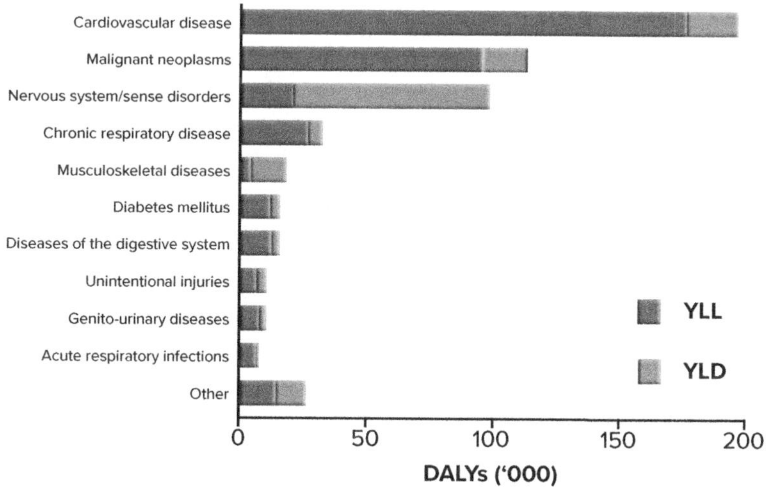

Figure 16: Leading causes of burden of disease and injury in women aged 65 years and over. YLD = Years Lost Due to Disability = Non-fatal burden of illness, i.e., chronic illnesses. YLL = Years of Life Lost due to premature death by the same illness. DALY = YLL + YLD = Total Burden (*Source: Australian Burden of Disease and Injury Study*).

CHAPTER 16

Disabilities

"I can't change the direction of the wind, but I can adjust my sails to always reach my destination".

– Jimmy Dean (1928-2010)

"Si jeunesse savait, si vieillesse pouvait. (If only youth knew, if only age were able)."

– Henri Estienne (1531-1598)

Disabilities may be approached in two different ways:

1. The actual practical impediment e.g., unable to turn on tap
2. The causative condition—e.g., arthritis

Causes of Disabilities by Age and Sex

There are many illnesses that, while they do not kill us, effectively turn us into invalids. A stroke may not be fatal but can leave us paralysed down one side and unable to talk. Obviously, preventing such disabilities is of prime focus.

But there are some amazing people who have coped with significant disabilities, too, from Franklin Delano Roosevelt who became the most powerful man in the world as President of the USA during the Great Depression and WW2 but had contracted polio, such that his legs were paralysed, to Stephen Hawkins, condemned to a wheelchair and microphone with Motor Neurone Disease but still one of the great brains of physics. Then, too, are the Paralympians.

Despite these examples of amazing people, there are also some conditions people regard as "worse than death" and many disabilities that see people effectively condemned to nursing homes. The whole mission of this book is for you to avoid any and all of these, and knowing about them may be motivational to look after yourself better.

Overall (All Age) Non-Fatal Burdens of Diseases

1. IHD (Ischemic Heart Disease)
2. Stroke
3. COPD (Chronic Obstructive Pulmonary (Lung) Disease)
4. Depression
5. Lung cancer
6. Prescription Drugs
7. Dementia
8. Diabetes
9. Colon Cancer
10. Asthma
11. Osteoarthritis
12. Suicide
13. MVA (Motor Vehicle Accident)
14. Breast Cancer

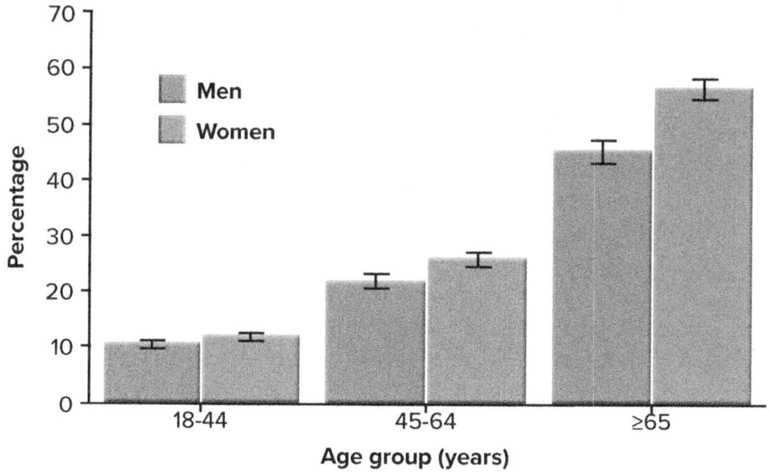

Figure 17: Percentage of adults aged ≥18 years reporting disability, by sex and age group – United States, 2005 (*Source: Morbidity and Mortality Weekly Report (MMWR) CDC*).

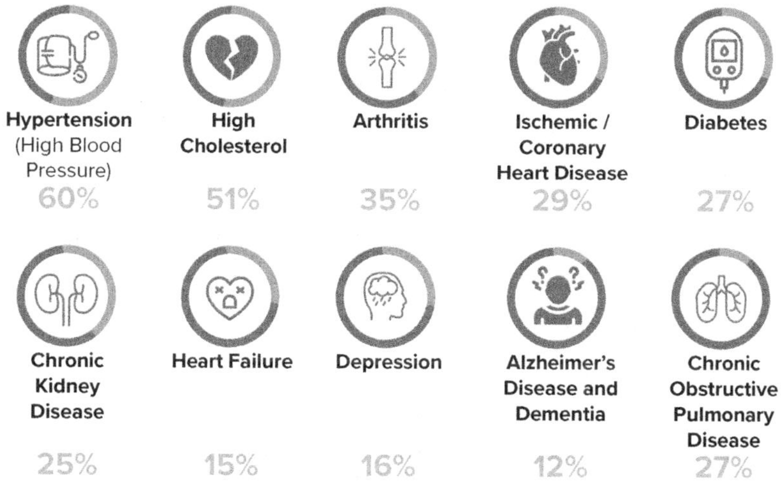

Figure 18: Ten common chronic conditions adults 65+ on Medicare (USA) were treated for in 2018 (*Source: Centers for Medicare & Medicaid Services. Chronic Conditions. Chronic Conditions Prevalence State/County*).

You should now get tested for all these (see Appendix).

The Most Helpful and Revealing Data Lists:

1. Actual Practical Impediment
2. Actual Medical Causative Conditions
3. USA Overall Causes of Disability in Men

It is highly recommended you read the following three tables to see just what becomes more and more difficult as we approach 65.

To live longer, we must actively fight the imposts of age, especially by staying mobile, flexible, and mentally alert.

These are official USA tables, and although they were created in 2005, they are the most profound source of age changes and remain perfectly relevant today. I have found them to be extremely useful as they, more than any data I have found, tabulate the changes age brings. This has alerted me to 'what's in store' so I can take measures to avoid or minimize problems.

Progression of Imposts and Disabilities with Age

These following lists not only show the progression of various disabilities with age but those we are most likely to encounter. Many of these are unvoiced. People are not likely to talk as to how they now find difficulty bathing, but from age 18 years to 65 years it has become 13 times more difficult! This was brought home to me when a 75-year-old patient complained how he "could no longer wipe his bottom"--hardly something he is going to tell his friends but, more's the point, something he could have avoided had he known, as you can now, what potential disabilities await.

Look at the 18-years-old column and then the 65-years-old column and see what disabilities show the greatest increases, viz: hearing, walking three city blocks, lifting 10 pounds, getting out of a chair, bathing, taking care of money, preparing meals, or light housework.

Most, if not all, of these can be avoided or considerably minimized. Each should now be addressed to assess your future potential predicaments and prevention, or minimization tactics now started.

As examples, I had a great friend who was twice the British Actor of the Year and a ferocious tennis competitor even though he was 15 years my senior. We would play five sets of tennis (and not "tip and giggle" but flat strap). One year, he showed me how he was now doing yoga and could grab both hands behind his back with one over his shoulder and the other behind his waist. I am sure he had no trouble wiping his bottom. He lived, working, to 89 years.

My neighbour uses noisy mowers and brush-cutters but doesn't wear earmuffs. Elsewhere, I noted my rock drummer friend and the teens at the traffic lights with their 12 surround speakers lifting their car into the ear with each beat... all destined for hearing losses but all preventable.

I am surprised at the fall-off in exercise capacity, but if we look at the next table, as to the actual medical causes, arthritis, spine problems, and heart troubles are the big three which may restrict some, but not all, such exercise.

These lists provide a valuable guide revealing what we are likely to be "in for" and how we can take avoiding action. Walking speed has been shown to be directly linked to longevity, and as can be seen, at age 18 to 24 years, only 2.9% of the population had difficulty walking three city blocks, yet 11.3% of those between 45 and 64 years old had trouble, rising to 31.7% for those over 65 years.

Resistance exercises are also good, in fact essential, for us; in the same survey, while only 2.3 % had trouble lifting 10-pound weights aged 18 to 44, this increased to 21.8% when older than 65 years.

1 in 4 of today's 20-year old's will be disabled before they retire.

The lessons to be taken from these surveys is to be conscious of walking quickly, doing resistance training, and attending to these other, mostly avoidable, disabilities of aging.

1. Actual Practical Impediment: Take Avoiding Actions

If we are aware of these otherwise inevitable age onsets, *Live Longer's* contention is we can fight back and institute prevention.[82]

Table 16: Actual practical impediment.

	% 18 - 44	**% 45 - 64**	**% 65 (+)**
Difficulty-specified functional activities	6.3	19.4	47.5
Seeing words/letters in newsprint	1.3	3.8	
Hearing normal conversation	1.1	3.6	11.2
Having speech understood	0.8	1.1	2.1
Walking three city blocks	2.9	11.3	31.7
Climbing a flight of stairs	2.8	11.4	30.2
Grasping objects	1.0	4.2	8.2
Lifting/Carrying 10 lbs	2.3	7.8	21.8
Difficulty-activities of daily living	1.0	4.1	12.5
Getting around inside home	0.4	1.8	6.4
Getting in/out of bed/chair	0.6	2.7	7.5
Bathing	0.6	2.2	7.9
Dressing	0.5	1.7	5.3
Eating	0.2	0.6	2.1
Toileting	0.3	1.0	3.6

82 CDC, 2009, *Morbidity and Mortality Weekly Report,* 1 May, Vol. 58, No. 16, www.cdc.gov.mmwr.

Difficulty with instrumental activities of daily living	2.2	6.0	19.1
Getting around outside of home	1.1	3.8	13.7
Taking care of money and bills	1.1	1.7	7.4
Preparing meals	0.8	1.8	8.0
Doing light housework	0.9	3.2	9.9
Managing prescriptions	0.7	1.6	6.2
Using the telephone	0.4	0.8	4.6
Reporting of selected impairments	5.6	6.9	8.1
A learning disability	2.2	1.3	0.6
Mental retardation	0.7	0.4	0.3
Other developmental disability	0.4	0.2	0.1
Alzheimer's disease/senility/dementia	0.3	0.6	3.8
Other mental/emotional disability	3.5	5.6	5.6
Use of assistive aid	1.0	4.6	19.2
Wheelchair	0.4	1.3	5.2
Cane, crutches, or walker	0.8	4.2	17.9
Limitation to work around the house	3.5	10.7	20.3
Limitation in ability to work at a job or business	4.5	11.3	

2. Actual Medical Causative Conditions[83]

Main cause of disability among civilian non-institutionalized U.S. adults aged ≥18 years with self-reported disabilities.

Table 17: Actual medical causative conditions (*Source: U.S. Census Bureau, 2004 Survey of Income and Program Participation, 2005*).

Conditions	Total %	Men %	Women %
Arthritis or rheumatism	19.0	11.5	24.3
Back or spine problem	16.8	16.9	16.8
Heart trouble	6.6	8.4	5.4
Lung or respiratory problem	4.9	4.9	4.9

83 *Ibid.*

Mental or emotional problem	4.9	5.2	4.6
Diabetes	4.5	4.8	4.2
Deafness or hearing problem	4.2	6.8	2.4
Stiffness or deformity of limbs/extremities	3.6	3.6	3.7
Blindness or vision problem	3.2	3.9	2.8
Stroke	2.4	3.1	1.9
Cancer	2.2	2.4	2.1
Broken bone/fracture	2.1	1.9	2.3
High blood pressure	1.9	1.6	2.1
Mental retardation	1.5	1.7	1.3
Senility/Dementia/Alzheimer's	1.2	1.0	1.3
Head or spinal cord injury	1.1	1.5	0.9
Learning disability	1.1	1.6	0.7
Kidney problems	0.9	1.2	0.7
Stomach/Digestive problem	0.8	0.7	0.8
Paralysis of any kind	0.6	0.7	0.5
Epilepsy	0.6	0.6	0.6
Hernia or rupture	0.5	0.6	0.5
Cerebral palsy	0.5	0.8	0.3
Missing limbs/extremities	0.5	0.8	0.2
Alcohol or drug problem	0.4	0.8	0.2
Tumor/Cyst/Growth	0.3	0.2	0.3
Thyroid problems	0.2	0.1	0.3
AIDS or AIDS-related	0.2	0.2	0.2
Speech disorder	0.2	0.1	0.2
Other	12.9	12.1	13.5
Total	**100.0**	**100.0**	**100.0**

Table 18: USA overall causes of disability in men.

Disability	**% Affected**
Back or spinal problems	16.9
Arthritis or Rheumatism	11.5
Heart trouble	8.4
Deafness or impeded hearing	6.6

Mental or emotional problems	5.2
Lung or respiratory problems	4.9
Diabetes	4.8
Vision problems or blindness	3.9
Stiffness or deformity of limbs	3.6
Stroke	3.1
Cancer	2.4
Fractures – broken bones	1.9

Table 19: Leading single causes of burden of disease and injury in men by age (*Source: Australian Burden of Disease Study 2022, 13 December 2022*).

Condition	DALYs	Per cent of total
25-44 years		
Suicide and self-inflicted injuries	23,296	10.3
Depression	16,827	7.4
Road traffic accidents	14,929	6.6
Alcohol dependence and harmful use	13,026	5.8
HIV/AIDS	10,250	4.5
All causes total	**225,873**	
45-64 years		
Isachaemic heart disease	57,521	16.7
Lung cancer	22,509	6.5
Chronic obstructive pulmonary disease	16,999	4.9
Hearing loss	15,861	4.6
Diabetes mellitus	15,711	4.6
All causes total	**345,095**	
65 years and over		
Isachaemic heart disease	113,681	21.7
Stroke	45,111	8.6
Lung cancer	36,206	6.9
Chronic obstructive pulmonary disease	30,348	5.8
Alzheimer's disease and other dementias	27,804	5.3
All causes total	**523,774**	

About 36 million women in the U.S. have disabilities, and the number is growing. About 44% of those aged 65 years or older are living with a disability. The most common cause of disability for women is arthritis or rheumatism.[84]

Women (24.4%) had a significantly higher prevalence of disability compared with men (19.1%) at all ages. For both sexes, the prevalence of disability doubled in successive age groups (18-44 years, 11.0%; 45-64 years, 23.9%; and ≥65 years, 51.8%).

By 2030, and that's closer than we think, the number of U.S. adults aged ≥65 years will approximately double from current numbers, as will be the case for the other first world nations (and worse for China, India, and other such nations). The implications of this growing number of older adults include unprecedented demands on public health and senior services and the nation's healthcare system. For example, greater numbers of trained professionals will be needed to expand the reach of effective community-based programs to mitigate the effects of disability.

Modifiable lifestyle characteristics, e.g., physical inactivity, obesity, and tobacco use, are the *major contributors* to the most common causes of disability and sometimes stem from a primary disabling condition.

People across the world are living longer but often spending more time in ill health as rates of non-fatal diseases and injuries decline more slowly than death rates. For example, while increases in rates of Diabetes have been substantial, rising by around 43% over the past 23 years, death rates from Diabetes increased by only 9%.

Just one in 20 people worldwide (4.3%) had no health problems in 2013, with a third of the world's population (2.3 billion individuals) experiencing more than five ailments. In the past 23 years, the leading causes of health loss have

84 *CDC Disability and Health Information for Women with Disabilities 2020*

hardly changed. Low back pain, depression, iron-deficiency anemia, neck pain, and age-related hearing loss resulted in the largest overall health loss worldwide. In 2013, musculoskeletal disorders (i.e., mainly low back pain, neck pain, and arthritis) and mental and substance abuse disorders (predominantly depression, anxiety, and drug and alcohol use disorders) accounted for almost half of all health loss worldwide.[85]

I find the label "Non-Fatal Burdens of Disease" (NFBD) cumbersome. I think we can just call them "Health Burdens", as it's hard to conceive a burden if we are dead. It would seem all of us are destined to be burdened in some way in our final years.

Increasing longevity is not necessarily indicative of good health; most age groups are now living longer, but some reports are for a disability or other health problem, increasing the length of a poor-quality life more than a good-quality life. The Baby Boomer generation, which is now reaching old age, is not seeing improvements in health similar to the older groups that went before them. Only for people aged 65 and older was there a "compression of morbidity" recorded—a reduction in the proportion of years spent with disability or ill health.

Different factors may affect disability at different ages. For instance, younger populations may have had an increase in disability because of a greater emphasis on mental health, increased diagnoses of autism and attention deficit hyperactivity disorders, and changes in drug use.[86]

---

85 Global Burden of Disease Study 2013 Collaborators, 2015, "Global, regional, and national incidence, prevalence, and years lived with disability for 301 acute and chronic diseases and injuries in 188 countries, 1990–2013: a systematic analysis for the Global Burden of Disease Study 2013", *The Lancet*, Vol. 386, No. 9995, pp. 743-800, https://doi.org/10.1016/S0140-6736(15)60692-4.

86 Lord, C., Elsabbagh, M., Baird, G. & Veenstra-Vanderweele, J. 2018, "Autism spectrum disorder", *Lancet*, Vol. 392, No. 10146, pp. 508-520, https://doi.org/10.1016/S0140-6736(18)31129-2.

Multiple Chronic Conditions (MCC) - Disabilities

Approximately 25% of U.S. adults have diagnoses of MCC. Data from the 2014 National Health Interview Survey (NHIS) were used to estimate prevalence of MCC (defined as two or more of 10 diagnosed chronic conditions) for each U.S. state and region by age and sex. Adults who reported a diagnosis of two or more of the following selected conditions were categorized as having MCC: arthritis, asthma, cancer, chronic obstructive pulmonary disease (COPD), coronary heart disease, Diabetes, hepatitis, hypertension, stroke, or weak or failing kidneys.[87]

Increased Disability Risks with Overweight & Smoking >17-38%[88]

A typical female, age 35, 5'4" (162.56cm), 125 pounds (56.7kg), non-smoker, who works mostly an office job with some outdoor physical responsibilities and leads a healthy lifestyle has the following risks:

A 24% chance of becoming disabled for three months or longer during her working career, with a 38% chance that the disability would last five years or longer and with the average disability for someone like her lasting 82 months.

If this same person used tobacco and weighed 160 pounds (72.57kg), the risk would increase to a 41% chance of becoming disabled for three months or longer.

A typical male, age 35, 5'10"(177.8cm), 170 pounds (77.11kg), non-smoker, who works an office job with some

---

87 Newman, D., Tong, M., Levine, E. & Kishore, S. 2020, "Prevalence of multiple chronic conditions by U.S. state and territory, 2017", *PLoS One*, Vol. 15, No. 5, https://doi.org/10.1371/journal.pone.0232346, erratum in *PLoS One*, Vol. 15, No. 9.

88 *Preventive Medicine*, Vol. 141, December 2020.

outdoor physical responsibilities and leads a healthy lifestyle has the following risks:

A 21% chance of becoming disabled for three months or longer during his working career, with a 38% chance that the disability would last five years or longer and with the average disability for someone like him lasting 82 months.

If this same person used tobacco and weighed 210 pounds (95.25kg), the risk would increase to a 45% chance of becoming disabled for three months or longer. There are a number of Personal Disability Quotient tables on the Internet which calculate your odds of an injury or illness.

The Centers for Disease Control and Prevention estimates that one in five adults in the United States is living with a disability. The National Organization on Disability says there are 56 million disabled people. Indeed, people with disabilities are the largest minority group in the United States, and as new disability categories such as neurodiversity, psychiatric disabilities, disabilities of aging, and learning disabilities emerge and grow, so does that percentage. These statistics are applicable to all first world countries and average 20% (one in five) of the population, increasing with age.

National Disability Rates

USA: Overall, there are about 42.5 million Americans with disabilities, making up 13% of the civilian noninstitutionalized population, according to U.S. Census Bureau data from 2021. This group includes people with hearing, vision, cognitive, walking, self-care, or independent living difficulties.[89]

UK: In 2021, across both England and Wales, the proportion of disabled people was 17.8% (10.4 million). The proportion of

89 Pew Research Centre, 24 July 2013

people that are disabled has decreased 1.7 percentage points from 2011, when it was 19.5% (10.0 million).[90]

Australia: Around one in six (18%) of people in Australia have a disability.[91]

With the aging population and the consequent reduction in such taxpayers, it would seem imperative we do not become disabled and are able to look after ourselves.

Conditions Patients Believe to be Worse than Death

While death may be considered the ultimate "adverse outcome" by doctors, many patients with serious illness consider some debilitating conditions to be even worse than death. The findings come from a study by the University of Pennsylvania that asked 180 patients with severe life-threatening illnesses to rate 10 different aspects of debility in comparison with their concerns about death.

The responses showed that six conditions were rated as bad as or worse than death by a significant proportion of patients:

1. Bowel and bladder incontinence
2. Relying on a breathing machine to live
3. Being unable to get out of bed
4. Being confused all the time
5. Having to rely on a feeding tube to live
6. Needing care all the time

Four more conditions that were rated as somewhat better than death were:

1. Living in a nursing home
2. Being at home all day

---

90 Office for National Statistics, 19 January 23

91 Australian Institute of Health and Welfare, 5 July 2022

3. Being in moderate pain all the time
4. Being in a wheelchair.[92]

As noted, a 2023 Norwegian study[93] found that the desire to live into advanced ages is significantly reduced by hypothetical adverse life scenarios, with the strongest effect caused by dementia and chronic pain.

92 Rubin, E. B., Buehler, A. E. & Halpern, S. D. 2016, "States Worse Than Death Among Hospitalized Patients With Serious Illnesses", *JAMA Internal Medicine*, Vol. 176, No. 10, pp. 1557-1559, https://doi.org/10.1001/jamainternmed.2016.4362.

93 Skirbekk, V., Langballe, E. M. & Strand, B. H. 2021, "Preferred life expectancy and the association with hypothetical adverse life scenarios among Norwegians aged 60+", *Age and Aging*, Vol. 50, No. 6, pp. 2012-2018, https://doi.org/10.1093/aging/afab113.

CHAPTER 17

Why Do You Go to the Doctor?

"What's Up, Doc?"

– Bugs Bunny, 1940

These statistics vary slightly from country to country and year to year (and pre-date Covid), but they show how patients' immediate concerns are different from long-term conditions (causes of death and disabilities). This, hopefully, highlights the fact that we are more interested in our immediate, rather than long-term, health.

This then leads to us neglecting our long-term health and not instituting preventive lifestyle programs or, paradoxically, overcompensating with the new longevity programs on offer.

Danger

The danger is that, by going to the doctor only when we are sick, we ignore the bigger health problems that prematurely kill or disable us, as they are asymptomatic and go unnoticed.

Prevalent Health Problems: Why We Go to the Doctor (%)

1. Dental caries
2. Hearing loss 16
3. Endentulism (loss of teeth) 7.6
4. Asthma 6.6
5. Periodontal Disease 5.6
6. Iron anemia 4
7. Alcohol abuse 4
8. Osteoarthritis 3
9. Chronic back pain 3.2
10. Depression 3
11. Diabetes 2 2.6
12. Slipped disc 1.9
13. Incontinence 1.7
14. Chronic Obstructive Pulmonary Disease (COPD) 1.6
15. Social phobia 1.6
16. Anxiety disorder 1.6
17. Burns/scalds 1.3
18. Benign prostatic hypertrophy 1.1
19. Peptic ulcer 1.0
20. Attention Deficit Disorder (ADD) 0.9
21. Cannabis abuse 0.9
22. Cataracts 0.9
23. Angina 0.9
24. Osteoporosis 0.8

Reasons for Attending the Doctor per 1000 patients

1. URTIs (Upper Respiratory Tract Infections) 2370
2. Dental Caries 594
3. Chronic back pain 330
4. Otitis media 56
5. Periodontal Disease 22
6. Depression 21
7. LRTIs 190 (Lower Respiratory Tract Infections)
8. Alcohol abuse 9
9. Peptic ulcer 9
10. Slipped disc 8
11. Hearing loss 6
12. Falls 20
13. Skin cancers 15
14. Diarrhea 205
15. Menstrual problems 6
16. Motor vehicle accident (MVA) 5
17. Diverticulitis 4
18. Anxiety disorder 4
19. Sports injuries 4
20. Asthma 4
21. Gall bladder disease 4
22. Stroke 3
23. Prostate hypertrophy 3
24. Interpersonal violence 3
25. Angina 2
26. Bipolar Disorder 0.7

Reasons for Attending the Doctor (%) – One Decade Later

1. Check-up 9
2. Prescription 7.1
3. Cough 4.5
4. Test results 3.6
5. Vaccination 3.1
6. Sore throat 2.5
7. Back complaint 2.3
8. Rash 1.9
9. Fever 1.5
10. URTI 1.4
11. Headache 1.4
12. Abdominal pain 1.3
13. Depression 1.3
14. Hypertension 1.2
15. Nasal problem 1.2
16. Ear pain 1.1
17. Diarrhea 1.0
18. Tiredness 1.0
19. Administrative 1.0
20. Knee complaint 0.9

Most Managed Problems by the Doctor (%)

1. Hypertension 6.1
2. URTI 4.4
3. Vaccination 3.2
4. Depression 2.4
5. Lipid disorder 2.1
6. Diabetes 2.0
7. Back pain 1.8
8. Bronchitis 1.8
9. Osteoarthritis 1.8
10. Prescription 1.4
11. Check-up 1.3
12. Oesophageal Disease 1.3
13. Female genital/pap 1.2
14. Sprain 1.2
15. Urinary tract infection 1.2
16. Sleep problems 1.1
17. Anxiety 1.1
18. Menopausal symptoms 1.0

Table 20: Most commonly reported long-term conditions (*Source: AIHW Analysis of Abs 2001 National Health Survey*).

Condition	Male %	Female %	Total %
Long-sightedness	20.4	24.3	22.4
Short-sightedness	18.3	23.5	20.9
Back pain/disc disorders	21.0	20.7	20.9
Hay fever/allergic rhinitis	15.1	15.9	15.6
Arthritis (all forms)	11.7	15.8	13.9
Asthma	10.5	12.6	11.6
Chronic sinusitis	8.9	12.4	10.5
Deafness (total/partial)	14.2	7.7	10.8
Hypertension	9.7	10.7	10.3
Presbyopia	9.1	9.0	9.0
Migraine	3.6	8.7	6.2
High cholesterol	6.5	5.6	6.1
Astigmatism	3.9	5.3	4.6
Anxiety disorders	3.4	5.6	4.5
Mood disorders	3.4	5.5	4.5
Bronchitis/emphysema	3.5	3.6	3.6
Diabetes (all forms)	3.0	2.9	3.0
GIT ulcers	2.8	2.7	2.7
Varicose veins	1.1	3.5	2.3
Hernia	2.5	1.6	2.0
Cataract	1.5	2.4	2.O
Tachycardia	1.7	2.1	1.9
Psoriasis	1.5	2.0	1.8
Neoplasms/cancers	2.0	1.4	1.7
Osteoporosis	0.6	2.5	1.6
Edema	1.0	2.1	1.6
Angina	1.6	1.2	1.4
Rheumatism	1.3	1.4	1.3
Anaemias	0.3	2.3	1.3
Haemorrhoids	1.0	1.2	1.1
Dermatitis/eczema	1.0	1.2	1.1

The immediate attention and treatment of even minor illnesses leads to better overall and long-term health. And so, knowing what "minor" illnesses are going around and what new illnesses seem to be evolving should persuade you to "get it seen, get it diagnosed, and get it better".

Vomiting and diarrhea, severe chest or abdominal pain, cuts, bleeding, possible fractures, fits, loss of consciousness, and acute dramatic episodes… any of these will alarm us and propel us to the doctor post-haste. But the laying down of cholesterol plaque in our coronary arteries, our greatest cause of death by a long shot, is painless and unrealized. This non-acute, slow deterioration of our bodies slithers along insidiously, without any dramatic symptoms to alert us.

Who would have thought hearing loss was the second most prevalent illness? Perhaps when we or our children are attending a rock concert, turning up the boom box, or jamming the earphones in and turning up the volume, we might try and arrange a conversation with an older, hearing-impaired person.

Hearing loss is isolating but also costly, even in middle-aged individuals: individuals with a diagnosis of hearing loss had 33% higher health care payments compared to patients without hearing loss. Age-related hearing loss affects more than 60% of US adults older than 70 years; the onset is gradual, with prevalence tripling from the age of 50 years to 60 years. Yet early, successful intervention may prevent future hearing-related disabilities and decreased quality of life. This finding indicates that negative health-related effects of hearing loss, a condition that many consider simply an unavoidable result of aging, may manifest earlier than is generally recognized and may affect use of health care across the continuum of care.

And who among us knew holes in teeth were the most prevalent health condition? The Loonies, Luddites and Leftovers rave against fluoride as they sail off the edge of their flat earth while not vaccinating their children. While polio can kill or lead to immediate limb paralysis, having rotten teeth is not as dramatic but can lead to heart disease, poor nutrition, and a shorter life in the long term.

The statistics on disabilities and death don't list alcohol abuse, but it is the seventh most prevalent condition (probably the first in Russia), and many acts of violence, causing death, are the direct result of its use, as well as work accidents and absenteeism. Unless controlled, it is a long-term time bomb. Ice and crystal meth are rapidly taking over—especially in remote and rural areas, but fentanyl is number one.

Having had to treat innumerable but avoidable domestic accidents, I urged my patients to 'child-proof' their homes. Pool fences are now mandatory where I live. Child-proof locks and climbable shelves are obvious, but the turning of handles of frying pans and saucepans into the wall prevents burns and scalds. Yet, when I visit homes, these handles are invariably sticking out, waiting to be hit.

Acute sunburn is a documented contributor to melanoma and skin cancers. People who live in sunbelt areas have more cataracts. Sunglasses are mandatory, even on kids, and don't leave them on the desk when you go to lunch.

Depression is being more widely recognized and treated—perhaps even over-diagnosed and over-treated. Try cognitive behavioral therapy.

Other conditions listed usually warrant investigation also: slipped discs, low back pain, asthma, urinary symptoms, and angina (too often brushed off as "indigestion"). Any chest pain lasting more than 30–40 minutes warrants investigating.

While some of these acute reasons for visiting the doctor may seem trivial, as pointed out with respect to deafness, the long-term effects are profound and lead to a shorter lifespan.

It is interesting how eyesight accounts for the greatest proportion of conditions in the top 20. Therefore, it should not be such a surprise that increased longevity and reduced disabilities are significantly improved by cheaper, more available, and quicker cataract surgery.

Most of us would not think, especially when we are young, that reduced vision would or could be a major cause of premature death or disabilities. But reduced vision is a daily impost to quality of life (QOL) and, therefore, is often a preventable cause of premature death or disability.

Conclusions

Thirty of these conditions can be prevented or treated, and many are curable if caught early enough. Many more illnesses than we think are preventable.

Initial neglect can see many of these acute, curable illnesses become long-term problems.

Now that we know what we are in for, how can we prevent these problems and optimize our health? Before we address the specific programs, there is an overall approach, with advice according to which personality type of patient (see Chapter: Need To Know) gets the best results. Then, the easiest analogy to understand preventive medicine is a comparison to how we look after our cars: Preventive Maintenance.

Preventive medicine is simply not practiced much or well. Patients do not want to pay for advice. They Google the latest fad diet and think they know more than the doctor—and maybe they do, since the doctor is too busy with the acute or hospital cases, and preventive medicine expertise by the medical profession has become a backwater. In addition, each country has its health services problems. In the USA, costs can be prohibitive. In the UK, the free NHS is simply overwhelmed.

It is hoped *Live Longer* helps solve both these problems by minimizing costs by age- and sex-specific illness analyses but also by giving improved dietary, nutrition, and lifestyle advice.

I don't wish to raise anyone's ire here, but it has always been a frustrating medical observation how some people claim they can't afford health services when they can afford to smoke, get tattoos, and buy the *latest* sneakers and mobile phones. Yes, I do understand that often these are the little luxuries that make their life tolerable, but I also wish some would get their priorities more toward their health.

Better longevity (preventive medical) lifestyles are either free or accessible, as per the Blue Zones.

Finally, some information as to trials and studies is offered: Researchers are desperate for funding, and so they publish dubious articles and make inflated claims—how do you know where the truth lies? Even the best medical journals have been fooled. Often lurking behind these trials are the drug companies making millions, if not billions, suppressing any bad results until many deaths are exposed, forcing them to come clean and withdraw their product. Be careful.

CHAPTER 18

Life Begins at 40?

"Life really does begin at forty. Up until then, you are just doing research."

– Carl Gustav Jung (1875-1961)

My, and many other doctors', observations conclude that physical declines begin sooner in life than typically detected. "Efforts to maintain basic strength and endurance should begin before age 50, when it's still possible to preserve the skills that keep people mobile and independent later in life." [94]

From the following graphs, we see they start even a decade before this research, and we should establish habits of physical effort even earlier than 40.

94 Hall, K. S., Cohen, H. J., Pieper, C. F., *et al.* 2017, "Physical Performance Across the Adult Life Span: Correlates With Age and Physical Activity", *The Journals of Gerontology: Series A*, Vol. 72, No. 4, pp. 572-578, https://doi.org/10.1093/gerona/glw120.

Conditions:

1. Cardiovascular disease
2. Blood pressure
3. Cholesterol
4. Diabetes
5. Cancer
6. Lung disease
7. Rheumatoid arthritis
8. Osteoporosis and Osteoarthritis
9. Eyesight
10. Weight

All get worse, or rather become symptomatic, around age 40.

These graphs need not be studied in minute detail. What they dramatically show at a glance is how most of the pathological changes that prematurely kill or burden us take off at the age of 40. Unfortunately, most of these changes start earlier, go largely unnoticed, and only become symptomatic or fatal later.

While these graphs show how these major illnesses dramatically and suddenly make their appearance from age 40, they have been asymptomatic, incubating for many years.

We have been "cultivating and incubating" disease conditions certainly since age 11, when we are meant to be at the peak of health. It is becoming increasingly likely that the process starts even earlier, with evidence suggesting it may even begin *in utero.*

It is common sense that if we continually abuse our bodies, the damage will be cumulative. Damage may be in small doses, but it is cumulative, so it *"suddenly"* breaks out when we hit 40.

1. Cardiovascular Disease Takes Off After 40

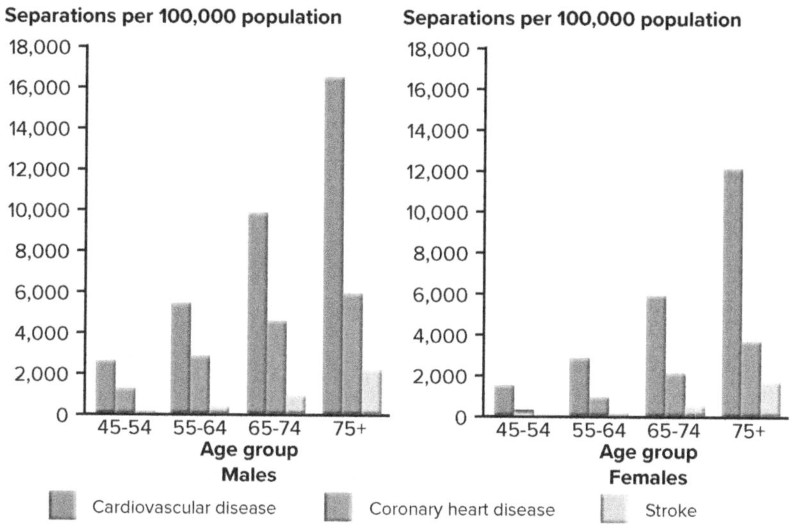

Figure 19: Hospital separations for cardiovascular disease, ages 45 and over (*Source: AIHW Analysis 2001 National Health Survey*).

2. Blood Pressure Takes Off After 40

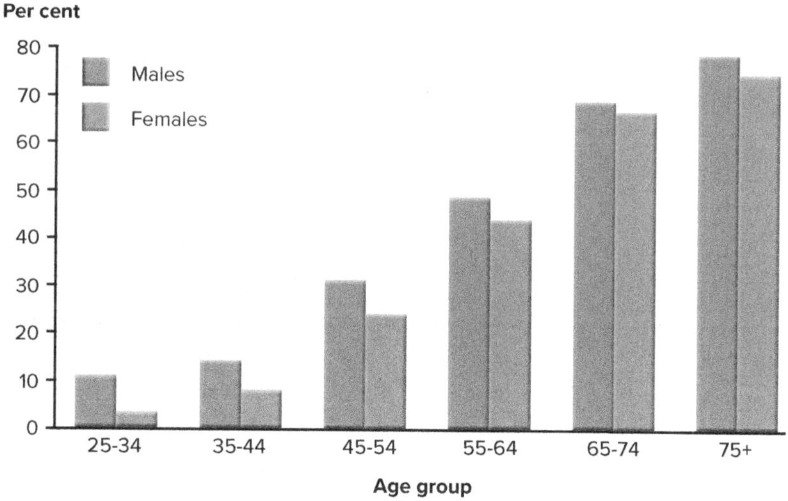

Figure 20: Proportion of people with high blood pressure. Based on WHO definition of high blood pressure (*Source: AIHW Analysis 2001 National Health Survey*).

3. Cholesterol Takes Off After 40

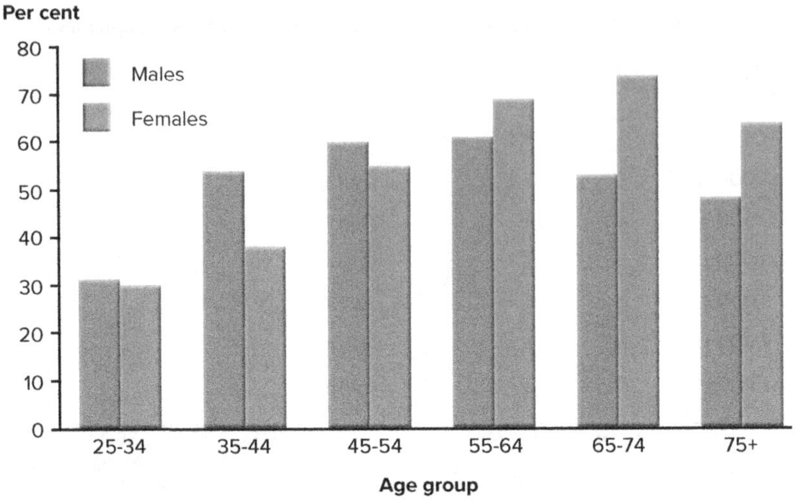

Figure 21: Proportion of adults with high blood cholesterol. High blood cholesterol is 5.5 mmol/L or more (*Source: AIHW Analysis 2001 National Health Survey*).

4. Diabetes Type 2 Takes Off After 40

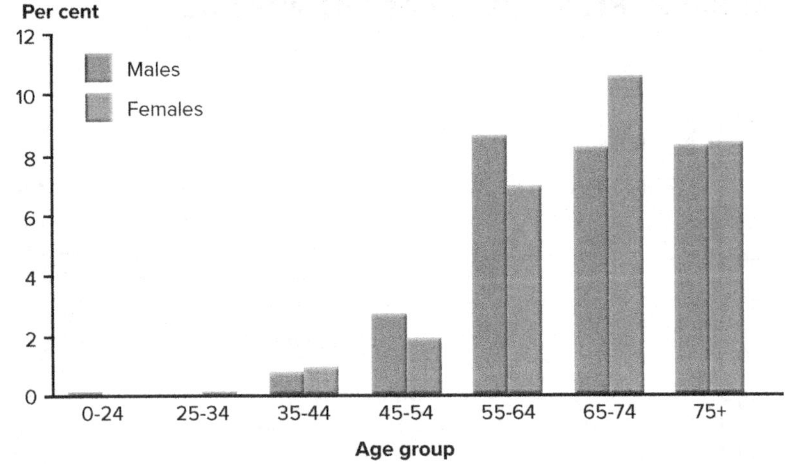

Figure 22: Age-specific prevalence of self-reported Type 2 diabetes. Estimates for males aged 0-24 and 35-44 and females aged 35-44 have relative standard errors of between 25% and 50% and should be used with caution. Estimates for males aged 25-34 and females aged 0-34 have relative standard errors greater than 50% and are considered too unreliable for general use (*Source: AIHW Analysis 2001 National Health Survey*).

5. Cancer Takes Off at 40

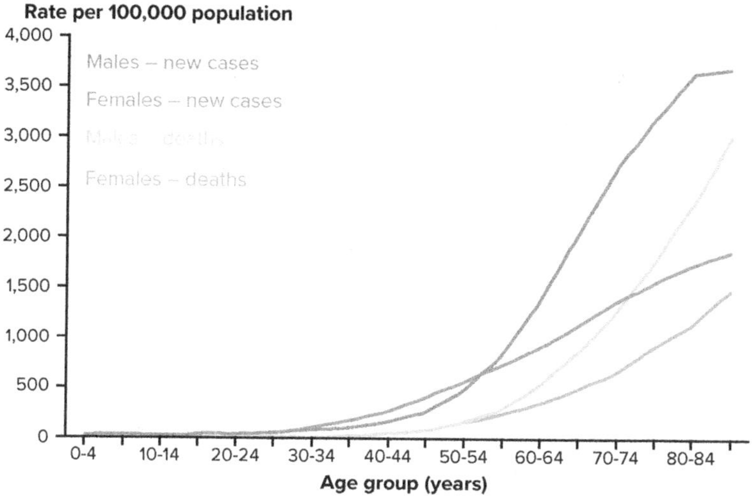

Figure 23: Age-specific incidence and death rates for malignant neoplasms by sex, excluding non-melanocytic skin cancer (*Source: AIHW Analysis 2001 National Health Survey*).

6. Lung Disease Takes Off at 40

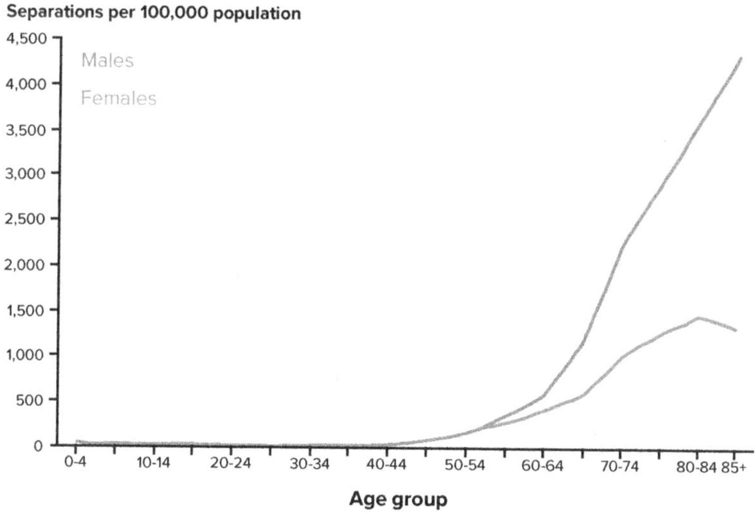

Figure 24: Age-specific hospital separations with COPD as the principal diagnosis (*Source: AIHW Analysis 2001 National Health Survey*).

7. Rheumatoid Arthritis Takes Off at 40

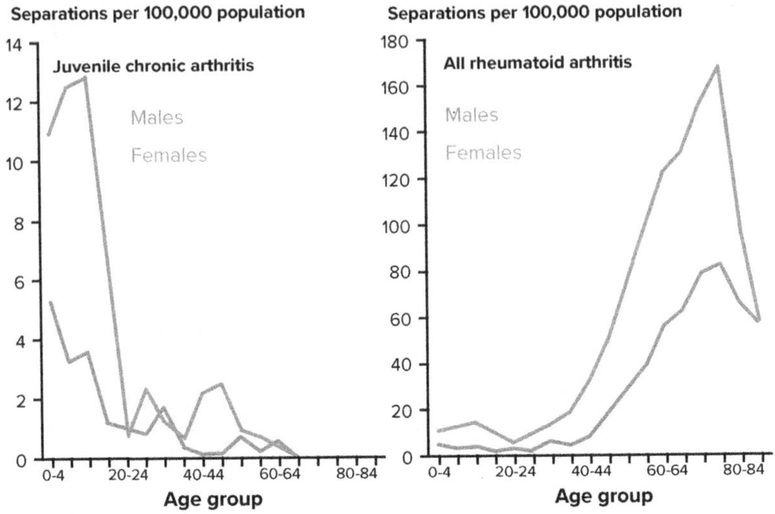

Figure 25: Age-specific hospital separations with principal diagnosis of juvenile chronic arthritis and rheumatoid arthritis (*Source: AIHW Analysis 2001 National Health Survey*).

8. Osteoporosis/Osteoarthritis Takes Off at 40

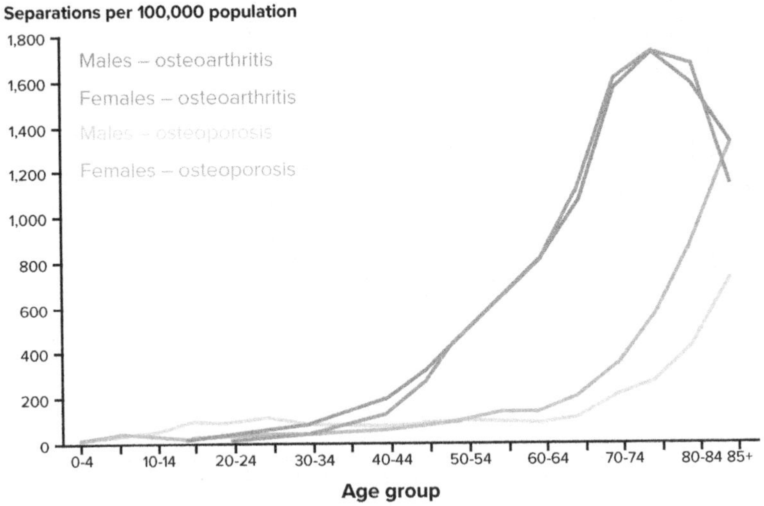

Figure 26: Age-specific hospital separations with principal diagnosis of osteoporosis and osteoarthritis (*Source: AIHW Analysis 2001 National Health Survey*).

9. Eyesight Deteriorates at 40

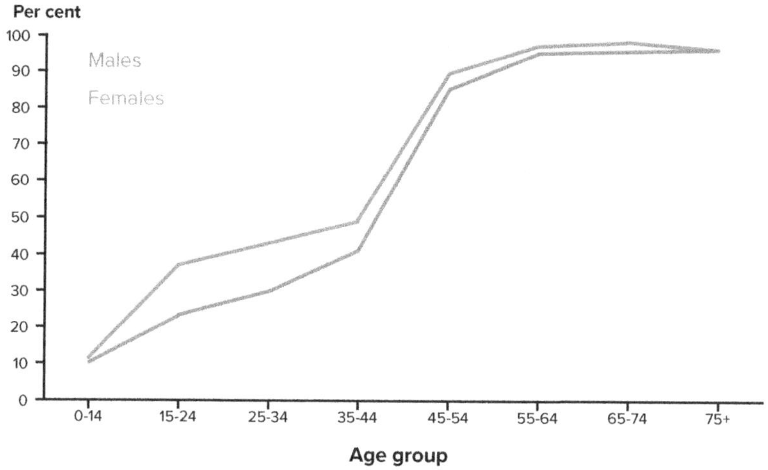

Figure 27: Self-reported prevalence of sight problems (*Source: AIHW Analysis 2001 National Health Survey*).

10. Weight

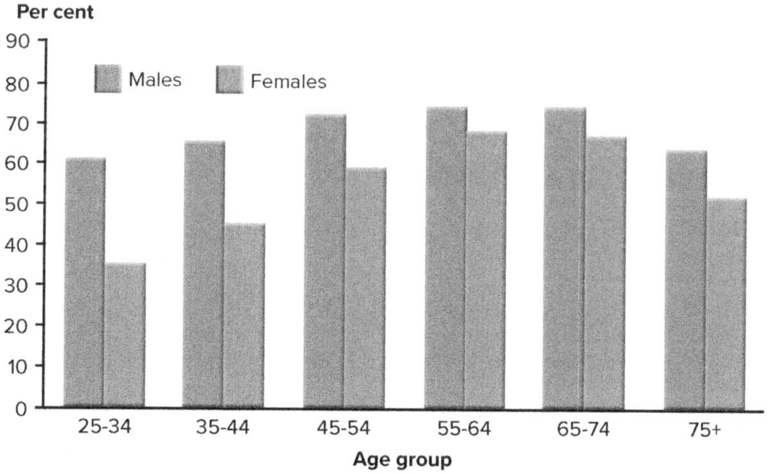

Figure 28: Proportion of people who are overweight, BMI of 25 or more. Based on measured data (*Source: AIHW Analysis 2001 National Health Survey*).

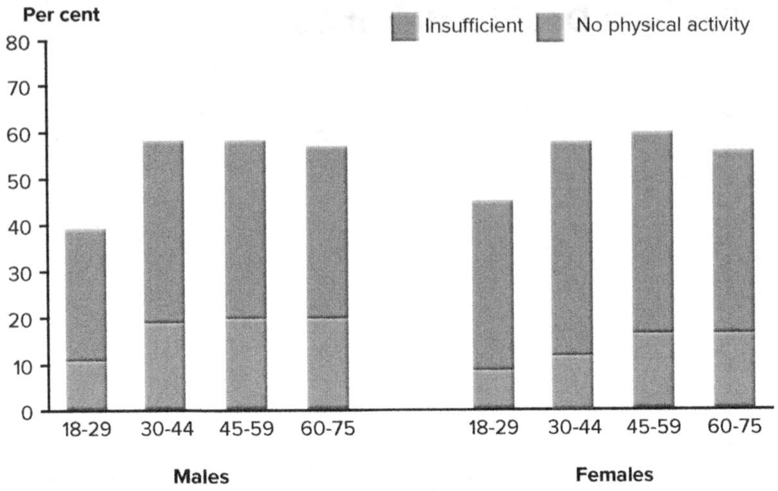

Figure 29: Proportion of adults undertaking insufficient or no physical activity. Age standardised to the 2001 Australian population. People aged 18-75 years. 'Insufficient physical activity' is less than 150 minutes or less than five sessions of physical activity in the previous week (*Source: AIHW Analysis 2001 National Health Survey*).

The weight graph above shows that even young people, aged 25 to 34 years (60% of males and 35% of females), are overweight. This is a significant finding, and perhaps the most revealing of all the graphs, as it is the only one where we can actually see that unhealthy practices are cumulative and gradually lead to a health problem, which seemingly takes off after 40. Most of the other illnesses which take off after 40 show no signs or symptoms, even though they have been `brewing" for years.

Weight gain, however, is visible at any age, even if we don't see it for ourselves. The second graph shows the amount of physical exercise undertaken by men and women across their lifespans. Not surprisingly, it mirrors the weight graph closely.

Exercise itself does not cause much weight loss, but people who exercise generally have a healthier lifestyle and diet.

Sun cancers and melanoma are at epidemic levels for Caucasians, and these, too, take off at 40.

Apocryphally, we start downhill at the age of 27. As these graphs demonstrate, there is a progressive degeneration only revealing itself at age 40. The obvious conclusion is that we should adopt healthy habits and lifestyle as soon as possible—certainly, I suggest, at age 30, if not before.

CHAPTER 19

Early Diagnosis & Treatment

"Get It Seen, Get It Diagnosed, Get It Fixed."

– *Live Longer* Dictum

Meticulous attention to our health provides benefits of which most of us will forever be unaware. This is the paradox of preventive medicine: "What you don't know, you'll never miss." If patients don't get ill, they ascribe it to their genes or even good luck, and while both may play a part, they may not make the connection to good, de facto preventive medical lifestyles.

We most often don't notice insidious changes, such as high blood pressure or cholesterol, that have long-term sequelae.

But even if patients follow most preventive recommendations, there is another very important facet that I vociferously advocate—getting every minor ailment attended to immediately. Many people are admirable stoics who don't complain about feeling ill or about what they consider a minor injury, but this oversight is fraught with danger.

Consider the following two animal studies:

The first was a documentary I watched, sited on the Mississippi River, where opossums were threatened with extinction from raccoons and other predators. They suffered scratches, bites, abrasions, and even open wounds. Of course, they couldn't treat themselves. The severe wounds became infected, and those opossums died, but others with even minor scratches didn't do too well either. They lost weight, their fur fell out, they looked sick, and they stopped breeding. This was mainly attributed to stress, and they recovered wonderfully when put on an island where there were no predators. While stress certainly played a big part, their wounds didn't heal as quickly or as well as they should have. Which came first, the chicken or the egg? Did the stress make the wounds and healing worse, or did the wounds make the stress worse? Whatever. The point is that these minor afflictions dragged down the overall health of these animals.

The second study[95] is research that showed mild infections without symptoms of illness can still lead to serious consequences by reducing the lifespan of the infected individuals. The "individuals" in this case were birds, and the infection was thought to speed up the aging process by shortening the telomeres (i.e., the chromosome ends) at a faster rate, thereby accelerating senescence. The researchers note, "Until now, the research community had believed that mild infections that do not produce symptoms of illness have no effect on survival and reproduction... If this is a general mechanism for any type of mild, chronic infection, which is quite possible, it will mean our study is of major interest to understand the impact that mild illnesses can have on other organisms, including humans."

95 Asghar, M., Hasselquist, D., Hansson, B. *et al.* 2015, "Chronic infection. Hidden costs of infection: chronic malaria accelerates telomere degradation and senescence in wild birds", *Science*, Vol. 347, No. 6220, pp. 436-438, https://doi.org/10.1126/science.1261121.

The small, non-measurable effects of the chronic disease appear to underlie the accelerated shortening of the telomeres. When the telomeres get too short, this has a fatal effect and causes premature death.

I have to agree, as for decades I have seen the detrimental effects that minor neglect has had on my patients who chose to ignore or minimize their healthcare.

Treat all conditions, no matter how minor. Treat them immediately and get them fully better.

There is a germ, which to the ordinary person is "just a sore throat", but which can strike fear and dread into the minds of doctors and, literally, the hearts (and kidneys) of the patients. It is clinically impossible to diagnose that it is so special. Ninety-nine times out of a hundred, indeed, it is just a sore throat. However, this awful germ identified more accurately as a beta-hemolytic streptococcus (Lancefield Beta Gp. 12, from memory), unlike other strep throats, causes an immune reaction in the patients' hearts and kidneys, leading, later in life, to heart valve problems and glomerulonephritis, or the equivalent of kidney shutdown. Some very famous people have had their lives or careers cut short by this germ, including one of the world's richest men, a national leader, a king, a pope, and one of the world's greatest composers, footballers, crooners, and even the Muppets founder.

Left untreated, glomerulonephritis and rheumatic heart disease can lead to heart or kidney transplants, but beta-haemolytic streptococcus is usually very susceptible to penicillin. Hence, the importance of treating, aggressively and immediately, even ostensibly "minor" ailments such as a sore throat or tonsillitis.

"Drug" is not necessarily a dirty word.

In pre-antibiotic days, people talked about how little Johnny had a "weak chest." Little Johnny never seemed to be without a cold, and it then developed into a productive cough. and then he was coughing up discoloured phlegm and was quite ill. Occasionally, you still see kids with green nasal discharge and a loose cough you can hear across a busy street. When discoloured sputum develops, and it may on top of a viral URTI, it means there is a secondary bacterial infection. Antibiotics are anti-bacterial and now should be prescribed. Like the previous examples of kids with the sore throats that ended up having heart or kidney transplants, their parents either considered it to be a trivial condition or they have been fed misinformation.

Many parents say they don't believe in antibiotics, and there is a worldwide movement to reduce their use. This is informed, good medical advice, as too many antibiotics have been used for viral colds they won't fix, and it causes antibiotic resistance. However, the pressure put on PCP/GPs not to prescribe antibiotics by the government and ivory tower "experts" is questionable in its theoretical approach. Often, a stitch in time saves nine. Patients may develop pneumonia or severe bronchitis and need buckets of antibiotics when prompt treatment would have cleared up the problem much more easily.

Once again, I emphasize being a clinician—a doctor who actually has to treat the patient and not hand down "advice" from a government office or a scientific research lab. If they were serious, as I proposed way back in 1964 as a medical student, they would stop the mega-doses of antibiotics being fed to cattle, chickens, and most domestic animals (including salmon and other farmed fish) who are not even ill but are fed these drugs as a preventive.

Then, there are the many countries where even the most powerful antibiotics can be bought over the counter without a prescription. No wonder there is increasing resistance…but not due to doctors overprescribing.

However, without the immediate repair antibiotic treatment provides, the little Johnnys of yesteryear were often doomed to a long-term burden of chronic problems, and in many cases, the result of the so-called `weak chest" was premature death.

Antibiotics administered correctly can remove this possibility.

Again, this advice is not meant to endorse the use of antibiotics in viral infections, like the common cold, where they don't work. Be reassured: antibiotics are nothing to fear, especially when prescribed by a good clinician. Used wisely, antibiotics are a miracle.

Even with good preventive maintenance, there are, unfortunately, many illnesses that we can't avoid despite our best efforts. However, there are also many illnesses we may think are unavoidable but that can, if diagnosed early, be prevented from developing into something very serious. Regular visits to your GP are an important part of the *Live Longer* plan.

Treat all conditions immediately.
Get them fully better.
Treat them no matter how minor.
Repair activates and optimizes health.

SECTION C

WHAT WE MOST FEAR

"You can conquer almost any fear if you will only make up your mind to do so. For remember, fear doesn't exist anywhere except in the mind."

– Dale Carnegie (1888-1955)

"God and the Doctor we alike adore
But only when in danger, not before;
The danger o'er, both are alike requited,
God is forgotten, and the Doctor slighted."

– Euricius Cordus (1486-1535)

The following chapters provide the current best information on what polls reveal are the illnesses we fear most.

1. Cancer
2. Alzheimer's Disease
3. Heart Disease
4. Stroke
5. Diabetes
6. Flu, COVID, Pneumonia

This was an Australian survey in 2023. As populations grows older, dementia keeps climbing to the top. Some polls now put Alzheimer's Disease as our greatest fear. Be that as it may, as emphasized, Cardiovascular is what actually kills most of us and most importantly, most is preventable. Accordingly, I have changed this order because CVD is our greatest killer, but also over 80% is preventable and preventing it is where to start.

Our Greatest Health Fears[96]

1. Dementia, voted greatest health fear by 51% of participants
2. Cancer, 46%
3. Heart attack, 41%
4. Parkinson's Disease, Liver failure, Diabetes, 31%
5. Vision loss, 31%
6. Osteoporosis, 28%
7. Hearing loss, 27%
8. Broken hips/bones, 26%
9. Wheelchair bound, 24%
10. Motor Neurone Disease, 17%

96 News Corp Growth Intelligence, 2023, *Centre Health of the Nation Survey*, November.

CHAPTER 20

Inflammation

"Pain is inevitable. Suffering is optional."

– M. Kathleen Casey (1961-)

Inflammation may not be "what we fear most" but, in fact, it underlies most of our serious illnesses. Knowing this and implementing anti-inflammatory practices and nutrition is essential. Inflammation is part of the body's defence mechanisms, where the immune system recognizes and removes harmful and foreign stimuli and begins the healing process. It is a physiological defence and repair process. It is acutely activated by infections, trauma, toxins, or allergic reactions. However, if it becomes chronic, inflammation can end up stimulating the developmental measures and determinants of diseases, such as cardiovascular disease, autoimmune disease, neurological disease, or cancer. Additionally, during aging, inflammation becomes increasingly more chronic.

While we mostly recognise what acute inflammation is, such as the redness around a splinter or a pimple, if and when it becomes chronic, it is often unrecognised and its systemic influence has now been progressively recognised as the basis of many, if not most, of our long-term health conditions.

Acute Inflammation

Acute inflammation arises from tissue damage due to injury, invasion by germs, or irritants. It can be localised, as with a boil, or spread more, as with cellulitis, or be systemic, as with acute bronchitis but usually subsides within two weeks.

Chronic Inflammation

Chronic inflammation lasts for several months to years and even a lifetime, which we may not notice, according to the cause.

It is now considered as often initiating many other illnesses, and therefore, it may provide an early warning system to prevent them. Some of these disorders involve the immune system as well as many major diseases, including cancer, heart disease, (atherosclerosis was previously considered a bland lipid storage disease), Diabetes, and Alzheimer's disease. It is thought that statins may reduce heart disease by reducing this inflammation.

Chronic inflammation has been shown to create successions of destructive reactions that damage cells, thus playing a major role in the development of age-related diseases such as cancer, heart disease, and dementia.

According to the Centers for Disease Control and Prevention (CDC),[97] seven of the top 10 causes of death in 2010 were chronic diseases, with heart disease and cancer accounting for nearly 48% of all deaths. The CDC also reports in that same year that 86% of all healthcare spending was for people with one or more chronic medical conditions.

Low-grade chronic inflammation is indicated by levels of the inflammatory marker C-reactive protein (CRP).

---

97 CDC/National Center for Health Statistics, last reviewed 17 January 2024

Some disorders associated with inflammation include:

- Acne vulgaris
- Allergies
- Asthma
- Atherosclerosis
- Autoimmune diseases
- Autoinflammatory diseases
- Cancer
- Chronic prostatitis
- Coeliac disease
- Glomerulonephritis
- Hypersensitivities
- Inflammatory bowel diseases
- Interstitial cystitis
- Myopathies
- Pelvic inflammatory disease
- Reperfusion injury
- Rheumatoid arthritis
- Sarcoidosis
- Transplant rejection
- Vasculitis

My simplistic view (as the actual pathological process is a complex cascade of chemicals, enzymes, blood cells, and hormones) is that most inflammation is caused by some irritant. Germs are obvious, but there are things we never really think about, such as harder-to-digest food. I feel that processed foods (containing goodness knows what additives and irritants) in prolonged, fermenting contact with our gastrointestinal tract, may lead to an inflammatory response and cancer. Non-processed foods, high in fiber and causing rapid transit, would seem to be what we are evolved to eat. The shorter gut transit time with fruit and vegetables is credited with causing less irritation and, hence, less cancers of the gut. Green, leafy vegetables also seem to have an endogenous, natural, sulfur-based chemical which may be anti-inflammatory.

Inflammation, as noted, is meant to be a protective response, but chronic inflammation can become an irritant itself. Smoking would seem to be a good example. The smoke contains a number of irritants which bathe the lung cells and are then absorbed into the blood vessels, inflaming all they come into contact with. The lung cells react to this irritant by overgrowing (i.e., cancer). The blood vessels react (inflame) by allowing fat to deposit on the injured surface (i.e., atherosclerosis).

The advent of chronic diseases follows successes in limiting infection and infant deaths during the late 19th and early 20th century. With changing lifestyles and an aging population, chronic diseases have become increasingly common and now cause most of the burden of ill health. The World Health Organization (WHO) ranks chronic diseases as the greatest threat to human health.[98] The prevalence of diseases associated with chronic inflammation is anticipated to increase persistently for the next 30 years in the United States. In 2000, nearly 125 million Americans were living with chronic conditions, and 21% had more than one. In recent estimates, nearly 60% of Americans had at least one chronic condition, 42% had more than one, and 12% of adults had five or more chronic conditions like Diabetes, cardiovascular disease, arthritis, chronic obstructive pulmonary disease, cancer, obesity and allergies. Worldwide, three out of five people die due to chronic inflammatory diseases.

---

98 Pahwa, R., Goyal, A. & Jialal, I. 2023, "Chronic Inflammation", *StatPearls [Internet]*, https://www.ncbi.nlm.nih.gov/books/NBK493173/

Risk Factors

1. Age
2. Obesity
3. Diet
4. Smoking
5. Low Sex Hormones
6. Stress and Sleep Disorders

Symptoms of Chronic Inflammation

- Body pain, arthralgia, myalgia
- Chronic fatigue and insomnia
- Depression, anxiety, and mood disorders
- Gastrointestinal complications like constipation, diarrhea, and acid reflux
- Weight gain or weight loss
- Frequent infections

Treatment / Management

Treatment is both general and cause-specific. Medical care accounts only for an estimated 10% to 20% of health outcomes, while our daily behaviours drive 36% of outcomes.[99]

According to the UN, the combination of maintaining a healthy weight, regular exercise, eating a healthy diet, and not smoking can reduce the risk of developing the most common and deadly chronic diseases by as much as 80%.[100]

99 Magnan, S. 2017, "Social Determinants of Health 101 for Health Care: Five Plus Five", *NAM Perspectives*, Discussion Paper, National Academy of Medicine, Washington, DC, https://doi.org/10.31478/201710c

100 Trovato, G. M. 2012, "Behavior, nutrition and lifestyle in a comprehensive health and disease paradigm: Skills and knowledge for a predictive, preventive and personalized medicine", *The EPMA Journal*, Vol. 3, No. 1, https://doi.org/10.1007/s13167-012-0141-2.

Diet

The *Newtrition* Diet (end of book), based on the Mediterranean diet and incorporating most known anti-inflammatory foods, should be adopted.

Lifestyle Changes

These may be helpful in removing inflammation triggers and reducing chronic inflammation, as listed below. The most effective is weight loss.

Physical Exercise

Drugs

All the following are anti-inflammatory:

- Metformin
- Statins
- Non-steroidal anti-inflammatory drugs (NSAIDs)
- Corticosteroids

Patient Education

- Diet
- Minimize antibiotics and NSAIDs.
- Maintain an optimum weight.
- Exercise regularly.
- Sleep longer.
- Stress less.

Laboratory tests: CRP, glucose, creatinine, liver function, serum protein electrophoresis, rheumatoid factor, complete blood count, and antinuclear antibodies may help diagnose underlying diseases.

In addition, tumor necrosis factor alpha (TNF-α) has been identified as a major regulator of inflammatory responses and is known to be involved in the pathogenesis of some inflammatory and autoimmune diseases. TNF-α is a crucial component for a normal immune response. That said, I have never yet tested for it.

Diagnostic and imaging studies

e.g., Colonoscopy

Complications

Chronic inflammation progresses silently, but it is the cause of most chronic diseases:

1. Cardiovascular diseases
2. Cancer
3. Diabetes
4. Rheumatoid arthritis
5. Allergic asthma
6. Chronic Obstructive Pulmonary Disease (COPD)
7. Alzheimer's Disease
8. Chronic Kidney Disease (CKD)
9. Inflammatory Bowel Disease (IBD)

What foods can help fight the risk of chronic inflammation?

I have done a great deal of research on nutrition and as noted. I have written a book *Super-Newtrition* (being revised).

It is firmly based on the Mediterranean diet, recognised as the best of all diets, but I went further by researching the micronutrients and which foods donated special benefits—hence the "Super" and the "New".

These are listed in the final chapter and are as anti-inflammatory as any diet possible.

My take on all this is that there are at least some 5,000 micronutrients and 13 vitamins in foods—*if* we get enough variety. And, I think, given these millions to 190,000 years it took for we humans to evolve, we did so while eating this variety. We needed citrus for its vitamin C, which our body can't make, but the orange has some 50 *other* micronutrients and, just from common sense, surely our bodies absorbed these and used them and needed them.

It is further plausible that diets rich in anti-inflammatory components attenuate neuroinflammation via several immune pathways within the brain and indirectly from the gut microbiome and systemic circulation.

Older people (whoops!) are more susceptible to chronic inflammation, so diets rich in fruits and vegetables, which contain polyphenols, protect against age-related inflammation and chronic diseases. Polyphenols are abundant micronutrients in our diet, and evidence for their role in the prevention of degenerative diseases such as cancer and cardiovascular diseases is already emerging. Their health effects depend on the amount consumed and on their bioavailability. They may help reduce the release of pro-inflammatory mediators in people at risk of chronic inflammation.

So, rather than packaged breakfast cereal, I have fruit and yoghurt for breakfast. My wife and I are completely flummoxed why anyone would eat cereals, bacon, eggs, sausages, or puff pastry croissants. If and when forced to (as when staying with people), I feel I can feel the cholesterol depositing in my coronary arteries.

But most often, we don't eat breakfast. Intermittent fasting would seem beneficial.

Eating less, caloric restriction (CR), may help us reduce inflammation and lead longer, healthier lives. A large, multicenter study reveals that a 25% reduction in calories can significantly lower markers of chronic inflammation without negatively impacting other parts of the immune system.[101]

Furthermore, certain foods, such as saturated fats, have pro-inflammatory activity.[102] An umbrella review provided compelling evidence that pro-inflammatory diets increase the risk of 27 chronic diseases and premature death and found clear evidence a pro-inflammatory diet is linked with an *increased risk* of developing certain chronic diseases and premature death.

The "Western diet", which consists of calorie-dense, ultra-processed foods, high in the trans and saturated fats that are found in commercially baked goods, fried foods, and fatty meats and is low in fruits, vegetables, and other plant-foods has been linked to higher levels of inflammation. Conversely, healthy dietary patterns have been linked to lower inflammatory markers. This includes the Mediterranean diet, which is high in fruits, vegetables, legumes, olive oil, and oily fish and low in ultra-processed, refined foods. With rheumatoid arthritis, the main conclusion is that anti-inflammatory diets resulted in significantly lower pain than ordinary diets.[103]

---

101 Meydani, S. N., Das, S. K., Pieper, C. F. 2016, "Long-term moderate calorie restriction inhibits inflammation without impairing cell-mediated immunity: a randomized controlled trial in non-obese humans", *Aging*, Vol. 8, pp. 1416-1431, https://doi.org/10.18632/aging.100994.

102 Trovato, G. M. 2012, "Behavior, nutrition and lifestyle in a comprehensive health and disease paradigm: Skills and knowledge for a predictive, preventive and personalized medicine", *The EPMA Journal*, Vol. 3, No. 1, https://doi.org/10.1007/s13167-012-0141-2 .

103 Schönenberger, K. A., Schüpfer, A. C., Gloy, V. L. *et al.* 2021, "Effect of Anti-Inflammatory Diets on Pain in Rheumatoid Arthritis: A Systematic Review and Meta-Analysis", *Nutrients*, Vol. 13, No. 12, pp. 4221, https://doi.org/10.3390/nu13124221.

According to the World Health Organization, chronic and noncommunicable diseases like heart disease, Diabetes, and respiratory diseases kill 41 million people each year.[104] By 2050, it is estimated that chronic diseases will be responsible for 86% of the 90 million deaths each year, a 90% increase in raw numbers since 2019. Worldwide, over 500 million people are living with Diabetes, and that number is expected to rise to 783 million by 2045. By 2040, the International Diabetes Foundation predicts that spending on Diabetes could exceed $800 billion a year.

There is no government or healthcare system in the world that can successfully manage this onslaught of chronic diseases. To repeat myself, you and I will have to do it ourselves, firstly through behavioural-lifestyle changes then by addressing specific age issues.

LIVE LONGER ORDER

1. Cardiovascular Disease, Heart Disease, and Strokes
2. Cancer
3. Alzheimer's Disease
4. Diabetes
5. Flu, COVID, Pneumonia

Note: Some of the following has been accessed from WHO publications Licence: CC BY-NC-SA 3.0 IGO: Cancer 3 February 2022, Dementia 15 March 2023, Diabetes 5 April 2023, Cardiovascular Disease 11 June 2021, Influenza 3 October 202.

104 Global Burden of Disease Collaborative Network, 2020, *Global Burden of Disease Study 2019 (GBD 2019) Results,* Institute for Health Metrics and Evaluation (IHME), https://vizhub.healthdata.org/gbd-results/.

CHAPTER 21

Cardiovascular Disease, Heart Disease, & Strokes

"There (s)he goes – a heart attack about to happen."

– Arguably the most heard observation
from my colleagues

This may well be the most important chapter in the whole book, as heart disease kills or cripples most of us and has done so for over 50 years, but 80% to even 90% is preventable.

Eighty-five percent of these cardiovascular disease deaths were due to heart attacks and strokes. Risk factors include unhealthy diets, low physical activity, smoking, alcoholism, and pollution.

As documented, I was appointed to the world's first coronary care unit and frequently worked 120 hours a week. I remember I never saw the sun for one stretch of 13 weeks in the middle of summer.

Speed was of the essence, so I bought a boiler suit and slip-on shoes and kept them laid out beside my bed so I could just 'run into them' and keep going to get to the patient. Like babies, heart attacks seem to occur at the most inconvenient times. Perhaps memories enhance or distort, but I seem to remember 4 am as being particularly 'popular',

We pioneered some advanced treatments for those days. I well remember injecting adrenaline/epinephrine directly into hearts of an otherwise dead patient, and, like a miracle, they revived and lived.

That said, some others didn't make it, and maybe I have PTSD, but I still grimace and softly shudder when I remember having to go out into the hospital corridor to tell the pretty young mother with two or three kids hanging onto her skirt that, "I'm terribly sorry, your husband didn't make it". I recall the look of complete disbelief, bewilderment, incomprehension, and confusion as she stood there, paralysed by this news.

I also remember most such fatalities were men in their 40s and 50s who were overweight.

This profoundly angered me as, even then, I figured such heart attacks were largely preventable. These patients stimulated me into researching how to do so.

I can't imagine medicine getting more high-powered than this, but I was called to what had morphed from CCU (Coronary Care Unit) to the ICU (Intensive Care Unit) when running another hospital. The patient has suffered a massive 'inferior' myocardial infarct—a severe heart attack. He was a bad diabetic with severe complications of keto-acidosis, and if that weren't enough, he had adrenal shutdown.

This was as bad and as complex as it gets. No, it got worse; his heart had stopped.

I was the new boy on the block, new to this hospital, and the advanced training I had received swung into action. I revived him with an injection straight through his chest wall into his heart ventricle and then set about normalising his keto-acidosis and adrenal shutdown. That hospital had never seen anything like it!

I would like to take credit, but in reality, I had been superbly trained and was 'just doing my job'.

I didn't find it at all remarkable, but the hospital sure did! For the next weeks, I was confused by nurses huddling and pointing at me (and not for the usual reasons!), but then the hospital superintendent called me to pay me a nice compliment and make me a very flattering offer.

If that were not enough, I then found out the patient, now home and well, was the father of one of my wife's best friends, who was extremely grateful.

Prevention: Where to Start

BLEDS or **B**lood Pressure, **L**ipids, **E**xercise, **D**iet, and **S**moking attention would prevent most heart problems, yet every day, I see fit young people sitting down, eating junk, smoking and slightly overweight, so I wonder what their cholesterol and BP are. They are living in a 'Fool's Paradise' with 20 years or more of this high-risk behaviour before experiencing crushing chest pain or blinding headaches and paralysis, if they live.

Again, longevity is not dying prematurely, and this is where you must start.

It is so tragically (yes, tragically) simple!

Just do it! Get tested.

Nine out of ten heart attacks can now be predicted. This finding suggests that approaches to prevention can be based on similar principles and have the potential to prevent most premature cases of myocardial infarction.

1. Blood Pressure (BP)

Suggested BP targets have varied with time and country, but the averaged recommendations are between 120 to 140 Systolic - SBP (upper) and 80-90 Diastolic -DBP.

Probably the lower the better.

It is sometimes written as 120/60 Hg. The Hg is the chemical symbol for mercury, which was what the original blood pressure machines (sphygmomanometers) used.

But the main point is to get it tested!

Millions of people simply don't know their BP. This is about as dumb as you can get, other than playing Russian Roulette with a loaded pistol.

The American Heart Association recommends that blood pressure screenings start at the age of 20 and be conducted every year.

Most agree it can be allowed to rise as we get older to 150/90 if over 80, but not this aged black duck! Somehow, I keep mine below 130 without medication.

The SPRINT Trial found, among patients at high risk for cardiovascular events but without Diabetes, targeting a systolic blood pressure of less than 120 mm Hg, as compared with less than 140 mm Hg, resulted in lower rates of fatal and nonfatal major cardiovascular events and death from any cause.[105]And this is what I aim for.

If your blood pressure is ever elevated or you are over 50, I highly recommend you buy a wrist blood pressure machine and self-monitor.

Combination of These 4 Traits May Increase Early Heart Attack Risk[106]

These, in effect, constitute the Metabolic Syndrome but each may only be slightly elevated and not noticed.

105 SPRINT Research Group, 2015, "A Randomized Trial of Intensive versus Standard Blood-Pressure Control", *The New England Journal of Medicine*, Vol. 373, No. 22, pp. 2103-2116, https://doi.org/10.1056/NEJMoa1511939, erratum in *he New England Journal of Medicine*, 2017, Vol. 377, No. 25, p. 2506.

106 European Society of Cardiology Meeting, 2023

1. Waist circumference of 102 centimetres or above for men and 88 centimetres or above for women. This equates to about 40.1 inches and 34.6 inches, respectively—maybe a fraction more if very tall.
2. High cholesterol levels measured at 6.1 mmol/l or above, which is roughly 236 mg/dL.
3. High blood pressure, specifically 130 mmHg or higher systolic blood pressure and/or 85 mm Hg or higher diastolic blood pressure.
4. High blood sugar levels with "fasting plasma glucose 5.6 mmol/l or higher," equating to about 101 mg/dL.

2. Lipids

Patients should get their cholesterol and triglycerides checked at least every five years—and more often if risk factors exist. See the specific tests and the note on cholesterol, as ApoB has been shown to be the best test for the damaging cholesterol particles. The standard cholesterol testing is arguably somewhat outdated because it doesn't check for particle size and particle number, and this information is what is needed to tell what's really going on with your cholesterol. Two commonly used advanced lipid tests are apolipoprotein B (apoB) and LDL particle number (LDL-P).

For most children, the National Heart, Lung, and Blood Institute recommends one cholesterol screening test between the ages of 9 and 11 and then suggests it be repeated every five years after that. Initially, if elevated, treatment is diet changes, exercise, and weight control.

There are other contributors than ApoB/LDL which are being investigated, but this is where to start. See the Appendix test and cholesterol section for the levels to be achieved to minimise your risk.

3. *Exercise*

See Specific Chapter

4. *Diet*

See *Newtrition* Chapter.

5. *Smoking*

Simply the worst thing you can do, tantamount to slow suicide.

Finally

If you do have hypertension (elevated blood pressure) or high lipids or a family history of heart disease or strokes, you should get a check by a cardiologist, who may recommend further testing. Remember CVD is the greatest cause of us not living longer, and this is where to start.

CHAPTER 22

Cancer

"I choose to make the rest of my life the best of my life."

– Louise Hay (1926 -2017)

Cancer is our greatest fear, according to polls.[107]

What is more, it peaks earlier and not late in life like our other killers. Moreover, it is now increasing in younger people, and we don't know why (but our altered Western diet is suspected). The rate of cancer diagnosis increased in adults in their 30s over the decade but remained stable in other under-50 age groups. At the same time, the rate of cancers in adults 50 and older is going down.[108]

Table 21:

Age	25-34	35-44	45-54	55-64	65-74	75-84	85+
% death	8%	13	23	30	31	24	12

107 Cancer Research UK, News, 15 August 2011

108 Koh, B., Tan, D. J. H., Ng, C. H. *et al.* 2023, "Patterns in Cancer Incidence Among People Younger Than 50 Years in the US, 2010 to 2019", *JAMA Network Open*, Vol. 6, No. 8, https://doi.org/10.1001/jamanetworkopen.2023.28171.

The Good News

Be that as it may, recent decades have been a "golden era" for cancer research and treatment that has resulted in over one million UK lives saved that would otherwise have been lost to the disease, according to a new data analysis from Cancer Research UK (CRUK), with UK cancer mortality rates falling by a quarter from their peak—meaning half of those who develop cancer now survive for at least 10 years.[109]

These results are applicable to other Western countries. A new global analysis highlights the substantial burden of premature deaths from cancer around the world—a burden that could potentially be averted through prevention, early detection, and timely treatment. According to the analysis, in 2020, over half of all cancer deaths occurred prematurely (before age 70), leading to a loss of roughly 183 million life-years from the disease worldwide. More than two thirds of premature cancer-related deaths—3.6 million, or 68%—were potentially preventable through lifestyle changes or early detection efforts, such as cancer screening, dietary changes, or smoking cessation, and about one third—1.65 million, or 31%—may have been treatable.

But two biostatisticians not involved in the study who took a deep dive into it urged caution in interpreting the data, noting that some proportion of these cancers could be prevented, and that percentage may be large, but the exact 70% estimate is very uncertain.[110]

Cancer is a generic term that includes malignant tumours and neoplasms for a number of diseases that can affect any part

109 Meredith, S. 2023, "A Million Lives Saved in 'Golden Era' for Cancer Research", *Medscape,* 1 September.

110 Brooks, M. 2023, "Experts Question Finding That 70% Cancer Deaths Preventable", *Medscape,* 27 October.

of the body. Their defining feature is the unrestrained overgrowth of abnormal cells that grow beyond their usual boundaries and can then invade or metastasise to adjoining parts of the body and spread to other organs. Metastases are the main cause of cancer death. Different tissue or organ cancers metastasise preferentially to different sites.

My approach is to prioritise which is most likely to affect us given our family history, sex, and lifestyles, then correct these, institute anti-cancer habits, and then investigate, as early diagnosis is often curative.

Your problem is then to change any bad habits and follow through.

These choices may sound simple and easy, but they are obviously not, such as giving up smoking, reducing booze, not eating junk food, losing weight, and exercising.

In fact, they are apparently the hardest things for us to do, but by giving you the evidence, this may be the motivation you need.

I really don't think any of us know how incredibly tough it is to break hard addictions such as smoking and alcohol (let alone opioid drugs), but what are also sinister are the 'soft' addictions of junk food and being sedentary. These seem to be issues we can easily fix… tomorrow.

Cancer[111],[112],[113] is a leading cause of death worldwide. The most common cancers in 2020 were:

---

111 Ferlay, J., Ervik, M., Lam, F. *et al.*, "Global Cancer Observatory: Cancer Today", International Agency for Research on Cancer, Lyon https://gco.iarc.fr/today, accessed February 2021.

112 de Martel, C., Georges, D., Bray, F. et al. 2020, "Global burden of cancer attributable to infections in 2018: a worldwide incidence analysis", *Lancet Global Health*, Vol. 8, No. 2.

113 World Health Organization, 2020, *Assessing National Capacity for the Prevention and Control of Noncommunicable Diseases: Report of the 2019 global survey*, Geneva.

- Breast
- Lung
- Colon and Rectum
- Prostate
- Skin (non-melanoma)
- Stomach

The most common causes of cancer death in 2020:

- Lung
- Colon and Rectum
- Liver
- Stomach
- Breast

Cancer arises from the transformation of normal cells into tumour cells in stages which are the result of the interaction between a person's genetic factors and three categories of external agents, including:

- Physical carcinogens, such as ultraviolet and ionizing radiation
- Chemical carcinogens, such as asbestos, components of tobacco smoke, alcohol, aflatoxin (a food contaminant), and arsenic (a drinking water contaminant)
- Biological carcinogens, such as infections from certain viruses, bacteria, or parasites.

The incidence of cancer rises dramatically with age, most likely due to a build-up of risks for specific cancers that increase with age. The overall risk accumulation is combined with the tendency for cellular repair mechanisms to be less effective as a person grows older.

Prevention

Between 30 and 50% of cancers can currently be prevented by avoiding risk factors and implementing existing evidence-based prevention strategies. The cancer burden can also be reduced through early detection of cancer and appropriate treatment and care of patients who develop cancer. Many cancers have a high chance of cure if diagnosed early and treated appropriately.

In a study of 110,799 individuals 40 to 75 years of age from the UK Biobank cohort, free of CVD or cancer between 2009 and 2012 who were followed up to 2021, it was found that a higher adherence to the Mediterranean lifestyle was associated with lower all-cause and cancer mortality in British middle-aged and older adults in a dose-response manner.[114]

Cancer risk can be reduced by:

- not using tobacco
- maintaining a healthy body weight
- eating a healthy diet, including fruit and vegetables
- doing physical activity on a regular basis
- avoiding or reducing consumption of alcohol,
- getting vaccinated against HPV and hepatitis B,
- avoiding ultraviolet radiation exposure (which primarily results from exposure to the sun and artificial tanning devices) and/or using sun protection measures,
- ensuring safe and appropriate use of radiation in health care (for diagnostic and therapeutic purposes),
- minimizing occupational exposure to ionizing radiation,

114 Maroto-Rodriguez, J., Delgado-Velandia, M., Ortolá, R. *et al.* 2023, "Association of a Mediterranean Lifestyle With All-Cause and Cause-Specific Mortality: A Prospective Study from the UK Biobank", *Mayo Clinic Proceedings*, Vol. 99, No. 4, pp. 551-563, https://doi.org/10.1016/j.mayocp.2023.05.031.

- reducing exposure to outdoor air pollution and indoor air pollution, including radon (a radioactive gas produced from the natural decay of uranium, which can accumulate in buildings, homes, schools and workplaces)
- exercise.

Treatment

Statins Boost Survival Rate of Cancer by Up to 47%[115]

In a 14-year follow up of people being treated with statins for high cholesterol, statins were associated with reduced mortality and improved survival in the four most common cancers, with lower risk of death in lung, breast, prostate, and bowel cancers:

- prostate: 47% lower risk of death (five year survival rates)
- breast: 43%
- bowel: 30%
- lung: 22%

Early Detection

Cancer mortality is reduced when cases are detected and treated early. There are two components of early detection: early diagnosis and screening.

Early Diagnosis

When identified early, cancer is more likely to respond to treatment and can result in a greater probability of survival with

115 Yang, J., Li, C., Shen, Y. *et al.* 2020, "Impact of statin use on cancer-specific mortality and recurrence: A meta-analysis of 60 observational studies", *Medicine,* Vol. 99, No. 14, https://doi.org/10.1097/MD.0000000000019596.

less morbidity, as well as less expensive treatment. Significant improvements can be made in the lives of cancer patients by detecting cancer early and avoiding delays in care.

Early diagnosis consists of three components:

- being aware of the symptoms of different forms of cancer and of the importance of seeking medical advice when abnormal findings are observed,
- access to clinical evaluation and diagnostic services, and
- timely referral to treatment services.

Early diagnosis of symptomatic cancers is relevant in all settings and the majority of cancers. Cancer programmes should be designed to reduce delays in, and barriers to, diagnosis, treatment, and supportive care.

Caution

Vitamin or mineral supplements could feed tumours and allow them to grow. Taken additionally, antioxidants such as vitamins A and C, selenium, and zinc can feed blood vessels in cancer.[116]

Screening

Screening aims to identify individuals with findings suggestive of a specific cancer or pre-cancer before they have developed symptoms. When abnormalities are identified during screening, further tests to establish a definitive diagnosis should follow, as should referral for treatment if cancer is proven to be present.

Screening programmes are effective for some but not all cancer types and, in general, are far more complex and resource-

116 Wang, T., Dong, Y., Huang, Z. *et al.* 2023, "Antioxidants stimulate BACH1-dependent tumor angiogenesis", *Journal of Clinical Investigation*, https://doi.org/10.1172/JCI169671.

intensive than early diagnosis as they require special equipment and dedicated personnel. Even when screening programmes are established, early diagnosis programmes are still necessary to identify those cancer cases occurring in people who do not meet the age or risk factor criteria for screening.

Screening for cancer also may *not* help to prolong life. The University of Oslo study, published in JAMA Internal Medicine,[117] found current evidence does not substantiate the conventional wisdom that cancer screening extends lifetime. Crucially, the researchers do not want screening abandoned but warned that patients need to be better informed of the associated risks and possible negative outcomes of screening.

This is, frankly, in my opinion, a not very helpful article, but also see Dr. Perry Wilson's analysis in the Appendix tests selection section. It is only included here for unbiased thoroughness.

I am sure many readers, and every clinician, know of many people who have had their cancers diagnosed early and treated successfully.

Patient selection for screening programmes is based on age and risk factors to avoid excessive false positive studies. Examples of screening methods are:

- HPV test (including HPV DNA and mRNA test), as preferred modality for cervical cancer screening.
- Mammography screening for breast cancer for women aged 50–69 residing in settings with strong or relatively strong health systems.

Quality assurance is required for both screening and early diagnosis programmes.

117 Welch, H. G. & Dey T. 2023, "Testing whether cancer screening saves lives: implications for randomized clinical trials of multicancer screening", *JAMA Internal Medicine*, https://doi.org/10.1001/jamainternmed.2023.3781.

High-Value Cancer Screening: American College of Physicians Recommendations

This section gives practicing clinicians a quick reference for evidence-based recommendations on cancer screening in asymptomatic, average-risk adults.

Breast: For women aged 40–49 years, mammography screening every two years should be offered if a woman requests it after a discussion of the potential benefits and harms. For women aged 50–74 years who are in good health, mammography should be encouraged every two years.

Cervical Cancer: While perceived as a disease of young women, more older women die from it than younger ones. Pap smears should be done until age 70, at least. For women aged 21–29 years, cytology testing is recommended every three years. For those aged 30–65, cytology plus HPV testing can be done every five years (instead of cytology alone).

The 9-valent human papillomavirus vaccine can potentially prevent 80% of cervical cancers if given to all 11- or 12-year-old children before they are exposed to the virus. The study also found the 9-valent vaccine, under the trademark of Gardasil-9, has the potential to protect against an additional 8% of oropharyngeal cancers, which include the base of the tongue and tonsils. This disease is the second most common HPV-associated cancer.

Ovarian: Screening isn't recommended, and the removal of fallopian tubes is debatable (it was thought it was preventive). This should be discussed with your oncologist, and maybe get a second opinion.

Colorectal: For patients aged 50–75 years, one of the following strategies should be encouraged: high-sensitivity fecal occult blood testing (FOBT) or fecal immunofluorescence testing (FIT) annually; sigmoidoscopy every five years;

combined high-sensitivity FOBT or FIT every three years, plus sigmoidoscopy every five years; or optical colonoscopy every 10 years.

Using data from a meta-analysis of randomized controlled trials, it was concluded that reductions in cancer-specific mortality take about a decade to become apparent, so less screening, or none at all, might be better in people with limited life expectancy. In a linked editorial, however, it was argued that this conclusion rests on the "questionable assumption" that absolute improvements in colorectal cancer mortality in older adults are similar to those in middle-aged adults;[118] in fact, the risk of such mortality increases sharply in older age with a corresponding increase in the benefits of screening. The time to benefit from screening "might be substantially shorter" than the study estimates, especially for adults who have not previously been screened. So, less screening is not necessarily better.

In 2001, the then director of the Center for Disease Control in Atlanta, USA (the NASA of medicine) declared (with respect to colon cancer): "Screening saves lives... 90% are cured if diagnosed and treated early enough."

Prostate: For men aged 50–69 with a life expectancy of at least a decade, discuss screening's benefits and risks. If patients prefer screening, do prostate-specific antigen and K4Scoretesting once every two–four years. But if any problems or symptoms arise, get an MRI, which is far more accurate.

118 Zheng, S., Schrijvers, J. J. A., Greuter, M. J. W. *et al.* 2023, "Effectiveness of Colorectal Cancer (CRC) Screening on All-Cause and CRC-Specific Mortality Reduction: A Systematic Review and Meta-Analysis", *Cancers*, Vol. 15, No. 7, pp. 1948, https://doi.org/10.3390/cancers15071948.

Breast Cancer

Risk Factors

Certain factors increase the risk of breast cancer, including increasing age, obesity, harmful use of alcohol, family history of breast cancer, history of radiation exposure, reproductive history (such as age that menstrual periods began and age at first pregnancy), tobacco use, and postmenopausal hormone therapy. Approximately half of breast cancers develop in women who have no identifiable breast cancer risk factor other than gender (female) and age (over 40 years).

One in 10 are linked to alcohol. Two units a day increases risk by 9%, six units a day increases risk by 60%; 2%-10% linked to inactivity; 8-13% are linked to overweight. One in 20 breast cancers could be avoided by breast-feeding.[119]

Family history of breast cancer increases the risk of breast cancer, but most women diagnosed with breast cancer do not have a known family history of the disease. Lack of a known family history does not necessarily mean that a woman is at reduced risk.

Certain inherited high-penetrance gene mutations greatly increase breast cancer risk, the most dominant being mutations in the genes BRCA1, BRCA2 and PALB-2. Women found to have mutations in these major genes may consider risk reduction strategies such as surgical removal of both breasts. BRCA2 is, in fact, known as the Angelina Jolie gene, as she underwent a double mastectomy in 2013 based on a positive BRCA test.

Signs and Symptoms

Breast cancer can have combinations of symptoms, especially when it is more advanced. Most people will not experience any symptoms when the cancer is still early.

119 *The Lancet Breast Cancer Commission*, 15 April 2024

Symptoms of breast cancer can include:

- a breast lump or thickening, often without pain
- change in size, shape or appearance of the breast
- dimpling, redness, pitting or other changes in the skin
- change in nipple appearance or the skin surrounding the nipple (areola)
- abnormal or bloody fluid from the nipple.

People with an abnormal breast lump should seek medical care, even if the lump does not hurt.

Most breast lumps are not cancer. Breast lumps that are cancerous are more likely to be successfully treated when they are small and have not spread to nearby lymph nodes.

Breast cancers may spread to other areas of the body and trigger other symptoms. Often, the most common first detectable site of spread is to the lymph nodes under the arm, although it is possible to have cancer-bearing lymph nodes that cannot be felt.

Over time, cancerous cells may spread to other organs, including the lungs, liver, brain, and bones. Once they reach these sites, new cancer-related symptoms such as bone pain or headaches may appear.

Cervical Cancer

HPV and Cervical Cancer

A large majority of cervical cancer (more than 95%) is due to the human papillomavirus (HPV).[120]

HPV is the most common viral infection of the reproductive tract. Most sexually active women and men will be infected at

120 Burd, E. M. 2003, "Human papillomavirus and cervical cancer", *Clinical Microbiology Reviews*, Vol. 16, No. 1, pp. 1-17, https://doi.org/10.1128/CMR.16.1.1-17.2003.

some point in their lives, and some may be repeatedly infected. More than 90% of the infected populations eventually clear the infection.

HPV Vaccination

There are currently four vaccines that have been prequalified by the WHO, all protecting against HPV types 16 and 18, which are known to cause at least 70% of cervical cancers. The 9-valent vaccine protects against five additional oncogenic HPV types, which cause a further 20% of cervical cancers. Two of the vaccines also protect against HPV types 6 and 11, which cause anogenital warts.

Clinical trials and post-marketing surveillance have shown that HPV vaccines are safe and effective in preventing infections with HPV infections, high grade precancerous lesions, and invasive cancer.

HPV vaccines work best if administered prior to exposure to HPV. Therefore, to prevent cervical cancer, adolescents and young adults are recommended to receive the 9vHPV vaccine from nine years of age and onwards. The optimal age for HPV vaccination is around 12–13 years, prior to exposure to HPV. People who have not received HPV vaccine by 14 years of age can still receive the vaccine up to 25 years of age.[121]

Some countries have started to vaccinate boys, as the vaccination prevents HPV related cancers in males as well as females. HPV vaccination does not replace cervical cancer screening. In countries where the HPV vaccine is introduced, population-based screening programmes are needed to identify

121 Information about human papillomavirus (HPV) disease, vaccines and recommendations for vaccination from the *Australian Immunisation Handbook*.

and treat cervical pre-cancer and cancer to reduce cervical cancer incidence and deaths.

In high-income countries, programmes are in place which enable girls to be vaccinated against HPV and women to get screened regularly and treated adequately. Screening allows pre-cancerous lesions to be identified at stages when they can easily be treated.

Symptoms of early-stage cervical cancer may include:

irregular blood spotting or light bleeding between periods in women of reproductive age

postmenopausal spotting or bleeding

bleeding after sexual intercourse

increased vaginal discharge, sometimes foul smelling

As cervical cancer advances, more severe symptoms may appear including:

- persistent back, leg, or pelvic pain
- weight loss, fatigue, loss of appetite
- foul-smell discharge and vaginal discomfort
- swelling of a leg or both lower extremities

Colorectal Cancer

Key Facts

- Colorectal cancer is the third most common cancer worldwide, accounting for approximately 10% of all cancer cases, and is the second leading cause of cancer-related deaths worldwide.
- It predominantly affects older individuals, with the majority of cases occurring in people aged 50 and above.
- Several lifestyle factors contribute to the development of colorectal cancer, such as a high intake of processed meats and low intake of fruits and vegetables, sedentary

lifestyle, obesity, smoking, and excessive alcohol consumption.
- Colorectal cancer is often diagnosed at advanced stages when treatment options are limited.
- The incidence and impact of colorectal cancer can be significantly reduced by implementing primary prevention strategies such as adopting a healthy lifestyle, avoiding risk factors, and practicing early detection through screening.

Common symptoms include diarrhoea, constipation, blood in the stool, abdominal pain, unexplained weight loss, fatigue, and low iron levels.

Many people will not have symptoms in the early stages of the disease.

The risk of colorectal cancer can be reduced by eating a healthy diet, staying physically active, not smoking tobacco, and limiting alcohol. Regular screenings are crucial for early detection.

Incidence rates of colorectal cancer have been decreasing in high-income countries, largely as a result of effective screening programmes. The prognosis for colorectal cancer varies depending on the stage at diagnosis. Early-stage cancers have higher survival rates than advanced-stage cancers. Timely diagnosis, appropriate treatment, and regular follow-up care are important for improving survival rates and quality of life.

Risk Factors

Factors that may increase the risk of developing colorectal cancer include:

- Age: the risk of developing colorectal cancer increases with age, with most cases occurring in individuals over 50 years old.

- Family history: a family history of colorectal cancer or certain genetic conditions, such as Lynch syndrome and familial adenomatous polyposis (FAP), can increase the risk.
- Personal history: individuals who have had colorectal cancer before or certain types of polyps are at a higher risk.
- Lifestyle factors: unhealthy lifestyle choices, such as a diet high in processed meats and low in fruits and vegetables, sedentary behaviour, obesity, smoking, and excessive alcohol consumption can increase the risk.

Common Symptoms Include:

- Colorectal cancer often has no symptoms in the early stages, but
- changes in bowel habits such as diarrhoea, constipation, or narrowing of the stool,
- blood in the stool (rectal bleeding), either bright red or dark and tar-like,
- abdominal cramps, pain, or bloating that won't go away,
- unexplained weight loss that is sudden and losing weight without trying,
- feeling constantly tired and lacking energy, even with enough rest,
- iron deficiency anaemia due to chronic bleeding, causing fatigue, weakness, and paleness can all be symptoms.

Prevention

Lifestyle changes and regular screening can help prevent colorectal cancer.

Lifestyle changes to help prevent colorectal cancer include:

- eating a healthy diet rich in fruits and vegetables,
- not smoking tobacco,
- keeping an active lifestyle,
- limiting alcohol consumption, and
- avoiding exposure to environmental risk factors.

Regular screening for colorectal cancer (secondary prevention) is the best way to catch the disease early.

Stool-based tests are non-invasive screening methods used to detect the presence of colorectal cancer or precancerous polyps in the stool. The common type of stool-based test is the fecal occult blood test (FOBT). FOBT detects hidden blood in the stool, which can be an indicator of colorectal cancer or polyps. It involves collecting a small sample of stool and sending it to a laboratory for analysis. If blood or abnormal findings are detected in the stool, further diagnostic procedures, such as a colonoscopy, are usually recommended to confirm the presence of colorectal cancer or polyps.

Stool-based tests are convenient, non-invasive, and can be effective in detecting colorectal cancer at early stages or identifying pre-cancerous polyps.

Individuals with a family history of colorectal cancer or certain genetic conditions may benefit from genetic counselling and genetic testing to assess their risk and determine appropriate screening measures.

Diagnosis

Diagnostic methods for colorectal cancer include physical examination, imaging (such as abdominal ultrasound, computed tomography scans, and magnetic resonance imaging), examination of the inside of the colon using colonoscopy or sigmoidoscopy, taking a sample of tissue (biopsy) for histopathology examination, and molecular testing to identify specific genetic mutations or biomarkers to guide the best treatment option.

Lung Cancer

Key Facts

- Lung cancer is the leading cause of cancer-related deaths worldwide, accounting for the highest mortality rates among both men and women.
- Smoking is the leading cause of lung cancer, responsible for approximately 85% of all cases.
- Lung cancer is often diagnosed at advanced stages when treatment options are limited.
- Screening high risk individuals has the potential to allow early detection and to dramatically improve survival rates.
- Primary prevention (such as tobacco control measures and reducing exposure to environmental risk factors) can reduce the incidence of lung cancer and save lives.

Overview

Lung cancer is a type of cancer that starts when abnormal cells grow in an uncontrolled way in the lungs. It is a serious health issue that can cause severe harm and death.

Symptoms of lung cancer include a cough that does not go away, chest pain, and shortness of breath.

It is important to seek medical care early to avoid serious health effects. Treatments depend on the person's medical history and the stage of the disease.

The most common types of lung cancer are non-small cell carcinoma (NSCLC) and small cell carcinoma (SCLC). NSCLC is more common and grows slowly, while SCLC is less common but often grows quickly.

Lung cancer is a significant public health concern, causing a considerable number of deaths globally. GLOBOCAN 2020 estimates of cancer incidence and mortality produced by the International Agency for Research on Cancer (IARC) show that lung cancer remains the leading cause of cancer death, with an estimated 1.8 million deaths (18%) in 2020.[122]

Smoking tobacco (including cigarettes, cigars, and pipes) is the primary risk factor for lung cancer, but it can also affect non-smokers. Other risk factors include exposure to second-hand smoke, occupational hazards (such as asbestos, radon, and certain chemicals), air pollution, hereditary cancer syndromes, and previous chronic lung diseases.

Symptoms

Lung cancer can cause several symptoms that may indicate a problem in the lungs.

The most common symptoms include:

- cough that does not go away,
- chest pain,
- shortness of breath,
- coughing up blood (haemoptysis),
- fatigue,
- weight loss with no known cause, and
- lung infections that keep coming back.

Early symptoms may be mild or dismissed as common respiratory issues, leading to delayed diagnosis.

---

122 Sung, H., Ferlay, J., Siegel, R. L. *et al.* 2021, "Global Cancer Statistics 2020: GLOBOCAN Estimates of Incidence and Mortality Worldwide for 36 Cancers in 185 Countries", CA: A Cancer Journal for Clinicians, Vol. 71, No. 3, pp. 209-249, https://doi.org/10.3322/caac.21660.

Prevention

Not smoking tobacco is the best way to prevent lung cancer.

Other risk factors to avoid include:

- second hand smoke
- air pollution
- workplace hazards like chemicals and asbestos.

Early treatment can prevent lung cancer from becoming worse and spreading to other parts of the body.

Prevention of lung cancer includes primary and secondary prevention measures. Primary prevention aims to prevent the initial occurrence of a disease through risk reduction and promoting healthy behaviour. In public health, these preventive measures include smoking cessation, promoting smoke-free environments, implementing tobacco control policies, addressing occupational hazards, and reducing air pollution levels.

Secondary prevention for lung cancer involves screening methods that aim to detect the disease in its early stages, before symptoms become apparent and can be indicated for high-risk individuals. In this population, early detection can significantly increase the chances of successful treatment and improve outcomes. The primary screening method for lung cancer is low dose computed tomography (LDCT).

Diagnosis

Diagnostic methods for lung cancer include physical examination, imaging (such as chest X-rays, computed tomography scans, and magnetic resonance imaging), examination of the inside of the lung using a bronchoscopy, taking a sample of tissue (biopsy) for histopathology examination and definition of the specific subtype (NSCLC versus SCLC), and molecular testing to identify specific genetic mutations or biomarkers to guide the best treatment option.

Prostate

The medical observation I was taught is that all men, if they reach 90, will develop prostate cancer—but few die from it.

Before cancer, men develop Benign Prostate Hypertrophy (BPH), which is it just enlarging. The first symptoms are frequency—having to void, well, frequently. Then nocturia or having to get up (hopefully) to void during the night.

Where BPH transitions into cancer is very difficult to diagnose. The only blood test is Prostate Specific Antigen (PSA) which is, at best, only 50% suggestive. Then a biopsy via the rectum was mostly done, and, in my experience, either missed the cancer or gave the patient an infection. So, it's a wretchedly difficult or troublesome diagnosis. My personal 'difficult diagnoses' are it and Cancer of the Pancreas, which we used to call 'the Hidden Cancer'.

In Chapter 9 Men 45-64 and the Appendix, I go into the diagnosis and treatment in more detail.

While we may all get it if we live long enough, and few die from it, there is, like most cancers, a most aggressive form that spreads to the bones such that a spontaneous fracture is often the only clue to the diagnosis.

As for prevention, I download the Johns Hopkins advice, with which I agree:

Things You Can't Change: Age, Race, and Genes

Prostate cancer is primarily a "disease of aging". As you get older, your chances of developing prostate cancer increase. Race and genetics also play a significant role. If you are African American, your chances of developing prostate cancer are double those of white American men. If your father, brother, or multiple blood relatives had prostate cancer, you are more likely to get it, too.

Preventing prostate cancer might be difficult if you have these risk factors, but screening early and often can help ensure that if you do get cancer, it's diagnosed and treated as soon as possible.

Things You Can Change: Diet and Lifestyle

Men in Western countries have much higher rates of prostate cancer than men in Asia. While no one can definitively explain this phenomenon, experts suspect differences in Eastern and Western diets are to blame. Poor eating habits and diets that heavily rely on fats and animal proteins can cause DNA damage and lead to cancer.

Even men who are already at greater risk due to age, race, or genetics can reduce their chances of developing prostate cancer by dopting healthy diets and lifestyles.

Improve Your Diet

Researchers don't completely understand the relationship between diet and prostate cancer prevention, but studies suggest that certain eating habits may help.

- **Reduce fat intake**. Eat less trans fats and saturated fats. Focus on healthy fats such as omega-3 fatty acids from nuts, seeds, and fish.
- **Eat more fruits and vegetables**. Incorporate a wide variety of produce, including plenty of leafy greens. The antioxidant lycopene, which is plentiful in cooked or processed tomatoes, has been shown in some studies to slow the growth of prostate cancer cells. Cruciferous vegetables (e.g., broccoli and cauliflower) contain a compound called sulforaphane that may protect against cancer.
- **Add green tea and soy**. Clinical trials have suggested that soy may lower PSA levels and that green tea may

help men who are at high risk for prostate cancer lower their risk.

- **Avoid charred meat**. Charred meat, from frying or grilling at high temperatures, may produce a chemical compound that leads to cancer.

Maintain a Healthy Weight

Obesity can be a risk factor for developing more aggressive prostate cancer. In general, losing weight and maintaining a healthy weight as you age can help reduce your risk of cancer and many other health problems.

Get Regular Exercise

In addition to helping you achieve a healthy weight, exercise can reduce inflammation, improve immune function, and fight some of the negative health effects of a sedentary lifestyle—all of which can help prevent cancer.

Stop Smoking and Drink Less

Quitting smoking can improve your health in many ways, including lowering your cancer risk. And if you drink, do so in moderation. Some studies suggest that red wine has antioxidant properties that may benefit your health.

Increase Your Vitamin D

Most people don't get enough vitamin D. It can help protect against prostate cancer and many other conditions. Vitamin D-rich foods include cod liver oil, wild salmon, and dried shitake mushrooms. Since the sun is a better, more readily available source of vitamin D, many experts recommend getting 10 minutes of sun exposure (without sunscreen) every day.

Doctors often recommend vitamin D supplements. However, you should talk to your doctor before taking any vitamin or supplement.

Stay Sexually Active

Two studies appear to show that men who have a higher frequency of ejaculation (with or without a sexual partner) were up to two-thirds less likely to be diagnosed with prostate cancer. Studies are ongoing, but some experts theorize that ejaculation clears the body of toxins and other substances that could cause inflammation.

My only addition is that when I was researching nutrition for *Newtrition*, I read an article that suggested orange bell peppers, or Capsicums, as having some protective effect—and just for you (and me) I've found it again.[123] It concludes that "these results suggest that Reactive Oxygen Species (ROS)-mediated capsaicin-induced autophagy blockage contributes to antiproliferation in prostate cancer cells, which provides new insights into the anticancer molecular mechanism of capsaicin." So, it would seem all bell peppers and chillies may offer some protection. And to translate, the peppers induce ROS or oxygen that causes the cancer cells to die (autophagy).

The five-year relative survival rate for most people with local or regional prostate cancer is nearly 100%. For people diagnosed with prostate cancer that has spread to other parts of the body, the five-year relative survival rate is 32%.[124]

123 Ramos-Torres, Á., Bort, A., Morell, C. *et al.* 2016, "The pepper's natural ingredient capsaicin induces autophagy blockage in prostate cancer cells", *Oncotarget*, Vol. 7, No. 2, pp. 1569-1583, https://doi.org/10.18632/oncotarget.6415.

124 2005-2024 American Society of Clinical Oncology (ASCO)

Throat (Oro-Pharyngeal) Cancer[125]

Throat cancer is caused by the HPV virus. Of the more than 100 types of HPV, about 40 types can spread through direct sexual contact to genital areas, as well as the mouth and throat. Oral HPV is transmitted to the mouth by oral sex, or possibly in other ways.

There is no test, just a visual examination.

Prevention

Vaccination prevents it. Get vaccinated!

125 Bloom, J. C., Kaufmann, N., Koss, S. *et al.* 2023, "Deciphering Knowledge and Opinions of Human Papillomavirus and Human Papillomavirus Vaccination for Facilitation of Point-of-Care Vaccination in Adults", *JAMA Otolaryngology Head & Neck Surgery,* Vol. 149, No. 10, pp. 870-877, https://doi.org/10.1001/jamaoto.2023.2073.

CHAPTER 23

Dementia & Alzheimer's Disease (AD)

"O! let me not be mad, not mad, sweet heaven;
Keep me in temper; I would not be mad!"

– William Shakespeare King Lear, Act 1, Scene 5

I so vividly remember looking down the microscope in my second-year medicine histology exam and seeing this obvious brain tissue but with blotches of red, gel-like substance obliterating the normal neuronal architecture—as if it had been carpet bombed. I was stupefied, horrified and transfixed, so much so the supervisor had to yell at me to 'move on'!

I was horrified, as here was the human brain, the organ I held most sacred in humans, being so assaulted and damaged. I was stupefied because, even then, over 60 years ago, I fully realised what a terrible impact this infiltration and accumulation of this red gel, this amyloid (Aβ), could have, effectively turning the functioning brain into just being a lump of gel itself.

Amyloid, or Aβ, is a *normal product of the cellular metabolism, but pathologically,* it clumps into plaques between neurons.

It is not the only factor in Alzheimer's-related brain changes, which may result from a complex interplay among abnormal tau and beta-amyloid (Aβ) proteins and several other factors. It appears that abnormal tau accumulates in specific brain regions involved in memory.

A 2023 report from the Alzheimer's Association estimates that one in three Americans older than 85 have Alzheimer's disease, the most common form of dementia. Little wonder it is of such concern.

But AD is not the only cause of dementia. There are a number of cognitive degenerative disorders, including:[126]

1. Alzheimer's Disease
2. Cerebrovascular Disease
3. Frontotemporal Degeneration (FTD)
4. Hippocampal Sclerosis (HS)
5. Lewy Body Disease
6. Mixed Pathologies
7. Parkinson's Disease
8. Chronic Traumatic Encephalopathy (CTE)

The fear that comes with the increasing incidence of dementia, mainly from AD, is leading, in my experience, to reciprocal frustration in how to prevent or avoid it. No one has the answers, just observational suspicions such as not smoking, eating a good diet, keeping fit, avoiding 'forever chemicals' and pollution, exercising our brain, sleeping well, avoiding stress and... oh, really? Same old; same old.

And who, in their 20s or 30s, will adopt such a specific regime? Do we move to the country, avoid the farmers' pesticides, only eat organic and drink 0.5 micron filtered rainwater, play chess and bridge, do crosswords, jog, and do resistance weights in the hope we may avoid it?

126 Alzheimer's Association, 2023, "2023 Alzheimer's Disease Facts and Figures", *Alzheimer's & Dementia*, Vo.l. 19, No. 4, https://doi.org/10.1002/alz.13016.

Well, to a great degree, I do... now. But that is by default, and well after, I should have developed AD. It is not a conscious, dementia-avoiding, calculated choice, and my past history of playing jazz, sometimes every night, for 17 years in a row, in smoky clubs, is hardly a good example.

And, even now, when I cook, the tins of tomatoes are lined with what I am told is PCP leaking plastic. Microplastics are in every bottle of bought water.

As I said, no one has the answers (yet), and all you can do is the best you can, plus the regular checks as per the Appendix. We (my wife and I) have a lovely friend who has just been diagnosed with AD. But, for years, we thought she was (clinically) hyperthyroid. She was, however, 'alternative', and we soon got the message that any suggestion of getting tested was not acceptable.

So, get tested.

Prevention

It is estimated that 40% of worldwide dementia could be theoretically prevented if the population shifts to a healthy lifestyle.[127]

A healthy lifestyle may provide a cognitive reserve to maintain cognitive abilities independently of common neuropathologies of dementia.[128] A healthy lifestyle score was developed based on self-reported factors, including noncurrent smoking, at least 150 minutes of physical activity per week, limiting alcohol consumption, a Mediterranean-DASH

127 Livingston, G., Huntley, J., Sommerlad, A. *et al.* 2020, "Dementia prevention, intervention, and care: 2020 report of the Lancet Commission", *Lancet*, Vol. 396, No. 10248, pp. 413-446, https://doi.org/10.1016/S0140-6736(20)30367-6

128 Dhana, K., Agarwal, P., James, B. D. *et al.* 2024, "Healthy Lifestyle and Cognition in Older Adults With Common Neuropathologies of Dementia", *JAMA Neurology*, Vol. 81, No. 3, pp. 233-239, https://doi.org/10.1001/jamaneurol.2023.5491.

Intervention for Neurodegenerative Delay (MIND) diet score higher than 7.5, and a late-life cognitive activity score higher than 3.2. The lifestyle score ranges from zero to five, with higher scores reflecting a healthier lifestyle.

I have banged on for years about using EVOO – Extra Virgin Olive Oil and recommended ingesting at least 20 ml a day. Now my advice has been vindicated: "Eating at least 7 g of olive oil daily -- about a half tablespoon -- was tied to an adjusted 28% lower risk of dementia-related death (pooled hazard ratio compared with never or rarely consuming olive oil for women but not men)".[129]

In another study, the data found a strong correlation between the daily consumption of processed food and meat items in AD patients.[130]

Physical activity is associated with better late-life cognition, but the association is weak.[131]

Dementia prevention is a complex topic, as there are many factors that may contribute to the risk or progression of the condition. According to some experts, the best way to prevent dementia is to adopt a healthy lifestyle that includes physical, mental, and social activities. However, there is no definitive evidence that any specific activity, such as learning a musical instrument, a language, or playing bridge, can prevent dementia.

---

129 Tessier, A., Cortese, M., Yuan, C. *et al.* 2024, "Consumption of Olive Oil and Diet Quality and Risk of Dementia-Related Death", *JAMA Network Open,* Vol. 7, No. 5, https://doi.org/10.1001/jamanetworkopen.2024.10021.

130 Ahmed, T., Zhang, P. & Kumar, K. 2024, "Australian Imaging Biomarkers and Lifestyle Flagship Study of Aging. Equilibrium of Dietary Patterns Between Alzheimer's Disease Patients and Healthy People: A Comprehensive Analysis Using Multiple Factor Analysis and Classification Modeling", *Journal of Alzheimer's Disease*, Vol. 97, No. 2, pp. 777-790, https://doi.org/10.3233/JAD-230634.

131 Iso-Markku, P., Aaltonen, S., Kujala, U. M. *et al.* 2024, "Physical Activity and Cognitive Decline Among Older Adults: A Systematic Review and Meta-Analysis", *JAMA Network Open*, Vol. 7, No. 2, https://doi.org/10.1001/jamanetworkopen.2023.54285.

Some studies have suggested that these activities may have some benefits for cognitive function, but the results are not consistent or conclusive. Therefore, it is important to consult your doctor before starting any new activity or intervention for dementia prevention.

Some of the factors that may reduce the risk of dementia are:

- Monitoring and controlling your blood pressure and cholesterol
- Exercising every day
- Eating a balanced diet with plenty of fruits and vegetables
- Maintaining a healthy body weight
- Avoiding tobacco products and limiting alcohol use
- Protecting your head from injury by using seat belts, helmets, and other protective equipment
- Staying mentally alert by learning new hobbies, reading, or solving crossword puzzles
- Staying involved socially by attending community activities, church, or support groups
- Managing chronic conditions such as Diabetes, thyroid problems, or depression

Most of the following, therefore, is FYI.

Keeping Sharp

The combination of exercise and cognitive training provided modest benefit in a small, randomized trial. Various interventions, including aerobic or resistance exercise and cognitive training, benefit patients with mild cognitive impairment (MCI).[132]

---

132 Bloom, J. C., Kaufmann, N., Koss, S. *et al.* 2023, "Deciphering Knowledge and Opinions of Human Papillomavirus and Human Papillomavirus Vaccination for Facilitation of Point-of-Care Vaccination in Adults", *JAMA Otolaryngology Head & Neck Surgery*, Vol. 149, No. 10, pp. 870-877, https://doi.org/10.1001/jamaoto.2023.2073.

A 2019 study from Blue Cross Blue Shield found that millennials were finding their mental and physical health decline faster than the previous generation and predicted they could see mortality rates climb by more than 40% compared with Gen-Xers at the same age. This is, in part, because millennials have higher levels of depression, substance abuse, hypertension and high cholesterol. Notably, deadly strokes and heart attacks have been increasing among young adults over the past decade. Is 30 the new 50?

A study in the Journal of the American Medical Association[133] found that seniors with higher levels of perceived stress were more than 50% more likely to experience cognitive impairment, even after adjusting for differences in socio-economic and lifestyle factors such as exercise and alcohol use, as well as chronic health conditions.

Use of prescribed PPIs for > 4.4 years by individuals ages 45 years and older is associated with a higher incidence of newly diagnosed dementia.[134]

Regular internet users experienced approximately half the risk of dementia than non-regular users.[135]

---

133 Kulshreshtha, A., Alonso, A., McClure, L. A. *et al.* 2023, "Association of Stress With Cognitive Function Among Older Black and White US Adults", *JAMA Network Open*, Vol. 6, No. 3, https://doi.org/10.1001/jamanetworkopen.2023.1860.

134 Northuis, C. A., Bell, E. J., Lutsey, P. L. *et al.* 2023, "Cumulative Use of Proton Pump Inhibitors and Risk of Dementia: The Atherosclerosis Risk in Communities Study, *Neurology*, Vol. 101, No. 18, https://doi.org/10.1212/WNL.0000000000207747.

135 Cho, G., Betensky, R. A. & Chang, V. W. 2023, "Internet usage and the prospective risk of dementia: A population-based cohort study", *Journal of the American Geriatrics Society*, Vol. 71, No. 8, pp. 2419-2429, https://doi.org/10.1111/jgs.18394

People 60 and older who spent more time being sedentary—passively watching TV, for example—had a higher risk of incident all-cause dementia.[136]

Higher concentrations of total $PM_{2.5}$ were associated with greater rates of incident dementia. In single-pollutant models, $PM_{2.5}$ from all sources, except dust, were associated with increased rates of dementia, with the strongest associations for agriculture, traffic, coal combustion, and wildfires.[137] (PM stands for particulate matter, and the 2.5 refers to matter that has a diameter of 2.5 micrometres or smaller).

Diet

A sample of 9543 Dutch participants for a mean of 14.5 years showed that a higher intake of dietary nitrate from vegetable sources was associated with an approximately 8% lower risk of developing dementia. No association was found, however, for nitrate from non-vegetable sources. Analyses were extensively adjusted for sociodemographic, lifestyle, and dietary variables, as well as for *APOE* ε4 status (a major genetic risk factor for Alzheimer›s disease).[138]

A higher dietary nitrate intake from vegetable sources was associated with a lower risk of dementia. No evidence was found that this association was driven by vascular brain health.[139]

---

136 Raichlen, D. A., Aslan, D. H., Sayre, M. K. *et al.* 2023, "Sedentary Behavior and Incident Dementia Among Older Adults", *JAMA*, Vol. 330, No. 10, pp. 934-940, https://doi.org/10.1001/jama.2023.15231.

137 *Ibid.*

138 *The American Journal of Clinical Nutrition*, Vol. 118, No. 3, pp. 487-734.

139 de Crom, T. O. E., Blekkenhorst, L., Vernooij, M. W. *et al.* 2023, "Dietary nitrate intake in relation to the risk of dementia and imaging markers of vascular brain health: a population-based study", *The American Journal of Clinical Nutrition*, Vol. 118, No. 2, pp. 352-359, https://doi.org/10.1016/j.ajcnut.2023.05.027

In the present study, higher biomarker-validated diet inflammatory index (DII) scores (indicating greater proinflammatory diet potential) were associated with an increased risk for incident dementia.[140]

Tests

Blood tests for dementia and AD are mooted as not being too far away, but, at present, the diagnosis of dementia is a clinical one.

These tests are usually only done in specialised neurological units.

1. Amyloid-β

Plasma amyloid-β 42/40-Aβ 42/40, neurofilament light chain-NfL, progranulin

The amyloid-β (Aβ)42/40 ratio in blood plasma has turned out to be a good biomarker of the cerebral amyloid pathology associated with Alzheimer's Disease (AD). I don't know if this test is widely available, so you may wish to check with your own doctor if you have any concerns.

Plasma neurofilament light chain (NfL) and progranulin (PGRN) levels are associated with cognitive and physical impairment in older individuals, and again, these tests may not be readily available.

2. Nutrition

Erythrocyte docosahexaenoic acid, eicosapentaenoic acid, omega-3 index; plasma homocysteine-Hcy, 25 hydroxyvitamin D.

Eicosapentaenoic acid (EPA) is an omega-3 fatty acid that is found along with docosahexaenoic acid (DHA) in cold-water

140 Charisis, S., Ntanasi, E., Yannakoulia, M. *et al.* 2021, "Diet Inflammatory Index and Dementia Incidence: A Population-Based Study," *Neurology,* Vol. 97, No. 24, https://doi.org/10.1212/WNL.0000000000012973.

fish, including tuna and salmon. EPA prevents the blood from clotting easily, reduces triglyceride levels in the blood, and has effects that might reduce pain and swelling.

The erythrocyte (our red blood cells) membrane content of eicosapentaenoic acid (EPA) and docosahexaenoic acid (DHA), which constitutes the omega-3 index (O3I), predicts cardiovascular disease mortality.

Red blood cell levels of eicosapentaenoic acid (EPA) and docosahexaenoic acid (DHA) are a reflection of tissue levels of metabolism and nutrition. Low red blood cell (RBC) membrane content of EPA and DHA, i.e., the omega-3 index (O3I), and elevated RBC distribution width (RDW) are risk factors for all-cause mortality.

The inference here is that EPA and DHA are very beneficial to our overall health and may, therefore, offer some preventive benefits against brain degeneration.

3 Inflammation

Plasma tumor necrosis factor receptor 1-TNFR-1, monocyte chemoattractant protein 1-MCP-1, interleukin 6-IL-6.

TNFR1 plays a major role in maintaining immune homeostasis by promoting apoptosis, cell survival, differentiation, and inflammation.

MCP-1 levels were significantly higher in frail individuals compared to nonfrail. These data support the conclusion that MCP-1 can be used as a measure of mammalian biological age that is responsive to interventions that extend healthy aging.[141]

141 Yousefzadeh, M. J., Schafer, M. J., Noren Hooten, N. *et al.* 2018, "Circulating levels of monocyte chemoattractant protein-1 as a potential measure of biological age in mice and frailty in humans", *Aging Cell*, Vol. 17, No. 2, https://doi.org/10.1111/acel.12706.

Interleukin-6 (IL-6): Astrocytes, microglia, and neurons express the cytokine interleukin-6 (IL-6), which in the brain has been suggested to reduce food intake, inhibit memory and learning, cause neurodegeneration, and exacerbate sickness behavior induced by other cytokines.[142]

Again, I do not know if these tests are widely available or even desirable at this stage.

4. *Cellular Stress*

Plasma growth differentiation factor 15-GDF-15.

Increased levels of growth differentiation factor-15 (GDF15) are associated with cachexia, cardiovascular disease, and all-cause mortality.

Social Isolation

Social isolation has been linked to declining cognitive function and late-life depressive symptoms. In a study of 9000 older adults (≥65 years) living in Japan who had undergone brain MRI scans, it was also associated with lower total brain volume and a higher burden of white matter lesions. Brain regions affected included those known to be involved with memory, mood, and cognition.[143]

Again:

1. Projects
2. Purpose
3. Participate – socialise

142 Godbout, J. P. & Johnson, R. W. 2004, "Interleukin-6 in the aging brain", *Journal of Neuroimmunology*, Vol. 147, No. 1-2, pp. 141-144, https://doi.org/10.1016/j.jneuroim.2003.10.031.

143 Hirabayashi, N., Honda, T., Hata, J. *et al.* 2023, "Association Between Frequency of Social Contact and Brain Atrophy in Community-Dwelling Older People Without Dementia", *Neurology*, Vol. 101, No. 11, https://doi.org/10.1212/WNL.0000000000207602.

Prevention

An international study led by researchers at the McCance Center for Brain Health at Massachusetts General Hospital devised and validated a Brain Care Score (BCS) card that makes it easy to total up what you're doing well and where you might do better. The prize is a healthier brain—specifically a lower risk for dementia and strokes.

Designed to predict how current habits might impact future brain health, the user-friendly scorecard is apparently the first of its kind.

Called the McCance Brain Care Score, the card tallies points from 12 physical, lifestyle, and social-emotional domains.[144]

Physical components relate to:

- blood pressure
- blood sugar
- cholesterol
- body mass index (BMI)

Lifestyle components include:

- nutrition
- alcohol intake
- smoking
- aerobic activities
- sleep
- social-emotional factors
- stress management
- social relationships
- meaning in life

---

144 Singh, S. D., Oreskovic, T., Carr, S. *et al.* 2023, "The predictive validity of a Brain Care Score for dementia and stroke: data from the UK Biobank cohort", *Frontiers in Neurology*, Vol. 14, https://doi.org/10.3389/fneur.2023.1291020

All these physical and lifestyle factors can contribute to the risk of dementia.

Alzheimer's Disease (AD)

AD is characterised by the accumulation of a sticky, gel-like protein plaque beta-amyloid (Aβ) outside the brain's neurons and with twisted strands of protein inside the neurons called tau. Death of the neurons follows with brain tissue damage. Inflammation and atrophy of brain tissue is also invariably present.

Recently, five different subtypes have been defined, which highlight the need for personalized medicine.[145]

When someone develops Alzheimer's before age 65, it's known as "early-onset Alzheimer's" or sometimes "younger-onset Alzheimer's" or "earlier-onset Alzheimer's." Less than 10% of all people with Alzheimer's develop symptoms this early.

Unfortunately, more than 100 years after the discovery of the disease, there is still no effective therapy for modifying the biology behind AD and nipping the disease in the bud. This state of affairs has made neuroscientists suspicious, so much so that for several years, the idea has gained ground that AD is not a direct neuropathological consequence taking place downstream of the deposition of the two toxic proteins, but rather a multifactorial disease, including mitochondrial dysfunction as an early event in the pathogenesis of AD, occurring even before clinical symptoms.[146]

Exercise is advocated as the key to keeping your mitochondria healthy. Endurance training enhances mitochondrial activity

145 *Nature Aging*, 9 January 2024

146 Atlante, A., Amadoro, G., Latina, V. & Valenti, D. 2022, "Therapeutic Potential of Targeting Mitochondria for Alzheimer's Disease Treatment", *Journal of Clinical Medicine*, Vol. 11, No. 22, https://doi.org/10.3390/jcm11226742.

and has been shown in mice to protect against brain atrophy. In studies with Alzheimer's patients, exercise increased blood flow to the brain, thickened the hippocampus, enhanced growth of new neurons, and improved cognitive performance. Alternatively, a sedentary lifestyle increased damaging reactive oxygen species, increased inflammation in the brain, and reduced mitochondrial activity.

To measure mitochondrial fitness, the best metric is VO_2max, which represents the maximum rate at which your body can use oxygen during exercise. Essentially, it reflects the body's ability to utilize oxygen for energy production (and remember, mitochondria are producing that energy). While a direct measure of your VO_2max requires special equipment, most fitness watches provide an indirect VO_2max estimate. In the Fitbit and Apple watches, this is called the "cardio fitness level". Numbers vary for men and women, but for best results, aim high.

Aside from exercise, mitochondrial health improves with an antioxidant-rich diet full of plants like blueberries, red beans, tomatoes, spinach, artichokes, and green tea. Studies show that calorie restriction and ketogenic diets may also be protective. And stay away from stress. In animal studies,[147] chronic stress, anxiety, low social status, aggression, social defeat, and fear all damage mitochondria.

Of course, even a person who follows this advice can still get Alzheimer's. But knowing that mitochondria appear to play a crucial role in its development will give scientists plenty to think about as they research new drugs to stave off this devastating disease.[148]

147 Ülgen, D. H., Ruigrok, S. R. & Sandi, C. 2023, "Powering the social brain: Mitochondria in social behaviour", *Current Opinion in Neurobiology*, Vol. 79, https://doi.org/10.1016/j.conb.2022.102675.

148 *Big Think Neuropsych*, 9 August 2023

Diagnosis

Diagnosis of dementia was largely a clinical diagnosis, based on symptoms of memory or thinking decline that were serious enough to affect someone's ability to live independently day-to-day, but now it is possible to measure evidence of Alzheimer's through the underlying proteins beta-amyloid and abnormal forms of tau protein using PET scans, cerebrospinal fluid tests, and now blood tests.

Symptoms and Signs

Warning signs include…

- Difficulty performing daily tasks like keeping track of bills and following a recipe while cooking
- Repetition, such as asking the same question over and over and telling the same story multiple times
- Struggling to find the right word
- Getting lost
- Personality changes, such as becoming more anxious, confused, afraid, or paranoid
- Confusion about time and place, especially if someone can't remember where they are or how they got there
- Misplacing items in unusual areas
- Trouble with hygiene
- Trouble with handling money
- Sudden loss of interest in family, friends, work, social events
- Forgetting old memories
- Increased anxiety and depression

Other symptoms of late-stage disease include:

- Cannot recognise family or friends.
- Extreme difficulty communicating

- Sense of self absent
- Extrapyramidal dysfunction might develop, including akathisia, parkinsonism, dystonia, bradykinesia, tremor, and tardive dyskinesia.
- Weight loss
- Seizures, skin infections, and difficulty in swallowing
- Groaning, moaning, and grunting
- Increased sleeping
- Lack of bladder and bowel control

Causes or Contributors

The cause is unknown, but risk factors have been noted:

- Advancing age
- Family history
- APOE4 genotype
- Obesity
- Insulin resistance
- Vascular factors
- Dyslipidemia
- Hypertension
- Inflammatory markers
- Down syndrome
- Traumatic brain injury
- Midlife hypertension (lower risk with treatment)
- Maybe education (lower incidence)
- NSAIDS (lower incidence long-term)
- Depression diagnosed in early, middle, or late life more than doubled the risk for subsequent dementia, a study of 1.4 million people in Denmark showed.[149]

149 Atlante, A., Amadoro, G., Latina, V. & Valenti, D. 2022, "Therapeutic Potential of Targeting Mitochondria for Alzheimer's Disease Treatment", *Journal of Clinical Medicine*, Vol. 11, No. 22, https://doi.org/10.3390/jcm11226742.

Most cases are sporadic. Familial forms account for some 25%. Early autosomal-dominant cases are < 5%.

Gene Variants

APOE4 increases the risk.

Ten years ago, researchers knew of only 10 genes linked with Alzheimer's. Today, more than 70 genetic regions associated with Alzheimer's have been identified.

Brief Microbiology if interested (or skip to 'Risks' below:

Basically, we are comprised of cells that contain a nucleus. The nucleus is effectively a cell's command centre—it instructs cells to divide, grow, or die. In each nucleus are chromosomes, deoxyribonucleic acid (DNA), double helix threads, which contain our hereditary material in genes. A chromosome contains hundreds to thousands of genes. Every normal human cell contains 23 pairs of chromosomes, for a total of 46 chromosomes.

Genes are chunks of DNA that contribute to particular traits or functions by coding for proteins that influence physiology.

Alleles are variant forms of a gene, each of two or more alternative forms of a gene that arise by mutation and are found at the same place on a chromosome. An individual's combination of alleles is known as their genotype.

Ribonucleic acid (RNA) is made in the nucleus then transported out, through the membrane, and can never re-enter the nucleus. mRNA, or messenger RNA evolved billions of years ago and is naturally found in every cell in your body. Its principal role is to act as a messenger (mRNA), carrying instructions from DNA for controlling the synthesis of proteins. However, it was recently developed to transport vaccines, first for the rabies vaccine, then Ebola, but most significantly, for Covid. mRNA is broken down quickly by the body. It cannot affect or combine with our DNA in any way to change our genetic code, despite the alarmist anti-vaxxers. mRNA vaccines were approved by the FDA for two COVID-19 vaccines, which demonstrated outstanding prevention efficacy as well as great safety profiles.

Major Genetic Risks

The major genetic risk modifier for Alzheimer's disease[150] and the greatest prognostic risk we can presently test for is the apolipoprotein E (APOE) gene.

APOE (sometimes written ApoE) is a gene involved in making apolipoprotein E, a protein that helps carry cholesterol and other fats in the bloodstream. It comes in three forms, or alleles:

- APOE2 decreases the risk of late-onset AD.
- APOE3 is thought to play a neutral role.
- APOE4 increases the risk.

APOE2

It is not known how APOE2 confers protection against AD. It is relatively rare.

It has also been identified as a longevity gene, suggesting a systemic effect of APOE2 on the aging process and protection against cognitive impairment in individuals over 90 years of age—even those who have high levels of Aβ in the brain.

APOE2/2 individuals and APOE2/3 (or APOE2 carriers) are more likely to be cognitively intact compare with APOE3/3 homozygotes among individuals with minimal Aβ pathology. Human studies show that APOE2 is associated with reduced Aβ

150 Li, Z., Shue, F., Zhao, N. *et al.* 2020, "APOE2: protective mechanism and therapeutic implications for Alzheimer's disease", *Molecular Neurodegeneration*, Vol. 15, https://doi.org/10.1186/s13024-020-00413-4

deposition in the brains of non-demented aged individuals and AD patients, suggesting that APOE2 reduces AD risk at least partially through Aβ-dependent pathways.

However, carriers exhibit increased risk of certain cerebrovascular diseases and neurological disorders with an increased risk of cerebral amyloid angiopathy (CAA), which often co-exists with AD pathology and is a major cause of haemorrhagic stroke. It is also associated with increased risk of certain neurological disorders such as post-traumatic stress disorder (PTSD), age-related macular degeneration (AMD) and supranuclear palsy (PSP).

APOE4

For some 30 years, it was realised there was an association with the APOE4 gene, but that Alzheimer's was not inevitable. Now, however, it has been found that over 95% of individuals over 65 years old who have two copies of the APOE4 gene—APOE4 homozygotes—show biological characteristics of Alzheimer's pathology in the brain or biomarkers of this disease in cerebrospinal fluid and PET scans. Also, individuals homozygous for APOE4 develop the disease earlier than those with other variants of the APOE gene. These findings suggest that having two copies of the APOE4 gene could represent a new genetic form of Alzheimer's disease.[151]

Generational links

Cases occur in at least three individuals in two or more generations, with two of the individuals being first-degree relatives.

---

151 Fortea, J., Pegueroles, J., Alcolea, D. *et al.* 2024, "APOE4 homozygozity represents a distinct genetic form of Alzheimer's disease", *Nature Medicine*, Vol. 30, pp. 1284-1291, https://doi.org/10.1038/s41591-024-02931-w.

Nutrition

Lately, processed foods have been implicated:

The findings from multiple-factor analysis (MFA) indicated that the diversity or equilibrium of daily diet might play a potential role in AD development. This study incorporated multiple-factor analysis (MFA) to evaluate dietary patterns and employed Random Forest (RF) classifier and Sparse Logistic Regression (SLR) for Variable Importance analysis.

The findings from multiple-factor analysis (MFA) indicated that the diversity or equilibrium of daily diet might play a potential role in AD development. They identified food items significantly associated with AD. Especially deli meats, and food made with meat items, are associated with AD.[152]

Overall, patients with Alzheimer's tended to eat a diet rich in "processed food and meat items". The foodstuff they regularly ingested included beef, meat pies, sausages, ham, hamburgers, and pizza—basically a mall food court's worth of delicious grub. Compared to the healthy cohort, they also tended to eat less fruits and vegetables and, intriguingly, drank wine at lower rates as well.

The reader is strongly recommended to an excellent article, "What Do We Know About Diet and Prevention of Alzheimer's Disease?", published by the NIH.[153]

---

152 Ahmed, T., Zhang, P. & Kumar, K. 2024, "Australian Imaging Biomarkers and Lifestyle Flagship Study of Aging. Equilibrium of Dietary Patterns Between Alzheimer's Disease Patients and Healthy People: A Comprehensive Analysis Using Multiple Factor Analysis and Classification Modeling", *Journal of Alzheimer's Disease*, Vol. 97, No. 2, pp. 777-790, https://doi.org/10.3233/JAD-230634.

153 National Institute on Aging, 2023, "What Do We Know About Diet and Prevention of Alzheimer's Disease?", https://www.nia.nih.gov/health/alzheimers-and-dementia/what-do-we-know-about-diet-and-prevention-alzheimers-disease, reviewed 20 November 2023.

Diagnosis

Diagnosis, in the absence of future blood tests, requires the finding of slowly progressive memory loss of insidious onset in a fully conscious patient. Alzheimer's disease cannot be diagnosed in patients with clouded consciousness or delirium. Toxic metabolic conditions and brain neoplasms must also be excluded as potential causes of the patient's dementia.

Laboratory tests can be performed to rule out other conditions, such as:

- cobalamin (vitamin B_{12}) level
- thyroid function tests
- CT or MRI of the brain

Additional investigations may include:

- Complete blood cell count (and B_{12})
- Liver function tests (LFT)
- TSH (thyroid-stimulating hormone) levels
- Rapid plasma reagin test to rule out syphilis
- Abnormalities in HIV serology and/or polymerase chain reaction assay to rule out HIV/AIDS
- Abnormalities in paraneoplastic antibodies to rule out autoimmune encephalitis.
- Abnormalities in cerebrospinal fluid proteins tau, P-tau, and 14-3-3 to rule out Creutzfeldt-Jakob disease.

Testing

The 'great debate' is whether to test or not when there is nothing or not much anyone can do, as yet, if the test results are APOE4/APOE4.

This is a personal decision, but I first did my lipids in 1968 and my ApoB and alleles in 1990 when there was not much known about them and little that could be done… but I am glad I did them.

I also see that one famous movie star, Chris Hemsworth, a patient of Dr. Attia's, revealed in an 'exclusive interview' with Vanity Fair how he was E4/E4 and how he was coping with the news. This is on the internet, and I would recommend you source it if you are undecided (or even if you are not), but it would seem he was glad he had the test.

If you are APOE2/2 and APOE2/3, you are more likely to live longer and not suffer from AD but could have a haemorrhagic stroke, macular degeneration, PTSD, and two rare neurological disorders (above).

If you are APOE3/APOE3, you run the average risks.

If you are APOE4/APOE4, you are at a higher risk, now thought to be a form of AD, and may choose to see a neurologist regarding protective/preventive measures against AD.

Three rare single-gene variants are also known to cause the disease:

- Amyloid precursor protein (APP) on chromosome 21
- Presenilin 1 (PSEN1) on chromosome 14
- Presenilin 2 (PSEN2) on chromosome 1[154]

Changes in these three genes result in the production of abnormal proteins that are associated with the disease. Each of these mutations contributes to the breakdown of APP, a protein that's function isn't completely understood. The breakdown of APP is part of a process that makes harmful forms of sticky amyloid fragments. These fragments cluster to form plaques in the brain, which is a hallmark of Alzheimer's.

In addition to the three genetic variants that are known to cause Alzheimer's, people with Down Syndrome have an extra

154 National Institute on Aging Alzheimer's Disease Genetics Fact Sheet

copy of chromosome 21, which carries the APP gene, and are at a higher risk of developing early-onset Alzheimer's. Estimates suggest that 50% or more of people living with Down Syndrome will develop Alzheimer's, with symptoms appearing in their 50s and 60s.

Genetic Testing for Alzheimer's Disease

Genetic tests are not routinely used in clinical settings to diagnose or predict the risk of developing Alzheimer's or a related dementia. APOE testing is available, and now that two copies of the APOE4 gene—APOE4 homozygotes— homozygous or E2/E2 pair, is thought to be a form of AD, no doubt it will become more sought.

Draft New Proposed International Guidelines

Blood tests and brain scans may soon replace memory tests for earlier and more accurate diagnosis of Alzheimer's disease with the development of excellent diagnostic blood biomarkers, some of which have been clinically proven. Initially, the draft criteria would largely be applied in research and trials.

This would call for Alzheimer's to be defined biologically rather than on clinical symptoms and highlight that early diagnosis will help people understand the cause of their cognitive challenges so they can make informed decisions about how they want to manage their lives.

Prevention

Sildenafil (Viagra)

Early studies did not find any benefit, but the latest study, which looked at more than 27,000 over-65s, found that the risk was

62% lower for men and 47% lower for women. Viagra boosts the blood supply to improve brain health, meaning that it has the potential to treat dementia. It also blocks an enzyme that has been found in the brain of those who suffer from the disease.[155]

Prior vaccination against tetanus and diphtheria, with or without pertussis (Tdap/Td), herpes zoster (HZ), better known as shingles, and pneumococcus are all associated with a reduced risk for developing Alzheimer's disease. People who received at least one influenza vaccine were 40% less likely than their unvaccinated peers to develop Alzheimer's disease.[156]

Metformin[157]

In a study of metformin users, terminating metformin treatment was associated with increased dementia incidence, corroborating prior observational research that initiating metformin was associated with reduced risk of dementia. But this study suggests that metformin cessation is associated with increased dementia incidence. To be clear, metformin reduces the incidence of dementia as it seems to have a (neuro)-protective effect; but, if stopped, this protection ceases, and there is then an increased dementia incidence.

---

155 Huo, X. & Finkelstein, J. 2023, "Using Big Data to Uncover Association Between Sildenafil Use and Reduced Risk of Alzheimer's Disease", *Studies in Health Technology Informatics*, Vol. 302, pp. 866-870, https://doi.org/10.3233/SHTI230291.

156 Harris, K., Ling, Y., Bukhbinder, A. S. *et al.* 2023, "The Impact of Routine Vaccinations on Alzheimer's Disease Risk in Persons 65 Years and Older: A Claims-Based Cohort Study using Propensity Score Matching", *Journal of Alzheimer's Disease*, Vol. 95, No. 2, pp. 703-718, https://doi.org/org/10.3233/JAD-221231.

157 Huo, X. & Finkelstein, J. 2023, "Using Big Data to Uncover Association Between Sildenafil Use and Reduced Risk of Alzheimer's Disease", *Studies in Health Technology Informatics*, Vol. 302, pp. 866-870, https://doi.org/10.3233/SHTI230291.

Treatments

Obviously, AD is high priority, and drugs have been, and are being, developed, but they are not yet curative. They only slow down the process.

Recommendations come and go as the passage of time reveals their worth or otherwise but underlining it all is keeping the brain connections connected. New mental challengers would seem optimistic, but there are conflicting and contradictory studies as to if learning a musical instrument, learning a language, playing bridge, doing crosswords, as well as investing in socialising or meditation can help. I, personally, observe how music seems to have the most profound effect, even on the most affected patients. So, maybe this is an area to concentrate on. But I would certainly encourage any activity that stimulates and uses the brain.

While the drugs have been clinically tested, I cannot vouch for the (following) breathing and antioxidant treatments. However, they certainly can do no harm.

Drugs

Lecanemab is the drug that has recently been approved as a targeted therapy for Alzheimer's. Donanemab slows disease by up to 60%, which offered some people at least a year of extra time without their disease progressing. The drug attacks and destroys build-ups of a protein called amyloid in the brains of patients with the disease.

Counterpoint

Focusing on drugs for Alzheimer's disease, with at best marginal efficacy, distracts from the use of drugs with clear benefits for Diabetes, hypertension, and depression. The treatment of these diseases is associated with a substantially decreased risk of developing Alzheimer's disease and other dementias (as well as many other diseases). According to a 2020 report[158] on preventable risk factors for dementia, interventions that target 12 modifiable risk factors could prevent or delay around 40% of cases. Hearing loss is the most prevalent preventable risk factor.

At present, drugs for Alzheimer's disease have unproven clinical benefits and proven harms. Billions of dollars spent on hearing aids, smoking cessation, encouragement of healthy lifestyles, and treatment of hypertension, Diabetes, and other modifiable risk factors may benefit patients more than spending on these drugs.[159]

Breathing Exercises

These brief breathing sessions had significant impacts: volunteers' heart rate variability increased during each exercise period, and the levels of amyloid-beta peptides circulating in their blood decreased over the four weeks of the experiment. These findings are from USC Leonard Davis School of Gerontology and are published in the journal *Nature Scientific Reports.*

The exercise was simple: inhale for a count of five, then exhale for a count of five. Do that for 20 minutes, twice a day, for four weeks.

Antioxidants

While multiple factors potentially play in the disease process, such as mitochondrial dysfunction, inflammation, and oxidative

158 Livingston, G., Huntley, J. Sommerlad, A. *et al.* 2020, "Dementia prevention, intervention, and care: 2020 report of the *Lancet* Commission", *The Lancet Commissions*, Vol. 396, No. 10248, pp. 413-446, https://doi.org/10.1016/S0140-6736(20)30367-6.

159 Molchan, S. & Fugh-Berman, A. 2023, "Are New Alzheimer Drugs Better Than Older Drugs?", *JAMA Internal Medicine*, Vol. 183, No. 9, pp. 902-903, https://doi.org/10.1001/jamainternmed.2023.3061.

damage, it has been found, in a small study,[160] that concentrations of lycopene, retinol, zeaxanthin, α-tocopherol, anhydrolutein, and lutein were all strikingly lower in brains with confirmed neuropathology characteristics of AD than in HE brains with no evidence of pathology.

As this study says, "Given the vulnerability of the brain to oxidative damage, constant generation of reactive species through normal brain functions, and limited antioxidant resources, it is reasonable to consider that brains with 40–50% lower levels of α-tocopherol and four carotenoids, and marginally lower levels in three of the four remaining brain carotenoids, would be more vulnerable to oxidative damage and inflammation. This new evidence of selective carotenoid and tocopherol deficiencies in the brains of subjects with AD add further support to the growing evidence (recently reviewed by Polidori et al.) that greater dietary intake of lutein, zeaxanthin, lycopene as well as α- and γ-tocopherols may slow cognitive decline prior to— and possibly following— a diagnosis with AD."[161]

It would not hurt, in my opinion, to ensure intake of these carotenoids and tocopherols, which are good for your eyesight, too.

All five micronutrients are antioxidants:

1. *Lycopene*—found in red fruits and vegetables like tomatoes, watermelon, red oranges, pink grapefruits, apricots, and guavas.
2. *Retinol*—found in foods like cheese, eggs, oily fish, milk, yogurt, and liver. Indirect sources include yellow, red,

160 Dorey, C. K., Gierhart, D., Fitch, K. A. *et al.* 2023, "Low Xanthophylls, Retinol, Lycopene, and Tocopherols in Grey and White Matter of Brains with Alzheimer's Disease", Journal of Alzheimer's Disease, Vol. 94, No. 1, pp. 1-17, https://doi.org/10.3233/JAD-220460.

161 *Ibid.*

and green leafy vegetables like spinach, carrots, sweet potatoes, and red peppers, as well as yellow fruits like mangos, papaya, and apricots.

3. *Lutein* is thought to protect eye tissue from sun damage and is found in egg yolks, spinach, kale, corn, orange peppers, kiwis, grapes, zucchinis, and squash.
4. *Zeaxanthin* is known to protect eye tissues from the sun and is found in eggs, oranges, grapes, corn, goji berries, mango, and orange peppers.
5. *Vitamin E* can be found in plant-based oils, nuts, seeds, fruits, and vegetables like sunflower oil, soybean oil, almonds, peanuts, spinach, pumpkin, red bell peppers, asparagus, mangoes, and avocados.

Hearing Aids

For the healthiest adults, who did not have other conditions such as heart failure, the hearing aids made no difference to their risk of dementia. But for those who already had signs of memory loss, or who had other underlying health conditions, using hearing aids made a big difference. Three-year cognitive change was 48% lower in the group given the hearing aids compared with the one that was not.

Regular Eye Tests

Getting your eyes checked regularly could reduce the chances of developing dementia in later life, a study suggests. The research, published in the journal *JAMA Ophthalmology*,[162] involved almost 3,000 people in their 70s and older in the USA. Overall, 12.3%

162 Tran, E. M., Stefanick, M. L., Henderson, V. W. *et al.* 2020, "Association of Visual Impairment With Risk of Incident Dementia in a Women's Health Initiative Population", *JAMA Ophthalmology*, Vol. 138, No. 6, pp. 624-633, https://doi.org/10.1001/jamaophthalmol.2020.0959.

of the participants showed signs of dementia, but rates were far higher in people who had visual problems when tested. For those with problems seeing things that were further away, the rate was 19.5%, and for those who had problems with closer vision, it was 21.5%. In a group of people classed as having moderate to severe visual impairment, or who were blind, the rate was 32.9 %.

Others

Growing evidence supports a protective effect of anti-inflammatory dietary patterns, especially the Mediterranean diet, against cognitive decline in older persons, but causal associations between diet and AD remain uncertain.[163]

Much research emphasises mitochondria fitness and ties this to overall fitness, recommending smart watch VO_2max apps.

Cerebrovascular Disease/Vascular Dementia

Brain tissue becomes injured when cerebral blood vessels are so damaged that not enough oxygen or nutrients are delivered. The brain is the most oxygen-dependent organ of the body. Vascular diseases contribute to approximately 25% of all diagnosed dementia. High blood pressure, high cholesterol, Diabetes, smoking, obesity, and sleep apnea are contributing, but modifiable, risk factors.

Frontotemporal Degeneration (FTD)

Neurons in the frontal and temporal lobes die, and the lobes shrink with accumulations of abnormal amounts of tau and transactive response DNA-misfolded binding protein (TDP-43).

163 McGrattan, A. M., McGuinness, B., McKinley, M. C. *et al.* 2019, "Diet and Inflammation in Cognitive Aging and Alzheimer's Disease", *Current Nutrition Reports*, Vol. 8, No. 2, pp. 53-65, https://doi.org/10.1007/s13668-019-0271-4.

Frontotemporal dementia is the most common type of dementia for people younger than 60 years old, but overall, it's not a very common form of dementia. The 67-year-old actor Bruce Willis has frontotemporal dementia, apparently with symptoms of aphasia in 2022.

Hippocampal Sclerosis (HS)

The hippocampal tissue shrinks and hardens with accumulation of the misfolded protein TDP-43.

Lewy Body Disease

Abnormal aggregations of the protein alpha-synuclein clump in the cortical neurons.

Mixed Pathologies

Are self-evident.

Parkinson's Disease (PD)

Parkinson's Disease is the fastest-growing neurological condition in the world and the most prevalent of neurodegenerative disorders. It is a progressive disorder caused by degeneration of nerve cells in the part of the brain called the substantia nigra, which controls movement. These nerve cells die or become impaired, losing the ability to produce the chemicals called dopamine, norepinephrine, and serotonin. These chemicals determine mood, energy, and motivation, leaving many in a state of depression.

While its cause is unknown, there is an abnormal accumulation of a protein called alpha-synuclein (Lewy bodies). There may be a 10 to 20% genetic input but no hereditary passing. Traumatic head damage is also a cause, and environmental toxins are suspect, but there is no current evidence to confirm the specific cause.

A recent study claims exposure to environmental toxicants is the principal reason and details three environmental toxicants that are likely among the main causes of Parkinson's disease—certain pesticides, the solvent trichloroethylene, and air pollution. All three environmental toxicants are ubiquitous, many affect mitochondrial functioning, and all can access humans via various routes, including inhalation and ingestion. It reaches the hopeful conclusion that most of Parkinson's disease is, thus, preventable.[164]

The diagnosis is Parkinson's Disease dementia when a person experiences dementia at least one year (and usually several years) after the onset of symptoms of Parkinson's Disease. Parkinson's symptoms may include a mask-like facial expression and changes in movement, like a tremor.

Exercise (dancing),[165] a healthy diet, and avoiding toxins such as herbicides, pesticides and the dry-cleaning fluid trichlorethylene (banned in many countries) may all help prevent Parkinson's disease. The Parkinson's Outcomes Project shows at least 2.5 hours a week of physical activity can slow PD symptom progression.[166] Dancing has shown impressive results.

The most useful drug, Levodopa, is 50 years old. I remember it being introduced, and we hailed it as a breakthrough, but it is concerning that there have been no further developments. Changes in movement detected passively by smartwatches can

---

164 Dorsey, E. R. & Bloem, B. R. 2024, "Parkinson's Disease Is Predominantly an Environmental Disease", *Journal of Parkinson's Disease*, Vol. 14, No. 3, pp. 451-465, https://doi.org/10.3233/JPD-230357.

165 Gyrling, T., Ljunggren, M. & Karlsson, S. 2021, "The impact of dance activities on the health of persons with Parkinson's disease in Sweden", *International Journal of Qualitative Studies on Health and Well-being*, Vol. 16, No. 1, https://doi.org/10.1080/17482631.2021.1992842.

166 Parkinson's Foundation

help flag Parkinson's disease (PD) years before symptom onset, new research shows.

An analysis of wearable motion-tracking data from UK Biobank participants showed a strong correlation between reduced daytime movement over one week and a clinical diagnosis of PD up to seven years later.

Retina changes may well pick up changes earlier.[167]

Physical activity has been tied to a significantly decreased risk of Parkinson's disease (PD) in women, results of a large, long-term prospective study show.[168,169]

Giving patients with Parkinson's disease and constipation a probiotic for three months improved not only their gut microbiome but also nonmotor symptoms such as sleep, fatigue, and constipation, results of a new randomized trial show. The probiotic used was a liquid formulation (Symprove) and contained four strains: *Lacticasei bacillus rhamnosus*, *Enterococcus faecium*, *Lactobacillus acidophilus*, and *Lactiplanti bacillus plantarum*.[170]

Parkinson's can strike tragically early: The actor Michael J. Fox was only 29 when diagnosed in 1991.

---

167 Zhang, Y., Zhang, X., Yue, Y. & Tian, T. 2021, "Retinal Degeneration: A Window to Understand the Origin and Progression of Parkinson's Disease?", *Frontiers in Neuroscience*, Vol. 15, https://doi.org/10.3389/fnins.2021.799526.

168 Anderson, P. 2023, "'Robust Evidence' That Exercise Cuts Parkinson Risk in Women", *Medscape*, 18 May 18.

169 Chahine, L. M. & Darweesh, S. K. L. 2023, "Physical Activity and the Risk of Parkinson Disease: Moving in the Right Direction", Neurology, Vol. 101, No. 4, pp. 151-152, https://doi.org/10.1212/WNL.0000000000207527.

170 Davenport, L. 2023, "Probiotics Improve Nonmotor Symptoms of Parkinson's", *Medscape*, 30 August.

Chronic Traumatic Encephalopathy (CTE)

CTE, "Punch Drunk", is a neurodegenerative disease linked to repeated trauma to the head. Symptoms can include behavioural and mood problems as well as issues with thinking, often leading to dementia.

Most cases have occurred in athletes, involving head trauma. The exact amount of trauma to cause it is not known. Despite this problem now being well known, men and women are still engaging in head trauma risk sports. Attempts to lessen head-high tackles are welcome but heads still make contact, helmets are of no use, and even soccer heading the ball is deleterious.

The deliberate ambition to damage another human's brain, I find reprehensible.

A definitive diagnosis of this disease can only occur at autopsy.

CHAPTER 24

Diabetes

"I do not love to work out, but if I stick to exercising every day and put the right things in my mouth, then my Diabetes just stays in check."

– Halle Berry

There are two types of Diabetes:

1. Type 1 (T1D), or Insulin dependent
2. Type 2 (T2D), mostly controlled by tablets or weight loss.

The cause of Type 1 is not known, but it is increasing dramatically in the countries with the highest standards of living.

Type 2 usually comes later in life and with weight gain.

T1D

T1D is an absolutely devastating illness which is increasing exponentially but lacks government or benefactor support.

There is nothing the child (usually) can do to prevent it yet. By contrast, HIV and Malaria are, to a large extent, preventable, but they attract immense funding.

This, in no way, is to begrudge them but certainly is a plea to better fund research into T1D, which effectively has not seen any real advance since 1921 when insulin was extracted from a pig's pancreatic cells—which is still the treatment today!

It is an auto-immune disease whence the beta cells of the pancreas which produce insulin are not recognised by the body as being 'self' and are destroyed by its immune system.

The recent advances are in a 'closed loop' system wherein a sensor, with a small needle-like probe, is stuck on the patient's body to constantly monitor the interstitial fluid glucose. This is linked to an insulin-loaded pump that feeds in the appropriate dose or is monitored by a smart phone.

These I consider mandatory, if you can afford one.

The best measure is the HbA1c, which since 2011 has been standardised around the world to read in SI Units, or mmom/mom. It averages the blood glucose (BG) over the previous 2-3 months. Keeping it below 7mmom/mom is recommended. T1D patients should be closely monitored by their doctor and/or and endocrinologist.

T2D

Type 2 Diabetes occurs when the body doesn't produce enough insulin to function properly or the body's cells don't react to insulin. This means glucose stays in the blood and isn't used as fuel for energy. Type 2 Diabetes is often associated with obesity and tends to be diagnosed in older people.

While there may be a genetic predilection, it is at epidemic proportions—an apt description because most is due to being overweight, arguably due to our ultra-processed, fast-food western Diet.

Exponential Increase—"You're Next"

From 2001 to 2020, Diabetes prevalence significantly increased among US adults 18 or older.

37.3 million people have Diabetes—that's 11.3% of the US population. 28.7 million people have been diagnosed with Diabetes. 8.5 million people who have Diabetes have not been diagnosed and do not know they have it.[171]

Total Pre-Diabetes

96 million US adults have Pre-Diabetes. 26.4 million adults 65 or older have Pre-Diabetes.

Cost of Diabetes

The total estimated cost of diagnosed Diabetes in 2017 was $327 billion, including $237 billion in direct medical costs and $90 billion in lost productivity. Excess medical costs associated with Diabetes were $9,601 per person in 2017.[172]

Unless you are aware of this pandemic, as it affects all Western countries, you will insidiously slip into being a Pre-Diabetic and soon progress to a T2D.

We all must take preventive measures *now.*

The Essential Gem of Prevention and Medical Advice:

- To avoid T2D, don't get fat.
- To remit T2D, lose fat.

171 "CDC By the Numbers: Diabetes in America", *National Diabetes Statistics Report 2023*

172 *2018-2019 National Health Interview Survey*

The Essentials of Prevention are:

- Good diet (see *Newtrition*)
- Weight control—measure waist
- Exercise
- Middle-age onset vs older-onset individuals possibly represent groups at different risk for the development of complications.
- Both hyperglycemia and hypoglycemia are related to an increased risk of geriatric syndromes, such as cognitive impairment, depression, falls, fractures, and functional disability in most observational studies.
- Other geriatric conditions such as muscle loss, mobility disability, and frailty are more prevalent in older patients with Diabetes.
- Treatment of Diabetes in older individuals includes lifestyle recommendations, when appropriate, and the use of pharmacologic therapies, which account for the presence of comorbidities, especially renal and hepatic impairment, as well as the physical and cognitive abilities of the patient, while seeking to minimize hypoglycemia.
- Clinical care needs to be individualized for the older adult with Diabetes, with simultaneous goals of management of hyperglycemia and prevention and treatment of both macrovascular and microvascular complications of Diabetes, avoidance of hypoglycemia, and preservation of quality of life.
- ADA: 2023 Standards of Care recommends screening all with Type 2 Diabetes for Fatty Liver Disease.[173]

173 *CDC: National Diabetes Statistics Report Estimates of Diabetes and Its Burden in the United States*

Can Exercise Erase the Genetic Risk for Diabetes?[174,175]

Exercise Is Good, More Exercise Is Better

Among 60,000 healthy, middle-aged adults, those who exercised the most—at least 68 minutes a day—were 74% less likely to develop Type 2 Diabetes. This was true even for those with a high "genetic risk score", those who were 2.4 times more likely to develop the disease due to their genes. Participants with a high genetic risk who were the most active had a lower risk of developing T2D than sedentary folks with *no genetic risk.*

Endurance exercise like running and cycling, when done long-term, can improve the way genes associate with metabolic health, which can help prevent diseases related to your metabolic function such as cardiovascular issues and type 2 Diabetes·

Participants with high genetic risk for Diabetes saw big improvements in body fat, blood lipids, and glycemic control after 12 weeks of strength training at a moderate intensity.[176]

It has been found that low-dose aspirin reduces the risk of type 2 Diabetes but the risk of gastrointestinal bleeds has to be considered.

---

174 Luo, M., Yu, C., Del Pozo Cruz, B. *et al.* 2023, "Accelerometer-measured intensity-specific physical activity, genetic risk and incident type 2 diabetes: a prospective cohort study", *British Journal of Sports Medicine*, Vol. 57, No. 19, https://doi.org/10.1136/ bjsports-2022-106653.

175 Chapman, M. A., Arif, M., Emanuelsson, E. B. *et al.* 2020, "Skeletal Muscle Transcriptomic Comparison between Long-Term Trained and Untrained Men and Women", *Cell Reports*, Vol. 31, No. 12, https://doi.org/10.1016/j.celrep.2020.107808.

176 Qadir, R., Sculthorpe, N. F., Todd, T. & Brown, E. C. 2021, "Effectiveness of Resistance Training and Associated Program Characteristics in Patients at Risk for Type 2 Diabetes: A Systematic Review and Meta-analysis", *Sports Medicine – Open*, Vol. 7, https://doi.org/10.1186/s40798-021-00321-x.

A study has suggested that depression could play a direct role in the development of Type 2 Diabetes.[177] Previous research has indicated that people with Type 2 Diabetes are approximately twice as likely to experience depression as those without Diabetes.

Also, people with depression were found to have a higher risk of developing Type 2 Diabetes. But which came first? Surely, the depression caused people to overeat, and being overweight contributed to the depression. I find it hard to envisage a single depression-T2D gene but, rather, reciprocal cause and effect.

Spirometry Predicts Mortality in Type 2 Diabetes

Among adults with type 2 Diabetes, the presence of preserved ratio impaired (PRISm) was significantly associated with increased risk of mortality and both macro- and microvascular complications, as well as increased mortality, based on data from more than 20,000 individuals.[178] Spirometry (PRISm) was significantly associated with increased risk of mortality and both macro- and microvascular complications, as well as increased mortality, based on data from more than 20,000 individuals.[179]

177 Maina, J. G., Balkhiyarova, Z., Nouwen, A. *et al.* 2023, "Bidirectional Mendelian Randomization and Multiphenotype GWAS Show Causality and Shared Pathophysiology Between Depression and Type 2 Diabetes", *Diabetes Care*, Vol. 46, No. 9, pp. 1707-1714. https://doi.org/10.2337/dc22-2373.

178 Splete, H. 2023, "Medical News Spirometry Predicts Mortality in Type 2 Diabetes", *Medscape*, 12 July.

179 Li, G., Jankowich, M. D., Wu, L. *et al.* 2023, "Preserved Ratio Impaired Spirometry and Risks of Macrovascular, Microvascular Complications and Mortality Among Individuals With Type 2 Diabetes", *Education and Clinical Practice: Original Research*, Vol. 164, No. 5, pp. 1268-1280, https://doi.org/10.1016/j.chest.2023.05.031.

CHAPTER 25

Flu, COVID, Chest Infections, and Vaccination

Make death wait – vaccinate!

I was surprised that the public nominated these as their sixth greatest concern, but they are right!

The flu pandemic of 1919 and the Covid pandemic of 2019 have been the greatest of world-wide killers.

For more than a century, the deadly 1918/19 flu had been the benchmark for pandemics in the US. Unfortunately, as of September 2022, the COVID-19 pandemic is officially the worst pandemic in American history.

The dedication to finding the genetic code of the 1918-19 flu is a medical saga of the highest order, and I would recommend it to all to read 'The Deadliest Flu: The Complete Story of the Discovery and Reconstruction of the 1918 Pandemic Virus' by Douglas Jordan, with contributions from Dr. Terrence Tumpey and Barbara Jester—see CDC's 1918 (H1N1 virus) website.

Such work has allowed the development of flu vaccines.

Normally, a typical vaccine development timeline takes five to 10 years, and sometimes longer, to assess whether the vaccine is safe and efficacious in clinical trials, complete the regulatory approval processes, and manufacture a sufficient quantity of vaccine doses for widespread distribution. But the incredible number of hospitalisations and fatalities from Covid saw an amazing speeding up of the process due to the already done research into m-RNA vaccines first tested as a flu vaccine in mice in 1990 and a rabies vaccine in humans in 2013, then later for the Ebola virus. Yet, it was not until Covid did they become commercially viable and necessary.

Covid will be seen to have the most profound effect on our lifestyles and health, and hence our longevity, and we should be alerted to these possible sequalae and attend to them.

History will surely consider 2020 as the most calamitous year in health since 1918, when influenza swept the globe. It will also be remembered as the worst economic crisis since the Great Depression. The social consequences of this pandemic will be felt for a long time to come. The pandemic affected everyone on the planet, directly or indirectly. By 2020, over 10% of the global population had been infected. With over 10,000 deaths per week, COVID-19 was now the third main cause of death globally.

Covid, as well as killing an enormous number of people world-wide, has left many disabled with Long-Covid but has also permanently altered our work and lifestyle practices.

Many are now working from home which, while fine for them, has seen previously fully-occupied office blocks throughout the world emptied out. The immediate effect of this is that the local businesses who depended on these office-workers are going broke, and while this may not immediately affect you or I, the downstream effect will. The lockdowns gave people more spending money for internet purchases while the big department stores and shopping centers became spookily empty. Interest rates went up, and this spending money has become increasingly scarcer.

To save money, in what has always been the great health paradox, people won't go to the doctor and won't, in many cases, even buy essential medicines. Paradoxically, they spend their money on 'little luxuries'. This, it would seem is human nature but also a harbinger of increasing avoidable illnesses.

What to do?

As to the economic sequalae of Covid, no one truly knows. The public and civil servants can be ordered back to work, but there is a universal reluctance. So, what can be done medically?

The response to the early days of Covid by most of the first world nations was tragic with the politicians disagreeing and duck-shoving. The UK's then Health Secretary, Matt Hancock, admitted at the enquiry in June 2023 that the UK's planning for a pandemic was "woefully inadequate" and that preparations were "completely wrong", "a calamitous state of affairs", and "a colossal scale of failure" by his own department.

The USA's story of COVID-19 is one of daunting scale, according to 'The United States' Response to COVID-19: A Case Study', which noted, "The U.S. epidemic dwarfed that of any other country. The U.S. reports almost 30 million cases and over 500,000 deaths, accounting for 25% of global cases and 20% of global deaths, despite comprising only 4% of the world's population. Life expectancy in the U.S. shrank by a full year in 2020. Had the U.S. responded with the swiftness and effectiveness of East Asia, over 428,000 American lives could have been saved".[180]

---

180 *London Telegraph,* 28 ?? 2023.

Looney theories from people without any qualifications were given publicity. It was as if their opinions regarding how to design a space-rocket engine could be similarly aired. But I would warn you that jade vaginal eggs won't protect you and injecting bleach is probably fatal, but that vaccination works—so I won't be listening to celebs, real-estate developers, tennis players, or politicians.

That is not to say some doctors have also disagreed, but the beauty of medicine is that eventually the truth, or the best way, is revealed by frank and open debate and trials. It is now urgent these various Covid controversies be ruthlessly examined and the best preventive plans, both nationally and individually, be sought.

Flu and Covid are viruses, and there are no really effective anti-viral drugs when compared to antibiotics, which are anti-bacterial.

Pneumonia was usually caused by bacteria, but now it is often caused by the Respiratory Syncytial Virus (RSV), and vaccines have already been developed.

It is my opinion that we should get every vaccination possible, as needed. There are, of course, many anti-vaxxers but not many who have seen polio cripples, diphtheria, typhoid and cholera deaths, deaf Rubella babies, Smallpox cases (we thought we had seen the last in the world, which I helped to treat, when I was in Edinburgh in the early 70s, but some people in places like Pakistan don't like vaccinations, so reservoirs still exist), and so on.

But from December 2020 through November 2022, it is estimated that the COVID-19 vaccination program in the U.S. prevented more than 18.5 million additional hospitalizations and 3.2 million additional deaths. Without vaccination, there would have been nearly 120 million more COVID-19 infections. The vaccination program also saved the roughly U.S. $1.15 trillion in medical costs that would, otherwise, have been incurred.[181] Overall, vaccine effectiveness against COVID-19 was around 84% to 94% in the general population.[182]

Vaccination

Resistance to vaccination is not a new problem, but the COVID-19 pandemic exacerbated it. It should be clear by now that neither persuasion nor coercion is sufficient to change the minds or the behavior of people who are determined to refuse vaccines. Education and research cannot defeat coordinated misinformation. And government efforts—at federal, state, and local levels—are stymied by a combination of inadequate power, insufficient political will, and a lack of perceived legitimacy by vaccine refusers. One of America's core lessons from the COVID-19 pandemic is that a heavy-handed response to vaccine refusal can make things worse.[183]

Finally, I am not my brother's keeper, but I do feel a responsibility to provide the best evidenced information. If then you want to base jump, go big-wave surfing, smoke, take ice, etc., it is my job to advise as to the known risks. One of my older colleagues, when he matriculated from school, went camping with three friends, two boys and a girl, and the four of them contracted polio. He escaped with a withered right arm, but the girl spent the rest of her short life in what was then known as an Iron Lung. She was apparently a very pretty and smart girl,

181 Fitzpatrick, M. C., Moghadas, S. M., Pandey A. & Galvani, A. P. 2022, "Two Years of U.S. COVID-19 Vaccines Have Prevented Millions of Hospitalizations and Deaths," Blog, Commonwealth Fund, 13 December, https://doi.org/10.26099/whsf-fp90.

182 Australian Government Covid-19 Vaccine Information

183 Navin, M. C. & Attwell, K. 2023, "The Anti-Vax Movement Isn't Going Away. We Must Adapt to It", *Time*, 7 September, https://time.com/6311276/antivax-movement-adapt-essay/.

destined to pursue a medical career, but, instead, was cocooned in a metal tube and paralysed from the neck down.

Vaccination could have prevented this.

As I said, he was older, but I grew up seeing people in callipers with withered limbs until ten years later. I got the Salk vaccine and now don't see any cases of polio, unlike one of my colleagues who, while in the Air Force a few years ago, was sent to Pakistan, where the Taliban murdered the nurses administering the anti-polio vaccine drops.

But as the TIME article said, "Education and research cannot defeat coordinated misinformation," and as Dunning and Kruger observed, "the less people know, the more they think they do".

Your call.

Note: I would not get the flu and COVID vaccines together due to some reported side effects. It was and is my policy to always give any and all vaccines separated by an interval, preferably a week so that any side effects can be located to the offending vaccine.

SECTION D

PRIORITIES

CHAPTER 26

Priorities-Preventive Maintenance

"The simplest explanation is preferable to one that is more complex."

– Occam's Razor

The first International Conference on Health Promotion, meeting in Ottawa on November 1986, presented a "Charter for action to achieve *Health for All by the year 2000 and beyond"*.

Each year, if not each month, subsequently, similar wish-list articles are published in some of the best medical journals.

I mean, seriously? Health for all (the world) by 2000?

As detailed elsewhere the UK, the NHS (National Health Scheme) has tried, but after 75years, it would seem in a terminal decline. In reality, while even third world countries can afford tanks, arms and munitions, no government or nation can or will ever provide free health services.

So, *individuals (you and I) will have to do this for ourselves.* You must now look after and assume responsibility for your health.

Preventive Medicine (PM)

Definition: "Approaches and activities aimed at reducing the likelihood that a disease or disorder will affect an individual, interrupting or slowing the progress of the disorder or reducing disability." (The World Health Organization).[184]

There are some more specific characterizations:

- *Primary prevention*, which reduces the likelihood of developing a disease or disorder.
- *Secondary prevention*, which interrupts, prevents or minimizes the progress of a disease or disorder at an early stage.
- *Tertiary prevention*, which halts the progression of damage already done.

The Concept of Preventive Maintenance

Scheduled, routine preventive maintenance for airplanes is well-understood and accepted. It is totally inconceivable to any of us that we would fly in planes that have not been regularly inspected, tuned, serviced, and tested. The wisdom of regular preventive maintenance of our cars is also appreciated. Why is it, then, that we don't extend the same preventive maintenance principles to our own bodies? It very often takes a health scare before we do anything about looking after ourselves properly. In fact, most of us spend more money on regularly servicing our cars and getting regular haircuts or beauty treatments than we do on our own health.

On the other hand, many spend huge amounts of money on trying to be healthy by buying vitamins, supplements, special dietary foods. and gym memberships. These strategies may or

184 WHO Global Forum IV on Chronic Disease Prevention and Control, 2004, *Final Report*, Ottawa, Canada, http://apps.who.int/iris/bitstream/handle/10665/43208/9241593164_eng.pdf.

may not be necessary—or even healthy. In any event, they can possibly be improved given the correct medical evidence rather than a commercial sales pitch.

Waiting until we are ill before we visit the doctor is simply the way it has always been. However, like any machine, different parts of humans wear out at different times; different illnesses affect us at different ages. This new information now allows us to match a patient's age with their age-specific illnesses. And while we may wait until we are sick to visit the doctor, this is rather like waiting for your car to break down before you get it seen to. There is a better way to look after our bodies and optimize our health—preventive medical maintenance—in the same way we look after our cars and planes.

The evidence from the advances in medical research is that regular but *focused, specific medical checks* can nip problems in the bud. This approach gives you the best chance of "curing most known diseases", optimizing our health and increasing our lifespan by up to 15 or more years. The intent is not only to look for illnesses but also to identify risks that can be minimized to help *prevent* them.

You can continue, like most people, to see a doctor only if you have a problem—but that works only after you have done your preventive maintenance. The human body does not remain as we were at 11 years of age. Ignorance is not medical bliss.

The illnesses or causes of death for a 20-year-old male are different from those of a man aged 60. Women have a different set of age-specific illnesses, sometimes nearly the same as for men but sometimes widely different, as the tables show.

In addition to age-specific preventive measures, there are also universal recommendations for optimizing our health and, therefore, our longevity, which apply to all of us at any time in the lifespan. These involve the correct nutrition or diet, the correct exercise and lifestyle. Above all, in my opinion, these should be pleasant and acceptable, not a rigorous, spartan imposition that only a few of us can maintain.

Two Pictures of the Same Model 1928 Rolls Royce

These analogies, equating car maintenance to our own body maintenance, may seem somewhat trite or childish, yet we willingly spend money on maintaining our cars and resent spending money on our health—unless it's some glamorous gym, unproven wellness programs, or a magical vitamins or supplement. Hopefully, this Rolls Royce analogy may motivate you to think along these lines and illustrates the basic principles of preventive health maintenance.

The car in the second picture has been regularly serviced and maintained; the other hasn't. Which one is most like you?

The successfully aged Rolls had the **best fuel and oil** put into it, which equates to the best **nutrition or foods** for a human.

An **engine** which has been regularly tuned and not stressed is the equivalent of us having our **heart** checked.

Clean **headlights** with new bulbs are the equivalent of looking after our **eyes.** Correct loading so the **suspension** has not been stressed is the equivalent of us keeping our **weight** down and not pushing beyond limits, so that we do not overly strain our spine and joints.

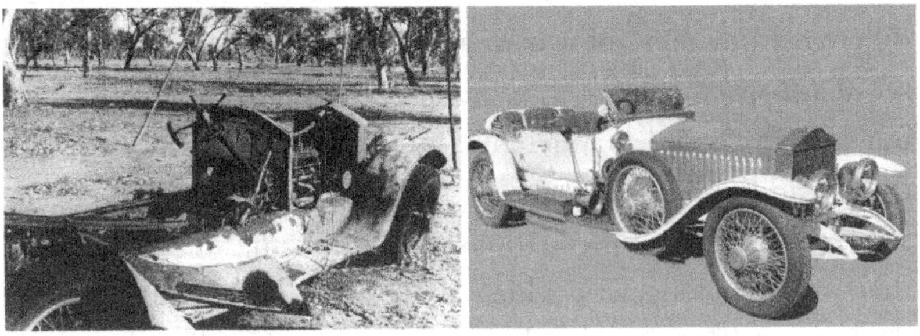

Figure 30: Two pictures of the same model 1928 Rolls Royce. Which one is most like you?

An **electrical system** that has been immaculately maintained is the equivalent of our **nervous system** being kept tuned and not poisoned with toxins such as alcohol and pollutants.

New **spark plugs** make the engine run smoothly—like a **pacemaker** or radiofrequency/freezing ablation for our aging hearts.

No **rust,** no **arthritis**: regular, full range of movements, gentle mobilization. **Tyres,** which are in splendid condition because the **air pressure** has been monitored and kept at the optimum level are equivalent to ensuring our **blood pressure** is checked on a regular basis so that our arteries will also be in good condition. Regular maintenance of the **air filter** and avoidance of airborne pollutants equates to similar care of our **lungs**. Having been kept garaged and out of the sun, the **upholstery** is not faded or cracked, but our **skin** is rarely given the same protection, and most of us have sun- and weather-damaged skin. A working **horn**, because it has not been overused is similar to our **voice** and **ears,** which will benefit from the same treatment.

Preventive maintenance and the early identification and repair of even trivial problems has resulted in this car remaining in great condition throughout its life due to, the principles of which can be transferred to our own care.

Continuing the analogy, the beautifully maintained car has only ever been serviced by qualified Rolls Royce mechanics familiar with the model. They have only used genuine spare parts when repairing the car and have never used additives or made modifications that haven't been proven to work for the car.

Yet, by contrast, we gobble down vitamins and supplements that we should not need and that may even damage us, or we try alternative therapies of unproven worth by unqualified "gurus" and influencers—the equivalent of unproven fuel additives and backyard mechanics. Few of us would treat our cars like that.

Human Applications

Finally, in cars, different systems are checked for each 5000 km or similar thresholds. Not every system is checked each time, and this analogy applies to humans. Since new evidence provides specific information for each decade and sex, a set of specific risks and appropriate tests and investigations can be recommended in place of the generic annual or corporate check-up. Regular, age-specific preventive medical maintenance optimizes and maximizes health, successful aging, and longevity.

The New & Previous Evidence

The objective of this book is dedicated to *not* dying or being disabled *prematurely* by optimizing our health to maximize our longevity and minimizing any illness.

Personal Responsibility

For optimum health, you have to be "health active and responsible". This means accepting responsibility for your own health and not expecting the government or someone else to look after you. It is your responsibility to exercise, eat healthy foods, and find out the known evidence for successful health and aging. It is your responsibility to study the death and disability tables, take specific avoidance actions, and get tested.

The problem, of course, is that processed junk food is cheaper than fresh foods and more convenient. However, as some compensation, people have never been healthier when food was restricted by rationing in the UK in WW2[185] and the

185 Hiltz, M. 2021, "How Wartime Rationing Helped The British Get Healthy", *War History Online*, 22 June.

USA embargo on Cuba in the 1960s.[186] It was not just the better quality of food (less junk) but increased exercise that helped.

Of course, I am not advocating this forced calorie restriction, but growing one's own fruit and vegetables is now a curiosity—even when people have ample back yards. I grow most of our own and make our own pasta, whereas none of my five kids do. They work long and hard, but times and attitudes have also changed.

I cannot change the world economics, but I can point out that an apple is better (far better) than a bought 'health' bar, and it does challenge my, and my colleagues' priorities when people can afford to smoke and do drugs or get tattoos but then complain they don't have money for fresh food.

This does not mean help is not at hand, but it does mean no one else can exercise or eat for you or cut out your high-risk behaviors. You can die prematurely or be disabled 20 years before you should, or you can adopt the world's best-evidenced medical advice. This is not a punitive, spartan, madly disciplined regime but, rather, proven and moderate (gentle) good sense.

The essence is to know what is bad and begin replacing it with what is good, knowing what illnesses are most likely for your age and how to avoid them.

The greatest obstruction to good medical prevention and health care is... you; especially if you are a male. Men don't go to doctors, and guess what? Men die four or more years before women. It used to be seven years. Men aren't improving, though—women are smoking more and indulging in higher risk behaviors.

Most people would prefer to spend their money on a new car, TV, holidays, restaurants, wine, their home, clothes, or

---

186 John, O. 2013, "Study: Economic Crisis Improved Cuba's Health During the devastating downturn of the 1990s, a new report shows, the average Cuban lost 11 pounds and was far less likely to be diagnosed with Diabetes", *Time*, 12 April.

even cigarettes and other drugs, all of which are certainly more pleasant than having a fiber-optic cable threaded up your colon, a finger up your rectum, or your breasts compressed between two steel plates.

And I am one of them! But we can't enjoy any of these things unless we are well!

No one knows how to inspire you to get these tests done (a heart attack is one of the best ways... if you survive). But if you commit to preventive maintenance, it will follow proven, evidenced guidelines for lifestyle improvements to maximize healthy longevity. There is no rebate for servicing or repairing your car or for cosmetic surgery. If you do have to pay for some of these tests for which there is little rebate, and the test results come back clear, then it would seem that this is money not just well spent, but best spent!

Of course, some people do not have the money for even these basic tests, as per the Appendix, but when influencers like Kim Kardashian recommend whole body MRIs costing $2,500, and it's not likely that insurance will pay even part of it[187] and longevity clinics in Singapore offer $100,000 programs, we are in trouble.[188] When only 10 % of these direct-to-consumer (DTC) tests, a few of which cost almost $2000, offer any potential clinical use[189] and the cost of a 6-day 5-MeO-DMT 'journey' at a Mexican retreat is $6995,[190] I am at least providing the evidenced

187 Thompson, D. 2023, "Kim Kardashian Just Got a Whole-Body MRI Scan. Should You?", *U.S. News*, 18 September.

188 Janin, A. 2023, "The Longevity Clinic Will See You Now—for $100,000", *The Wall Street Journal*, 10 July.

189 Shih, P., Ding, P., Carter, S. M. *et al.* 2023, "Direct-to-consumer tests advertised online in Australia and their implications for medical overuse: systematic online review and a typology of clinical utility", *BMJ Open*, Vol. 13, No. 12, https://doi.org/10.1136/bmjopen-2023-074205.

190 Tandava, https://www.tandavaretreats.com

lifestyle and dietary information to live longer, which doesn't cost more.

And the peasants in the Blue Zones, as follows, who allegedly live long are very poor but live inexpensive lifestyles.

CHAPTER 27

Who Live The Longest & What Can We Learn From Them

"I suppose real old age begins when one looks backward rather than forward."

– Mary Sarton

Oldest person ever

The oldest person to ever live was Jeanne Louise Calment (b. 1875, France), who died at the age of 122. She lived a fruitful life, taking up fencing in her 80s and continuing to cycle in her 100s. She claimed that her secret to long life was olive oil, port and chocolate; she quit smoking at the age of 120.

Since the turn of the century, 24 people have held the record for the oldest person (living) but only two have been male.

The Gerontology Research Group validated average old age, as at July 2023, at115 years 176 days.

Individual Longevity Top 100:

- The USA: 50
- Japan: 19
- UK: 8
- France: 6
- Spain: 3
- Italy: 2
- Australia: 1

National Life Expectancy Top 10 Countries:

Table 22: National Life Expectancy Top 10 Countries

	2013	2015	2023
1	Japan	Monaco	Hong Kong
2	Andorra	Japan	Japan
3	Singapore	Singapore	Macao
4	Hong Kong	Macau	Switzerland
5	San Marino	San Marino	Singapore
6	Iceland	Iceland	Italy
7	Italy	Hong Kong	Spain
8	Sweden	Andorra	Australia
9	Australia	Switzerland	Channel Islands
10	Switzerland	Guernsey	Iceland

By 2024, Hong Kong had surrendered its first place to Japan due to COVID-19.

The Paradox

While it can be seen the people in the Blue Zones (see below) live a life of fresh produce, exercise, and no pollution, it is Hong Kong and other heavily populated, crowded places that regularly top the longevity records. As will be seen, the authenticity of the Blue Zones has recently been queried.

People Who Live The Longer:

1. The Rich
2. Intelligence and Genetics
3. The Blue Zones
4. Seventh-Day Adventists of California
5. Individuals
6. Nations

1. The Rich

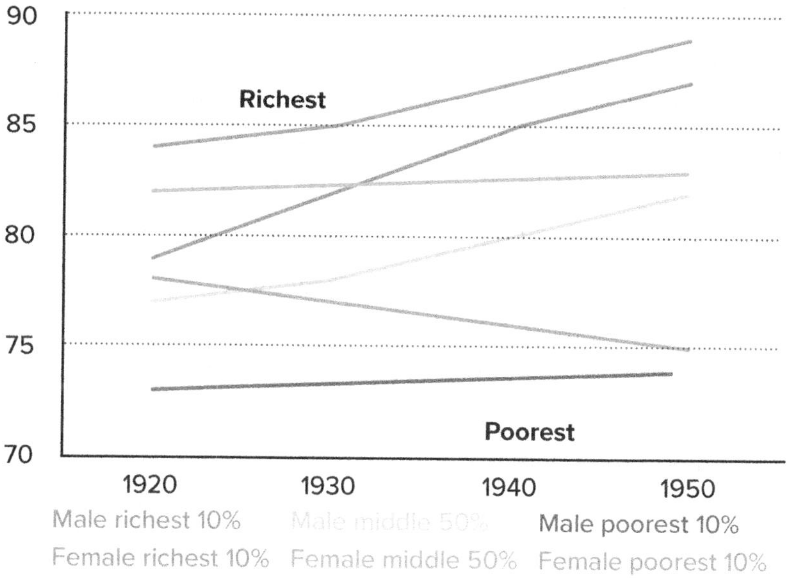

Figure 31: USA life expectancy at age 50 (*Source: Gapminder, 2015*).

The rich live longer than the poor, with an ever-widening dichotomy. Despite significant advances in medicine and technology, the longevity gap between high-income (socioeconomic classes 1 and 2) and low-income groups (socioeconomic groups 4 and 5) has been increasing sharply. In 2016 economists at the Brookings Institution found that the difference in life span after age 50 between the richest and poorest has more than doubled since the 1970s.[191]

In the United Kingdom, between 1930 and 1990, despite the best medical treatments, tests, investigations, medicines, hospitals and operations being offered and supplied *for free* from the late 1940s, the unskilled classes' health has become nearly three times worse than the health of the more affluent professional class. Access to free medical care does not, by itself, help you live longer. You need this new evidence, information and advice.

A 2016 *JAMA (Journal of the American Medical Association)* study provides a comprehensive look at income and life expectancy in the United States.[192] Using federal income tax and Social Security data from 1999 to 2014, researchers estimated mortality rates and calculated period life expectancy based on participants' taxable household income at age 40. Based on 1.4 billion person-years of data, researchers concluded:

Life expectancy increased continuously with household income. The discrepancy in life expectancy increased from 2001 to 2014: people in the top 5% of income increased their life expectancy by as much as 3 years, while the bottom 5% saw little change. Differences in lifespan were most pronounced in comparisons of the extremely wealthy and extremely poor. Compared with the bottom 1% of income distribution, men in the top 1% lived nearly 15 years longer, while women lived 10 years longer—a gap equivalent to the effect of a lifetime of smoking.

191 Burtless, G. 2016, "The growing life-expectancy gap between rich and poor", *The Los Angeles Times*, 22 February.

192 Chetty, R., Stepner, M., Abraham, S. *et al.* 2016, "The Association Between Income and Life Expectancy in the United States, 2001-2014", *JAMA*, Vol. 315, No. 16, pp. 1750-66, https://doi.org/10.1001/jama.2016.4226, erratum in *JAMA*, 2017, Vol. 317, No. 1, p. 90.

Be that as it may recent figures show life expectancy in the USA is falling and this was before Covid.

Americans' life expectancy is at a 20-year low. As a result, the gap in life expectancy between the United States and global peers is progressively growing wider, according to a new report in the *American Journal of Public Health.*[193]

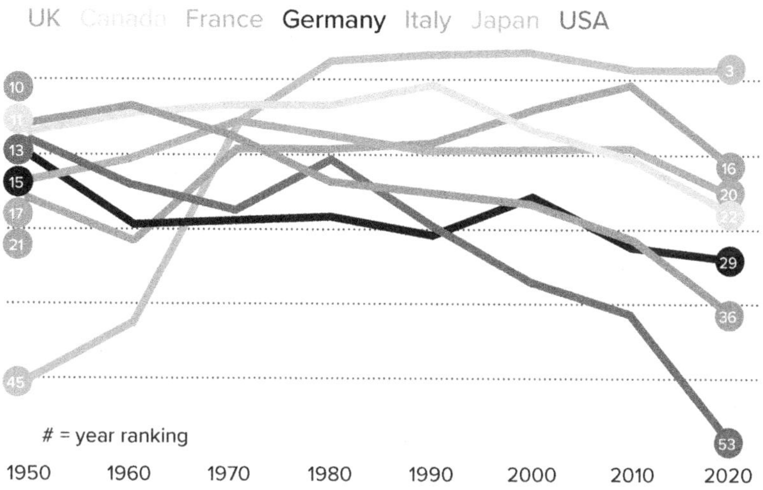

Figure 32: G7's international life expectance rankings (*Source: Satasta.com*).

But as Sally C. Pipes, president, CEO, and Thomas W. Smith fellow in healthcare policy at the Pacific Research Institute points out in her latest book *'False Premise, False Promise: The Disastrous Reality of Medicare for All'*[194] for years, progressives have blamed the lack of universal health coverage in the United States for this disparity. But that blame is misplaced. Americans are dying earlier

193 Ho, J. Y. 2022, "Causes of America's Lagging Life Expectancy: An International Comparative Perspective", *The Journals of Gerontology: Series B*, Vol. 77, Supplement 2, pp. S117-S126, https://doi.org/10.1093/geronb/gbab129.

194 Pipes, S. C. 2020, *False Premise, False Promise: The Disastrous Reality of Medicare for All,* Encounter Books.

because of social and cultural factors, not because of deficiencies in our healthcare system".

In other words, most are preventable.

American life expectancy was 77 years. The average across all high-income countries, by contrast, was more than 82 years.

Why is life expectancy so low in the United States when they spend 18% of gross domestic product on healthcare — about twice as much as the average developed nation? The answers are largely beyond the control of the healthcare system.

Consider car crashes, which took the lives of over 45,000 Americans in 2021 — nearly 14 deaths per 100,000 people. In Germany, by contrast, the motor vehicle death rate was just over three deaths per 100,000 people. Or take gun deaths. In 2019, the rate of firearm mortality was over 10 deaths per 100,000 people in the United States — roughly five times higher than the three next-closest countries: France, Switzerland, and Canada. The U.S. drug overdose death and suicide rates are also the highest in the developed world.[195]

These facts are tragic, but, as Pipe claims, they're by no means an indictment of the health system and she continues that in fact, there's no better place to get sick than the United States. For instance, their cancer death rates are among the lowest in the developed world. America's world-leading health system, Pipes argues, is saving countless lives — not shortening them.

Most of the variation in life expectancies observed across geographic areas was tied to differences in health behaviors, not healthcare access or other factors. Those in the low socioeconomic group suffered medical causes of death such as heart disease and cancer, after exhibiting obesity and behaviors such as higher

195 *CDC National Center for Health Statistics Accidents or Unintentional Injuries*, reviewed 5 November 2023.

rates of smoking and less exercise. These intrinsic causes were more prevalent than external causes, such as car crashes, suicide, homicide or lack of access to health care.

The conclusion is that the low socioeconomic groups do not look after themselves as well as the higher socioeconomic groups. This at least is the United Kingdom experience (see chart below), where free hospitals and medical treatments did not improve their lot, rather it became worse over time.

I have been admonished that, in the USA, "It's not as simple as 'do not'. It's more like 'are at an incredible disadvantage regarding time, money, and health education".

While this, of course, is also true, free treatment and free hospitals, as in the UK, did not see any improvement in the lower socio-economic groups' *health and* that money, at least, and indeed time and health education, when I worked in the UK, were not factors. It is a consummate frustration to most doctors to see how some sections of society seem hard-wired to high-risk behaviors. MY USA admonisher smoked and hinted at past drug and detrimental habits. She did not need time, money or health education to improve her long-term health and live longer.

I have long lost count of the endless nights I spent saving patients' lives, then counselling them about smoking (the main cause of their heart attack), only to see them walk out of hospital and immediately light up a cigarette.

Most, if not all doctors, will have encountered patients who 'can't afford' a treatment but have the latest iPhone, and watch and who smoke. My particular favourite, on whom I operated for free, was covered in whole of body tattoos which he told me had cost him $15,000 "so far".

I simply don't know how to get some people to prioritize their health as being most important which, essentially, is the equation.

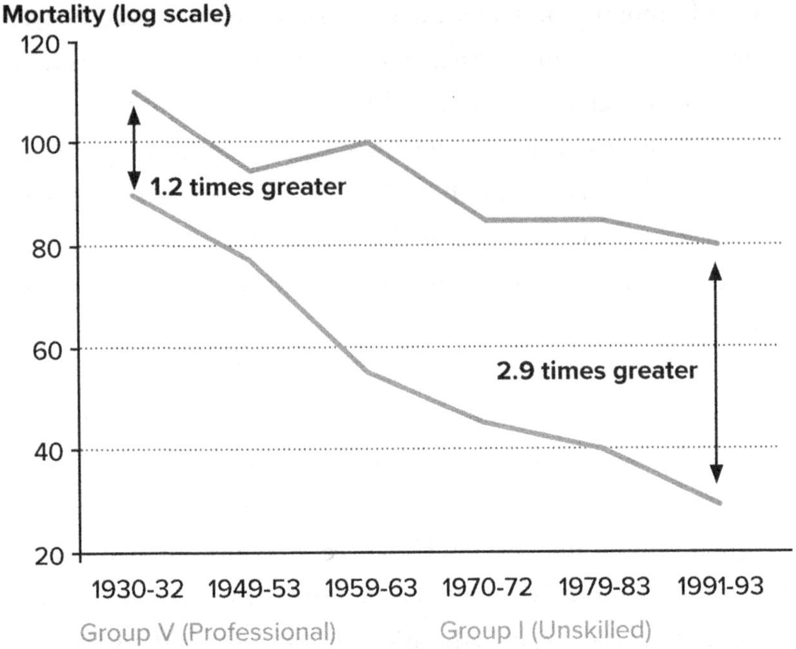

Figure 33: England and Wales mortality gap (*Source: Office for National Statistics*).

So, I totally agree it is not as simple as 'do not' but I would have thought the incredible crushing chest pain, the intubation, the drips, the disorientation, the catheters, the bedpans, the defibrillations, the drugs and the endless attention and care, may have had some salutary effect.

However, the forces assembled to extract your health dollar and disseminate false information as detailed elsewhere are immense, such as the Tobacco and Fast-Food Industries, and their advertising budget far exceeds that of many countries, buys off politicians, seduces and addicts the gullible.

Maybe my admonisher has the answer that has eluded the world's best medical efforts, but my contribution and all I can do is to inform you how to live longer, if that's what you want, based on the world's best trials, studies and evidence. Which is why I wrote this book...but I fully realize the people who need it most won't read it, let alone adopt the proven recommendations – even if they were given it for free.

The Diseases of Affluence

There is, however, a paradox with the development of the 'Diseases of Affluence'.

The rich who live longer do so by eating the best fresh produce and living healthy lifestyles.

This is most obvious if you go to the supermarkets in an affluent suburb and then in a poor suburb. The affluent shoppers are lean and often dressed in their gym gear. Their shopping trolleys are filled with fresh fruit and vegetables with little if any, processed foods. Whereas, in the poor suburb, the shopping trolleys are filled with sugar soft drinks, sodas, cookies, biscuits, cakes, precooked instant meals, sweets, snack bars and junk, junk, junk, and the shoppers are overweight and unkempt.

While we can, to a large extent, mimic the alleged Blue Zone conditions, the affluent West, with its promoted ultra-processed foods, cars, stressful long hours of work, and, paradoxically, increased loneliness, has introduced new illnesses that cause premature deaths.

In the West, cardiovascular disease is our greatest killer, but it is relatively unknown in Japan, as are our next greatest killers, breast, prostate and colon cancer. Even if we try to mimic the Japanese ways with diet and exercise, our Western way of life is so pervasive that we are still struck down with unexpected "Western" illnesses.

The diseases of affluence are mostly chronic non-communicable diseases (NCDs) viz: obesity, type 2 diabetes, asthma, cerebrovascular disease and hypertension, cancer, alcoholism, peripheral vascular disease, gout, some types of allergies, depression and other mental health conditions associated with increased social isolation and now, arguably, Alzheimer's.

Elsewhere, it is pointed out that the fast-food industry has the greatest (detrimental) influence on our health. They are not evil people but profit-driven businesspeople supplying a demand they have created, and because they create so much employment, the politicians won't stand up to them such that even kiddies' prime-time TV is saturated with ads for the latest sweets and junk.

2. Intelligence and Genetics

A study in 2015 analyzed the causes of the link between intelligence and longer lifespan.[196] It noted that many previous studies have found this correlation, but distinguishing the cause of the relationship is difficult. Common causes posited include socioeconomic status affecting intelligence and life expectancy, higher intelligence causing more healthy behavior choices, and shared genetic factors influencing intelligence and health. By analyzing three data sets of twins from the United States, Sweden and Denmark, the researchers determined that genetics contributed the most to the correlation between lifespan and intelligence.

In 1992 (USA), college graduates, on average, lived 2.6 years longer than those without a bachelor's degree. By 2019, the gap had more than doubled to 6.3 years. In 2021, it hit 8.5 years.[197]

Lower education was associated with lifetime CVD risk across adulthood; higher education translated to healthy longevity.

196 Hambrick, D. Z. 2015, "Research Confirms a Link between Intelligence and Life Expectancy", *Scientific American*, 22 December.

197 Case, A. & Deaton, A. 2023, "Accounting for the Widening Mortality Gap between American Adults with and without a BA", BPEA Conference Draft, 28-29 September.

Educational policy initiatives may be associated with long-term health benefits.[198]

3. The Blue Zones

"Blue Zones" are areas of the world that had been identified as where people lived longer – naturally – with more centenarians than elsewhere. This was thought to be due to factors like healthy diets, mostly homegrown and plant-based, exercising, restricted intake-fasting and integrated social support.

These areas were first identified by the demographer Michael Poulain, in 2000, in Sardinia and who then with a Sardinian doctor, Gianni Pes, put blue circles on a map around villages with the greatest number of very old people. Hence the identification as "blue zones".

Later, Dan Buettner, an American writer, expanded the term to areas in Greece, Japan, Costa Rica, and California and gained publicity from his Netflix series, *Live to 100 Secrets of the Blue Zones,* in 2023.

But these claims have recently been called "*a mix of soft science and comical anthropology strangely enduring against much evidence*" in an article in the *Daily Telegraph* (London)[199] by Ambrose Evans-Pritchard, who spent four years as a journalist in Central America and had great trouble believing the Costa Rican segment. He says how the original promotor of the Nicoya Blue Zone, the demographer Luis Rosero-Bixby, now says "new public administer records", in contrast to the earlier days, show that mortality rates are higher than average and that, therefore, the zone no longer qualifies.

---

198 Magnani, J. W., Ning, H., Wilkins, J. T. et al. 2023, "Educational Attainment and Lifetime Risk of Cardiovascular Disease", *JAMA Cardiology*, Vol. 9, No. 1, pp. 45-54, https://doi.org/10.1001/jamacardio.2023.3990.

199 Evans-Pritchard, A. 2024, "How they claimed areas where people live to 100 maybe a scam", *Daily Telegraph,* Wednesday 28 February.

Evans-Pritchard goes on to point out that, according to scientist Dr Saul Newman, now at Oxford University's Leverhulme Centre for Demographic Science, these pockets of extreme longevity seem to occur in areas with "greater poverty, higher illiteracy, higher crime rates, and worse population health" than the norm and "Whenever you get an investigation on the pension system, the rates of centenarians suddenly collapse. This is what happened in Greece after the financial crisis," said Dr Newman. In fact, data from the United Nations even suggests that Cambodia was a Blue Zone of sorts during the genocide of the Khmer Rouge.

The conclusions are that these hotspots can be chiefly explained by *welfare fraud, identity theft, namesaking and criminal abuse of the pension system - or confusion over dates or lack of birth certificates.*

Yet Newman's paper detailing these anomalies remains unpublished and sits on the Open Access roster of preprints visited 200,000 times, never systematically challenged, and unable to reach the publication stage of peer review. "The resistance was massive. I got emails of support, but nobody wanted to put their head above the parapet," he said.

It would seem we are all too willing to be seduced by the 'simple peasant, naturally achieving 100 without spending money or visiting the doctor' rather than engage in actual hard-nosed investigation or debate, as per Newman and made public by Ambrose Evans-Pritchard, who goes on to detail yet further anomalies, not just in the blue zones, but also in London and Ireland.

As Newman also notes, "Whenever you get an investigation on the pension system, the rates of centenarians suddenly collapse. This is what happened in Greece after the financial crisis." The Greek labour ministry concluded that 200,000 pensions were being paid to fraudulent claimants. In most of the countries, 9000 centenarians were dead.

The same thing happened in Japan in 2010 after the mummified corpse of Tokyo's oldest man was discovered. His family had drawn the pension from his bank account for 32 years. The inquiry discovered that 238,000 people listed as aged 100 or more were unaccounted for. Some had died in the Second World War.

Evans-Pritchard says, "The matter needs proper airing. We know what leads to a long life: affluent, good education, good health care, and a low GINI coefficient (indicative of income inequality). Add unsaturated lipids such as olive oil along with fresh greens, fiber, and Omega-3; go easy on red meat and fast-release carbs. *Telegraph* readers know the drill. The blue zones add little and take away much" and how "Buettner told the ZOE program that no superfood or pill will deliver extreme old age. That is true, but nor is there a miracle super zone that will do so either".

(The Zoe Health Study, formerly the COVID Symptom Study, is a health research project of British company Zoe Limited and developed by King's College London; Guy's Hospital; St Thomas' Hospital).

What I also found disturbing from this article is that while Dan Buettner created the Blue Zones LLC (Limited Liability Company), it is now owned by Adventist Health (who are very aggressive evangelists for vegetarianism). The *Telegraph* article, dated 28 February 2024, says that *The New York Times* reports that the enterprise has issued blue zone certificates to 80 towns and localities in the US for $3 million to $40 million each. But I could not locate this.

Be that as it may, I detail where these Blue Zones are and their claims, but I would recommend we keep an open mind and follow developments.

Blue Zones was coined to identify a demographic or geographic area where people live longer and evolved when demographers drew concentric blue circles on a map of villages in Sardinia's Nuoro province with the highest concentration of male centenarians.[200]

Five regions were identified in Buettner's book *The Blue Zones: Lessons for Living Longer from People Who've Lived the Longest*:

1. ***Sardinia***, ***Italy*** (particularly Ogliastra, Barbagia di Ollolai and Barbagia of Seulo): one team of demographers found a hot spot of longevity in mountain villages where an amazing proportion of men reach the age of 100 years. In particular, a village located in the Barbagia of Seulo, holds the record of 20 centenarians from 1996 to 2016, that confirms it is "the place where people live the longest in the world".
2. ***Okinawa***, ***Japan:*** another team examined a group that is among the longest-lived on Earth.
3. ***Loma Linda, California***: Seventh-day Adventists.
4. ***Nicoya Peninsula, Costa Rica:*** Average life expectancy is 85. Staples of the traditional Nicoya diet include homemade corn tortillas, black beans, white rice, a variety of squash, yams, papaya, bananas, and pejibayes. Meat, fish, and poultry only make up 5% of the usual diet. Meanwhile, the average individual from the United States ate 222.2 pounds of meat and poultry in 2018.[201] They also work hard manually.

200 Poulain, M., Pes, G. M., Grasland, C. *et al.* "Identification of a geographic area characterized by extreme longevity in the Sardinia island: the AKEA study", *Experimental Gerontology*, Vol. 39, No. 9, pp. 1423-1429, https://doi.org/10.1016/j.exger.2004.06.016.

201 *Seattle Times*, 2 January 2018.

5. ***Ikaria, Greece:*** has the highest percentage of 90-year-olds on the planet – nearly 1 out of 3 people make it to their 90s. Ikarians have about 20 percent lower rates of cancer, 50 percent lower rates of heart disease and almost no dementia.
6. ***Öland, Sweden:*** southern Småland and northeastern Skåne,
7. ***Acciaroli, Italy:*** one-third of its citizens (~ 300 persons) live at least 80 years.

Some earlier studies had identified **Abkhazia, Caucasia, Vilicanba, Ecuador** and the **Hunza Valley, Pakistan, as places where people also lived longer,** but these have been debunked as there were no reliable records and the elderly were prone to exaggerate their age. Nevertheless, their physical lifestyle, primitive plant-based diet and social integration are similar to the above, and maybe some are living longer.

Intelligence, or rather education, is not necessary in the Blue Zones. These are characterized by a "primitive" fresh produce diet with little meat, hard physical activity and good social integration.

So what is the cause of disparities in longevity, and how can we live as long as the rich? The examples of the Japanese where people live longer, would suggest that money is not the answer. It is their environment, lifestyle, nutrition and activities which optimize the conditions for longevity. But probably, more's the point, it is the bad lifestyles and diets of the Western World that shorten our lives.

Poor Lifestyles Lose Canadians (and therefore the rest of us) Six Years of Life.[202]

---

202 Manuel, D. G., Perez, R., Sanmartin, C. *et al.* 2016, "Measuring Burden of Unhealthy Behaviours Using a Multivariable Predictive Approach: Life Expectancy Lost in Canada Attributable to Smoking, Alcohol, Physical Inactivity, and Diet", *PLOS Medicin*, Vol. 13, No. 8, https://doi.org/10.1371/journal.pmed.1002082.

Smoking, poor diet, physical inactivity, and unhealthy alcohol consumption contribute to about 50% of deaths in Canada and are costing an estimated six years of life.

Research found:

- 26% of all deaths are attributable to smoking.
- 24% of all deaths are attributable to physical inactivity.
- 12% of all deaths are attributable to poor diet.
- 0.4% of all deaths are attributable to unhealthy alcohol consumption.

For men, smoking was the top risk factor, representing a loss of 3.1 years. For women it was lack of physical activity, representing a loss of 3 years.

Canadians who followed recommended healthy behaviors had a life expectancy 17.9 years greater than individuals with the unhealthiest behaviors.

4. Seventh-Day Adventists (of California)

On average Adventist men live 7.3 years longer and Adventist women live 4.4 years longer than other Californians.[203]

Five simple health behaviors promoted by the Seventh-day Adventist Church for more than 100 years (not smoking, eating a plant-based diet, eating nuts several times per week, regular exercise and maintaining normal body weight) increase our life span, and you needn't even be an Adventist.

5. Individuals

It is intriguing that, while the United States overall is poor for longevity, it has by far the greatest number of longest-living individuals of any nation. One can only assume they benefit from

203 Adventist Health Studies, Loma Linda University

access to the world's best and latest medical advice and care... if they can afford it.

6. Nations

As a nation, the Japanese live longest. This is thought to be because of their predominantly fish and seaweed diet. However, the Okinawans, some of allegedly the longest-living people, swear by purple sweet potato, eating up to 0.5kg a day, but recently disputed by Dr Newman (see before).

The Japanese diet—is rich in fish and lightly cooked vegetables, low in fat and served in modest amounts. The advice in the "Okinawa Way" is to stop eating before one feels full.[204] as well as my own observations that pride in one's appearance reflects our internal condition.

While the United States has more long-living individuals than any other nationality, the combined national average for longevity for the general population is in the mid-30s.

Different sources provide slightly different lists, which may account for some differences. It is extremely difficult to draw any conclusions except that Japan, with its traditional diet, and Iceland, with its pristine environment, are always in the top 10. But Hong Kong, Singapore and now Monaco are listed, three of the most densely populated places on earth. San Marino is a mountainous microstate surrounded by Italy, so in effect it is Italian for these purposes. Switzerland is also right up there. We might surmise that stable government provides security and less stress, and should therefore be conducive to longevity, but Hong Kong and Italy don't seem to provide it and make the list anyway.

---

204 Wilcox, B., Wilcox, C. & Suzuki, M. 2001, *The Okinawa Way: How to Reverse Symptoms of Ageing in Four Weeks*, Penguin.

The Hispanic Paradox: Latinos Age at a Slower Rate[205]

According to the Centers for Disease Control and Prevention, Latinos in the United States live an average of three years longer than Caucasians, with a life expectancy of 82 versus 79. At any age, healthy Latino adults face a 30% lower risk of death than other racial groups (two African groups, African-Americans, Caucasians, East Asians, Latinos and indigenous people who are genetically related to Latinos, the *Tsimané* or Chimane (as it is pronounced) of Bolivia), who aged even slower with minimal signs and very little evidence of the chronic diseases that commonly afflict modern society such as heart disease, diabetes, hypertension, obesity or clogged arteries, despite frequent infections.

The research also found that men's blood and brain tissue age faster than women's from the same ethnic groups. The discovery could explain why women have a higher life expectancy than men.

Social Support

Twins, Especially Male Identical Twins, Live Longer. It is thought this reflects the benefits of lifelong *social support.* The lifespan was extended more for identical rather than fraternal twins, which may reflect the strength of the social bond.[206]

Keep Your Friends Closer but Your Family Closer

Older individuals who have more family in their network, as well as older people who are closer with their family, are less

205 Horvath, S., Gurven, M., Levine, M. E. *et al.* 2016, "An epigenetic clock analysis of race/ethnicity, sex, and coronary heart disease", *Genome Biology*, Vol. 17, https://doi.org/10.1186/s13059-016-1030-0.

206 Sharrow, D. J. & Anderson, J. J. 2016, "A Twin Protection Effect? Explaining Twin Survival Advantages with a Two-Process Mortality Model", *PLOS ONE*, Vol. 11, No. 5, https://doi.org/10.1371/journal.pone.0154774.

likely to die;[207] no such associations were observed for number of or closeness to friends. But those who listed more non-spousal family members in their network—irrespective of closeness—had lower odds of death compared to those who listed fewer family members.

Public Health

Even so because of the advances in public health, such as pure water supply and vaccinations as well as the other medical advances in treatment, we are already living longer.

The 2014 Public Health Report from England documents that while life expectancy dropped in 2012 and 2013, it recovered in 2014 to be the highest ever recorded, making the maintenance of good health imperative; yet many are living longer in poor health.

Women aged 60 should expect to live a further 21 years on average. This means they are now likely to spend a quarter of their life in retirement. At 75 they can expect to live another 13 years, at 85 another 7 years and at 95 another 3 years.

Men aged 65 can look forward to another 19 years on average; at 75 another 12 years; at 85, six more years, while at 95 another 3 years.[208]

In 2016, Public Health England (PHE) stated that living healthily in midlife can double a person's chances of staying healthy aged 70 and older, with "simple and small" changes. A $7 million media campaign has been allocated, as the NHS spends more than $22 billion a year treating illnesses caused by the

---

207 Iveniuk, J. & Schumm, L. P. 2016, "Social relationships and mortality in older adulthood", 111th Annual Meeting of the American Sociological Association (ASA), 20-23 August, Seattle, Washington.

208 AIHW Deaths in Australia, web report, last updated 11 July 2023

effects of bad diet, lack of exercise, smoking and alcohol—with the direct cost of obesity and overweight being estimated at $12 billion a year, lack of exercise $1,800 million a year, and alcohol misuse $7 billion. Forty-two percent of midlife adults are living with at least one long-term health condition, which increases their risk of early death and disability.[209]

75 and Out?

Whetted by Dr Emanuel's not altogether curious age-75 deadline (see dedicated chapter), I checked at random to make it superficially statistically valid, the obituaries in *The New York Times* and found that only one person died aged 75! But out of 147 in all, some 110 lived (very well and successfully, according to their obituaries) beyond 75. The most 'popular' age of death, with 12 recorded, was 87, and there were 10 dying at 96 years of age.

In 1950, there were 97 centenarians in Japan; in 2015, there were 61,568, and as of September 2022, 90,500. In Britain, there were 295 centenarians in 1950, 14,450 in 2015, and in 2020, there were *15,384*. The number of Americans aged 100 and over increased from 50,281 in 2000 to 72,197 in 2014 to 89,739 in 2022.[210]

More Good News

And the whole of medicine is rocketing ahead with wonderful advances... if you know how to access them. Even so, the

209 Kirby, J. 2016, "Living healthily in middle age can double your chances of being healthy when you are 70, study finds PHE said evidence shows that living healthily in mid-life can double a person's chances of staying well aged 70 and older", *Independent*, Monday 7 March.

210 Buchholz, K. 2021, "Is 100 the New 80?: Centenarians Are Becoming More Common", *Statistia*, 5 February.

better you look after yourself *now*, any such interventions are minimized, and your recovery maximized. That said, there are, like greying hair, some inescapable imposts of age; but most are fixable. The progress of modern medicine is incredible and can only get better.

Again, to Look on the Bright Side

Many of the old-age imposts are eminently treatable. At 104 years old Edith Varley had a hip replacement;[211] her "terrible pain," according to her daughter, has been relieved and she is now able to walk with a frame. But she was not the oldest such patient; that was Gladys Hooper, 112 years old when she had her operation in 2015 at St Mary's hospital, Newport, UK.[212]

As before, I am not advocating aggressive or unnecessary interventions of the elderly but, as in these cases, if they are fit and such interventions bring a better QOL then they are obviously beneficial and old age need not be an exclusion to treatment.

2023: The Healthy Ageing and Prevention Index[213]

The International Longevity Centre (ILC-UK) is the UK's specialist think tank on the impact of longevity on society, and what happens next. It created a global index that ranked 121 countries against six indicators relating to healthy ageing and prevention: life span, health span, work span, income, environmental performance, and happiness.

211 *BBC News*, 7 March 2016

212 *Daily Mail*, 16 October 2015

213 International Longevity Centre UK, 2023, "Introducing the Healthy Ageing and Prevention Index", 2 May, https://ilcuk.org.uk/introducing-the-healthy-ageing-and-prevention-index-pdf/.

The Index brings together health, wealth and societal metrics in one place for the first time. This allows comparison of how sustainable different countries are, both in terms of longer lives and the extent to which their governments are investing in efforts to prevent ill health and support healthy aging.

The Real Imposts of Age

Silent atrial fibrillation (and other similar heart arrhythmias*)* is a potential epidemic but may be asymptomatic. are potentially fatal but also fairly easily treated. If not treated, the person nearly certainly will have a stroke or slide into heart failure. The person either dies a sudden death, is left a semi-paralyzed cripple or slowly suffocates to death—when it is treatable and preventable! It is now recommended that anyone over 65 should have an annual ECG/EKG, as this test enables the diagnosis.

Prime Minister (UK) Tony Blair was diagnosed in 2003 with supraventricular tachycardia (SVT), a different type of arrhythmia than atrial fibrillation (AF). He was treated with cardioversion and eventually underwent catheter ablation to restore his heart's natural rhythm, which continues to work. Sir Elton John received a pacemaker in 1999. Sir Roger Moore, the 007 actor, received a pacemaker after blacking out on stage in 2003. An overactive thyroid gland (hyperthyroidism) was reportedly the cause of the former president George H.W. Bush's atrial fibrillation episode in 1991. Former Vice President Dick Cheney missed campaign events in 2008 because of AF and his heart rhythm was restored with cardio version—a short electrical shock to the heart. The most common treatment today is a same-day radiofrequency ablation or cryosurgery (freezing) of the heart's short-circuiting malfunction, to restore normal rhythm thus reducing the incidence of crippling or fatal strokes.

Table 23: The top five G20 countries. G-20 comprises the G-8 countries (Canada, France, Germany, Italy, Japan, Russia, the United Kingdom and the United States) plus the European Union (Austria, Belgium, Bulgaria, Croatia, Republic of Cyprus, Czech Republic, Denmark, Estonia, Finland, France, Germany, Greece, Hungary, Ireland, Italy, Latvia, Lithuania, Luxembourg, Malta, Netherlands, Poland, Portugal, Romania, Slovakia, Slovenia, Spain and Sweden), Argentina, Australia, Brazil, China, India, Indonesia, Mexico, Saudi Arabia, South Africa, South Korea and Turkey.

Country	Life span (years)	Health span (years)	Work span (years)	Income GDP/ head ppp ($000s)	Environmental performance 0-100	Happiness 0-10
Australia	83.0	70.9	33.0	52.20	74.9	7.2
Canada	82.2	71.3	32.8	50.66	71.0	7.1
UK	81.4	70.1	31.5	48.51	81.3	7.2
Germany	81.7	70.9	30.6	55.89	77.2	7.0
Japan	84.3	74.1	31.2	42.20	75.1	5.9

Table 24: The countries ranked as the top five in the Index.

Country	Life span (years)	Health span (years)	Work span (years)	Income GDP/ head ppp ($000s)	Environmental performance 0-100	Happiness 0-10
Switzerland	83.4	72.5	34.0	73.11	81.5	7.7
Iceland	82.3	72.0	37.2	60.08	72.3	7.5
Norway	82.6	71.4	32.0	68.35	77.7	7.4
Sweden	82.4	71.9	32.2	55.07	78.7	7.4
Singapore	83.2	73.6	34.0	101.94	58.1	6.4

Increased life years free of disability

A Harvard study (June 2016) found that the increase in life expectancy in the past two decades has been accompanied by an even greater increase in life years free of disability.[214]

214 *The Harvard Gazette*, 7 June 2016

For the typical person, once you reach age 65, you can likely look forward to years of healthy activity and disability-free life. The Harvard study found that in 1992, the life expectancy of the average 65-year-old was 17.5 years, 8.9 of which were free from disability. By 2008, total life expectancy had risen to 18.8 years. In addition to the overall increase, the number of disability-free years increased, from 8.9 to 10.7, while the number of disabled years fell, from 8.6 to 8.1.

Driving those changes are two major treatment areas—cardiovascular health and vision treatment. There has been an incredibly dramatic decline in deaths and disabilities from heart disease and heart failure. Some of it is the result of people smoking less, and better diet, but it is estimated that as much as half of the improvement is because of medical care, especially statin drug treatment, which is both preventing heart attacks and improving people's recovery.

Much of the improvement in vision health can be summed up in a single word—cataracts. In the past, cataract surgery was very lengthy and technically difficult, whereas that same surgery today can be done in an outpatient setting so that complications and disability are significantly ameliorated.

While improved treatment for heart disease and vision problems have significantly added to disability-free life expectancy, some conditions—particularly dementia, neuro-degenerative disorders like Parkinson's disease and chronic-disabling conditions like diabetes—remain a concern.

CHAPTER 28

Patient Types for Best Outcomes

"Common sense is not so common."

– Voltaire

Patient Types and Outcomes

There are a great many studies as to patient types and outcomes, but from the table below, it can be seen that people who are most proactive achieve the best results:

Table 25:

Patient Type	**Response To Illness**	**Clinicians See Them**	**Health Outcome**
Type 1 Passive	Resigned	Unmotivated	Worst
Type 2 Concerned	Obedient	Cooperative but overly dependent	Average
Type 3 Health active, responsible	Involved, intense, self-directed	Motivated and demanding	Best

Socioeconomic Classes-used in medicine/health

Socioeconomic status is a combination of education, income, and occupation. A person may be a slum orphan but a business or scientific genius and so is considered as Class I, whereas some hereditary aristocrat may not be very bright and drops down the scale. One working system is:

- Class I: Professional and higher managerial
- Class II: Intermediate
- Class III: Small employers and own account workers
- Class IV: Supervisors, craft-related, skilled manual workers
- Class V: Working class, unskilled

Insurance Coverage[215]

The type and level of a person's health insurance affects access to screening. One American study reported that only 32.7% of uninsured people were screened for colorectal cancer versus 53.2% of those insured. A survey reported middle-aged English people were healthier than their American cohorts and inferred that access to Britain's free NHS was the reason. There may be a case for only doing colonoscopies on symptomatic patients, but a colonoscopy is a routine test for presidents of the United States and saved President Ronald Reagan's life.

Implementation Difficulties

Proof does not always ensure implementation, as we know from such ostensibly simple, achievable, effective, and evidenced pieces

---

215 Institute of Medicine, 2002, *Care Without Coverage: Too Little, Too Late*, The National Academies Press, Washington, DC, https://doi.org/10.17226/10367.

of preventive medicine as reducing salt below 7g a day in people with hypertension and minimizing sugar intake. The reduction in salt would have a large effect on reducing strokes and heart attacks in predisposed people, as excess salt represents the greatest preventable cause of worsening hypertension. Seventy-five percent of salt comes from processed food. Most of this is in bread and breakfast cereals but reducing it in processed food is unachievable on a large scale because of government reluctance to interfere with big business. After all, wars have been fought and empires lost over salt. Not all salt is bad; the problem is that it's being added to food and people are not really aware how much of it they are eating.

By using a lithium chloride marker to trace the use of salt in cooking and at the table, Sanchez-Castillo et al. (1987a, 1987b) found that only 10% of the salt came from the natural salt content of foods, 15% from salt added during cooking and at the table, and fully 75% from salt added during processing and manufacturing.[216]

Costs

When doctors in the United Kingdom were no longer paid to perform circumcisions, the procedure suddenly became a "mutilation", and any doctors who tried to point out the possible benefits were howled down. I know because I had done research into STDs, and when specializing in Edinburgh, the professor of pediatric surgery was incredibly rude and arrogant (and wrong) when I mildly suggested that circumcision may have some benefits. Some 50 years on, it has been found that circumcision

216 Sanchez-Castillo, C. P., Branch, W. J. & James, W. P. 1987, "A test of the validity of the lithium-marker technique for monitoring dietary sources of salt in man", *Clinical Science*, Vol. 72, No. 1, pp. 87-94, https://doi.org/10.1042/cs0720087.

significantly protects against HIV-AIDS, HBV (cervical cancer), other infections, and even cancer of the prostate. It will soon be "recommended", as it now is in South Africa, and is (and was) cost effective.

Most religious dictates are based on tribal survival, hence the Catholics fish on Fridays which donated iodine to diets preventing cretinism (despite other alleged reasons), the Jews banning pork to avoid *ascaris lumbricoides,* the killer pig worm, and bottom feeding fish which also transmitted diseases. and the Muslims and Jews and Australian Aboriginals who practiced circumcision—a hygiene ritual of desert people where water was in short supply.

Complementary and Alternative Medicine (CAM)

All these impediments to good medicine have opened the door for the entrepreneurs, charlatans, mountebanks, and misguided zealots who seized the preventive health high ground with vitamins, minerals, health foods, and weight clinics as well as the fringe anti-aging medicine of growth hormones, unproven therapeutics, and now the longevity clinics—which could do a good job, but I fear are run for profit and patient indulgence, not medicine.

Western medical graduates were perceived as not providing "holistic" (a Western medicine word) care. Whereas Complementary Alternate Medicine (CAM) promoted so-called "natural" cures. Sixty percent of people now admit to using alternate therapies, but much is a waste of money. Large, international, very well-conducted trials have found that not only do multivitamin and antioxidant supplements not work, but they can also shorten our lives. Vitamins *are necessary* if we are malnourished, and a lot of the elderly are. In these cases, a multi-vitamin does seem to help with preserving cognition, but

I repeat, if you are eating a variety of fresh fruits, vegetables, fish, and a little meat, you don't need them.

It is always tragically amusing to me to see advocates of "natural medicine" taking unnatural vitamins and supplements made in a factory. There are some 83,000 health supplements on sale in the United States. Only 13 vitamins are necessary for our health, and all of these are available from food or our environment (fruit, vegetables, meat, and sunshine) in the correct dose. The National Health Statistics Report reveals that Americans spent up to $34 billion per year on complementary alternative medicine in 2016. I can't find any later figures.

I have an open mind—or try to. After all, aspirin came from the bark of the willow tree and digitalis from the foxglove, while penicillin was a mould on bread, fruit, and even the saddles of the Arabs. These may well be considered 'natural' and 'alternative', but the difference is that they have been subjected to extraction of the pure active substance and then endless animal experiments and trials before the correct dose and side effects were determined and released to the public.

I even learned acupuncture from the London doctor, Felix Mann, who brought it out of China and first introduced it to the West. It works on selected cases and, for some, quite remarkably well. However, CAM is mostly a waste of money, allowing the quacks and charlatans to sell snake oil or its equivalents. Unlike Western medicine, there are no evidenced trials, and of course, the placebo effect is about 60% positive.

I recently listened to a remarkable talk on my car radio. It was a woman writer who had a wonderful, enviable style that captured me and prevented me from changing stations. It came out that she was poor, suffering some illness, and despite her apparent dogged resilience, she bemoaned the fact that she had spent so much, a small fortune, on useless alternative therapies such as paw-paw (papaya) wraps. The announcer came on after the program to identify her and say she died from multiple sclerosis in 2009.

I am suffused with disgust and loathing for these scam artists who so defraud such vulnerable people while seducing them with false hopes. Paw-paw oil is just a meat tenderizer enzyme, papain. It had a big vogue in the 60s for treating slipped discs. The FDA banned it, so Americans flocked like lemmings up to Canada where the scam-doctors made a fortune injecting their spinal discs. The FDA was correct—it doesn't work.

Older Better? Younger Smarter?

When the older generation of medical practitioners studied medicine, it was before antibiotics and "modern medicine" and, hence, mainly based on nutrition, hygiene, and healthy behaviors. While they later saw the advances of modern medicine, they were also able to observe the downsides of some of the new trends that my generation grew up with.

Junk food is one outstanding example. In their day, there was no fast-food—drive-thrus, take-aways, instant meals, home-delivered pizzas, super-sized sodas—which we have come to accept as normal. So, scientists and doctors could compare the "before and after" effects. This more complete overview allowed them a wider choice of optimal health practices. They knew fruit and vegetables supplied essential vitamins, fiber, and micronutrients, and the doctors of that era strongly recommended such a diet. But as Western civilization has progressively offered more processed, ultra-processed, and junk foods, our ingestion of these essential nutrients has been replaced.

The newer factory foods are high in calories but low in essential nutrients, and we now have an epidemic of obesity and the "Diseases of Affluence" such as type 2 Diabetes, hyperlipidaemia, coronary heart disease, cerebrovascular disease, peripheral vascular disease, obesity, hypertension, cancer, alcoholism, gout, and some types of allergy. They may also be considered to include depression and other mental health conditions. asthma, coronary heart disease, cerebrovascular disease, peripheral vascular disease, obesity, hypertension, cancer, alcoholism, and gout. They may also be considered to include depression and other mental health conditions.

Our Western diet has reduced our intake of fiber, but findings indicate that a high intake of dietary fiber is associated with a reduced risk of several types of cancer, including esophageal, gastric, colon, rectal, colorectal adenoma, breast, endometrial, ovarian, renal cell, prostate, and pancreatic cancers.[217]

We cannot process ultra-processed foods.

In the previous era, meat preserving was usually done just with salt, whereas today the shops are full to overflowing with delicious sausages and preserved meats that are full of chemical preservatives, some of which are suspicious for causing colon cancer. We think of sausages, bacon, and ham as "traditional" good foods… but maybe their modern processing is not.

Since WW2, chemicals can be introduced with few restrictions. These additives are only withdrawn after severe or fatal side effects are proven. Meanwhile, there are some 80,000 (now 100,000) chemicals in "approved" daily use—except no one has approved them.

When I Googled this, the report stated: "Of these 100,000 chemicals, the EPA has only taken action to reduce the risk of

217 Hu, J., Wang, J., Li, Y. *et al.* 2023, "Use of Dietary Fibers in Reducing the Risk of Several Cancer Types: An Umbrella Review", *Nutrients*, Vol. 15, No. 11, https://doi.org/10.3390/nu15112545.

over 3,600 chemicals, and it has banned or limited the production or use of only 5. It has not actually regulated a single chemical in the United States since the mid-1980s".[218]

I hasten to say that this is not a trip into the "good old days", as modern medicine has so much more to offer. In fact, one of the most common additives was introduced to prevent food poisoning. Each year, the FDA estimates some 48 million Americans—that's one in every six—become sick from contaminated food, of whom 128,000 are hospital and 3,000 die.[219] Some cases of irritable bowel syndrome can now be traced back to episodes of food poisoning, so the benefits of this additive far outweigh any suspected side effects.

I do think it is time to pause and make sure we have not thrown the baby out with the bath water, to rediscover old wisdoms while selecting the best modern medicine has to offer. The older generation of doctors saw how unprocessed food actually saved peoples' lives.

Sick Army Officers but Healthy Chickens

The story of rice is one where the outer brown layer of rice was taken off ("polished") because white rice appealed more to the consumer. This outer layer contained an essential vitamin, and so people eating white rice suffered a vitamin deficiency, resulting in heart and nerve diseases (beriberi and peripheral neuropathy). This condition was only deduced when chickens suffered these same illnesses when fed white rice left over from a military hospital in the Netherlands but recovered when fed natural,

218 Perro, M. & Adams, V. 2017, "What's Making Our Children Sick?: How Industrial Food Is Causing an Epidemic of Chronic Illness, and What Parents (and Doctors) Can Do About It", Chelsea Green Publishing.

219 FDA, *What You Need to Know about Foodborne Illnesses*

unprocessed brown rice (after some military martinet banned "civilian" chickens from eating the officers' "military" white rice). The missing, and then mysterious, compound was called a "vital amine", which came to be shortened to *vitamin*. Later, it was discovered that the outer layer of rice was rich in this vitamin B1—known as thiamine.

Other vitamin deficiencies were due to impoverished diets, such as in the slums of Glasgow where cod liver oil, rich in vitamin D, "miraculously" prevented rickets in the children whose families couldn't afford good food and who never saw much sun. My father was brought up in this era and saw these actual miracles of vitamins come to light.

Today, such poor diets with vitamin deficiencies should only be found in those who cannot afford good food, in an institution where the food preparation destroys the vitamins, or among some food faddists. These are the only people who would now need vitamin supplements.

My father's generation also knew the importance of personal hygiene. Ebola, MERS, and especially Covid have somewhat woken us up to the importance of personal hygiene and washing our hands—and have alerted us to the dangers of coughing and airborne infections. With the advent of antibiotics, we have become blasé and careless about these fundamental prevention techniques, as well as more advanced and sophisticated ones.

As already mentioned, my father saw all this and what older medicine had to offer but never sat me down to lecture me. Rather, it was bits and pieces of information dropped here and there to alert me. Now what's old is new again, and it amuses me to watch medical documentaries where my father's recommendations have been "rediscovered" as cutting-edge modern medicine. He used to open the windows and drive with the car windows down, even in winter. And with Covid, guess what? Yes, the 'latest' advice is to open the windows! Today, however, atmospheric pollution can be a problem.

"Holistic" is not an alternative medicine word but a legitimate Western medicine word defined as "characterized by the treatment of the whole person, taking into account mental and social factors, rather than just the symptoms of a disease."[220] To me, even this definition does not go far enough. While the whole person is being considered, he or she is still being treated for an illness. Whereas my philosophy, backed by 50 years of clinical experience, would prefer to keep you healthy by preventing illnesses.

Hayes Laws

Some years ago, I jotted down "Hayes' Laws of Medicine"—about how to aspire to be a good doctor. There was no superior knowledge or arrogance in this. I just tabulated what patients have to go through that many doctors are not aware of, as they haven't gone through it themselves. My goal was to, hopefully, make us more aware and prevent them. They are not relevant here, but, as an example, in running the world's first coronary care unit, my registrar and I noted how, when patients woke from their comas, they were totally disoriented and alarmed. The clock might read 12 o'clock—but in this closed unit, was that 12 a.m. or p.m., and where were they? As such, we arranged for 24-hour clocks, and I tried to get patients to windows as soon as possible, where the sun and sound of birds had a marvellously beneficial effect on their morale and recovery.

While excellent doctors may pass on excellent advice, only those who have visited "the other side" can truly offer the best firsthand advice. My long and varied experience also has provided

220 *Cambridge Dictionary, Merriam-Webster Dictionary*

me with the overall balance of covering most of life's foibles, problems and illnesses. I assure you I have not led a low-risk lifestyle. But underlying it all was a protective diet, an awareness of what illnesses were likely and how to avoid or prevent them, and the desire to investigate and find the very best medical treatment when things go awry.

Elsewhere, I have noted the observations on longevity of doctors who are older than 90 but still practicing, and I have to say I detect a great deal of wisdom in their advice, which may seem simplistic… but isn't.

Nor, by any means, am I claiming I stick rigidly to the best possible advice if and when it sets too difficult a standard. Most targets can be modified to acceptable levels with nearly as beneficial results. The Mediterranean diet, which forms the basis for good eating, is pleasant and easy to adopt. Knowing which exercises are best also helps, but since some are an effort, more gentle substitutes are recommended. What lifestyles optimize aging are easy to determine; and what illnesses are most likely for your age should make you keep a weather eye out.

The incredible impost of "information overload" is causing concern that room for this new information has to be made by pushing out earlier wisdoms. What is worse is that there is now a plethora, if not an epidemic, of predatory publications hiding behind legitimate-sounding names and flatteringly inviting academics. These academics, who are often judged by the number of publications in their CV, are duped into supplying an article—and worse is to follow. These articles are not properly scrutinized (peer-reviewed), and when nonsense articles are submitted, they are speedily published, complete with spelling errors.

One scientist fed up with this practice wrote a spoof claiming to have discovered weight-losing ingredients in chocolate. Of course, the media took up this faux revelation and presented it as a scientific breakthrough on talk-fest breakfast shows.

Other health books I've checked are about keeping fit or offering general health advice. While some are good, these fitness/diet titles ignore the fact that all of us are prone to and usually get certain illnesses at certain ages. Theirs is almost a philosophy of denial as if heart attacks and cancers don't exist in their super-fit, super-supplement world. On the other hand, others are "illness" books that concentrate on one illness and advocate strange alternative "cures". They tell you how to recover and beat your Diabetes, heart attack, cancer, or whatever but invariably offer false hopes, based on unproven recommendations, to a frightened and terribly vulnerable group.

The recommendations in this book come from the world's best trials and studies. They are peer reviewed and from the world's top 10 or so recognized medical journals.

Some information is given here which has not been conclusively proven but appears to have some basis in research; for example, cocoa and walnuts having a potential beneficial effect on the lining of our arteries. But now cocoa and chocolate have been found to contain heavy metals, such as lead and cadmium, which the manufacturers knew about! You are urged to be sceptical but keep an open mind about such suggestions. Similarly, I am a great fan and user of Extra Virgin Olive Oil (EVOO), but an article in 2007 in *The New Yorker*, by Tom Mueller alerted me to how much is adulterated. Now, I select mine from authentic sources.

Healthy foods are never labelled "healthy". If a supermarket has a "Healthy" or "Health" food section, what does that make the rest of the foods? The advertising industry assures us this or that breakfast mix is "healthy", and the fast-food industry makes its products delicious and, therefore, preferable to unprocessed, natural foods. Meanwhile, it's just a pity about the high sodium, sugar, and fat content that makes it so delicious (but deadly). And so, the fast-food chains, the vitamin and supplement manufacturers, and so on are pandering to (and exploiting) a demand. They are not the moral or health guardians of society.

In my book *Super-Newtrition*, I list the micronutrient content of an orange, which would blow your mind. From memory, there are some 46 micronutrients. as well as vitamin C. I suggest that these micronutrients adds to our health and welfare, but people go and buy 'pure' vitamin C tablets made in a factory with chemically processed corn or wheat.

CHAPTER 29

The Forces Against You: Who Is Trying to Prevent Your Longevity?

"With such a force arrayed against us, it's time to discuss other options."

– Braveheart 1995

First, the Bad News

There is an almost universal lack of official government programs to address this problem with evidenced prevention. Karelia in Finland, where government intervention reduced the highest rate of heart attacks to the least in Europe, is one of the very few I can find.

So, it can be done, but usually, all that happens are oodles of conferences attended by delegates paid to wring their hands over the fact that the health of society is getting worse or promoting their own bias, as with the Eat-Lancet Commission 2019 Norway

Conference Stockholm, which produced an amazingly beautiful report in several languages that delivered their 'planetary health diet'. It purported to make the world sustainable. But it seemed, to me, a vegetarian's wish-world advocating the culling of cattle and, when analyzed, was found to be methodically flawed, deficient in a number of vitamins, the "destruction of millennial healthy diets".

And, the Italian Minister for Health, Giulia Grillo, called it (the EAT-Lancet 2019 Norway Conference) "science fiction" in a letter to the World Health Organization (WHO). She expressed her concerns about the impact of the EAT-Lancet recommendations on people's health and livelihoods, especially in the Mediterranean region. She also questioned the scientific evidence and the conflicts of interest behind the EAT-Lancet initiative.[221]

The frightening scenario that we all see is society succumbing to the diseases of affluence to follow this inexorable, predictable sequence: Affluence—greater leisure—affordable junk food—obesity—arthritis/back pain—increasing sedentary behavior—Diabetes 2—heart disease—atrial fibrillation—depression—Alzheimer's… all of which the drug companies and the health scammers are only too eager to exploit. The costs are absolutely incredible… as are the profits to Big Pharma.

"Health" has now become big business and is referred to as a "product". Patients are now "consumers or clients". It is predicted to be the next trillion-dollar industry—if it's not already. As such, there is enormous competition for the health dollar, *your dollar,* from the following health-interested parties:

221 Torjesen, I. 2019, "WHO pulls support from initiative promoting global move to plant based foods", *BMJ*, 9 April, https://doi.org/10.1136/bmj.l1700.

Who wants your health dollar?

In order…

1. Governments
2. Insurers
3. Hospitals
4. Drug Companies/Big Pharma
5. Food Industry
6. Tobacco Industry
7. Media
8. Doctors
9. Allied Health Professionals
10. Health Workers
11. Patients (now "consumers")
12. Complementary and Alternative Medicine (CAM) and Longevity Mail-Order Tests and Supplements
13. Lifestyle/Longevity Clinics. Pop-up Labs
14. Businesses
15. Supply and Service Companies

I apologise, but I can't find my reference(s) for this list. I researched it well over a decade ago, but it still looks reasonable to me.

Of these, somewhat remarkably and surprisingly, the fast-food industry, with a US turnover in the trillions of dollars—bigger than the GDP of most countries—has arguably the most direct influence on our health.

The fast-food industry cannot be blamed entirely for the obesity pandemic and its sequela of metabolic syndrome, but given that our food has changed more in the last 60 years than in the previous 60,000, it must certainly be considered a prime suspect.

We now live in a toxic food environment where some 4,000 to 6,000 calories a day are produced for every man, woman, and child—when we need less than 2,000.

It is a somewhat frightening realization that the patient and the doctor have practically the least say in how we are being manipulated by most of the above.

It has been said that "society progresses on the backs of middle-class morality." Now, it is sustained by the taxes of those paying for this epidemic of diabetic drugs, blood glucose testers, arthritis pills, cardiovascular disease medications, statins, PPIs, hospitalizations, heart tests, anticoagulants, pacemakers, antidepressants, and the expenses of caregivers and nursing homes. Meanwhile, the hospital doors, examination/operating tables, and airplane seats have to be widened and reinforced.

Many of the patients I see are on 10 different drugs when, arguably, if they were lean and ate correctly, they may not need any!

If you think I am being severe, please see what American cardiologist John Mandrola said in "Heart Disease and Lifestyle: Why Are Doctors in Denial?":[222]

> "I know that exercise, diet, sleep, and finding balance in life are the key components of success. It is the same in cardiology… but… Bulging waistlines, thick necks, sagging muscles, and waddling gaits have begun to look like normal. I rarely click on "normal" (for the) physical exam. The general appearance is abnormal—either overweight or obese. New anticoagulant drugs are easy. Ablation technology is easy. Statins are even easier. The truth—nutrition, exercise, and balance in life—is hard".

222 Mandrola, J. 2015, "Heart Disease and Lifestyle: Why Are Doctors in Denial?", *Medscape*, 12 January.

Where the Health Budgets Go

If the health systems stay the same, the aging population will increase the health expenditure on this age group to a third of the total. Even now, a 75-year-old costs some $500 more each year than a 70-year-old.

The problem is multifactorial, with each "factor" pursuing their own ends and, to a degree, vested interests. In my observation, this has led to an explosion in hospitals as the main cause of health cost blowouts. Politicians love them, as they are often claiming them as monuments to their tenure and dubious achievements. Specialists love them, as it gives legitimacy to procedures such as expensive joint replacements in the very old: the surgeon earns money, the hospital earns money, the surgical supply company earns money, the hospital nurses, wardsmen, clerks, engineers, gardeners, and laundry staff all get paid from these operations and procedures.

Then there are the end-of-life chemotherapies, which are not necessary, or even contra-indicated, and the politician, where the governments subsidize health care and hospitals, bathes in the reflected glory, claiming to have delivered health to his or her constituency.

As pointed out in the 2015 report on the inquiry into skin cancer in Australia,[223] "early treatment following early diagnosis can reduce the cost of treatment from $3000 in a public hospital to $300 in a skin cancer clinic." In other words, a private skin clinic is 10 times more cost-efficient.

By my estimate (eight years ago), just to be admitted overnight and sit on a hospital bed without anything being done

223 House of Representatives Standing Committee on Health, 2015, *Skin Cancer in Australia: Our National Cancer,* tabled in Australian Parliament on 24 March.

costs between $1000 and $4000. It has been said that "the most expensive bed in the world is a hospital bed".[224]

While there are obviously certain procedures that can only be done in hospitals, the exploitation or misuse of GPs and primary care doctors worldwide, combined with the increase in medical litigation, has resulted in doctors simply sloughing many problems, no matter how minor, to the hospitals, whose legal bills are simply incredible. I know because the lawyer for one very big teaching hospital is a patient of mine, and a recent news article says the same about NHS hospitals in the UK. The result is a desperate world-wide shortage of GP/primary care doctors.

The blowout in medical litigation has forced defensive medical practices such as ordering a CT scan for a headache just to placate a patient. It has become so ridiculous that any disturbed person can make a frivolous and mischievous complaint about a doctor who then has to spend inordinate stressful time defending him or herself while the complainant is not penalized if found to be frivolous.

One excellent doctor I know had a complaint because a patient demanded he do an operation then and there. While this complaint was eventually thrown out, the stress was such that my colleague had a heart attack and retired from medicine.

The worldwide denigration and exploitation of primary care has simply resulted in passive resistance by GPs and the resultant unchecked expansion of unchecked hospital costs.

Meanwhile, back at primary care, where most people go to get health advice, there would seem from my reading the news and journals from the USA and UK, to be the worst predicaments now with the doctors having to see as many patients as possible in a day with insurers and governments paying more for six minutes than for any other schedule.

224 Alleged, but false, deathbed statement by Steve Jobs.

This is also why preventive medicine is not practiced, let alone pursued and updated, as are all other advances in medicine.

Hitting the Targets but Missing the Point

All is not well in the hospitals either: Two of our most vital industries, health care and education, have become increasingly subjected to metrics and measurements. Of course, we need to hold professionals accountable. But the focus on numbers has gone too far. We're hitting the targets but missing the point.

A study found that the electronic health record (EHR) (An electronic health record is the systematized collection of patient health information in a digital format. These records can be shared across different health care settings.) enforces the centrality of market principles in clinical medicine, redefining the clinician's role to be less of a medical expert and more of an administrative bureaucrat and transforming the patient into a digital entity with standardized conditions, treatments, and goals, without a personal narrative.[225]

Another 2013 study found that emergency room doctors clicked a mouse 4,000 times during a 10-hour shift.[226] The computer systems have become the dark force behind quality measures. In medicine, doctors no longer made eye contact with patients as they clicked away. Thoughtful and limited assessment can be effective in motivating improvements and innovations, but we need to tone down the fervor and think harder about the

---

225 Hunt, L. M., Bell, H. S., Baker, A. M. & Howard, H. A. 2017, "Electronic Health Records and the Disappearing Patient", *Medical Anthropology Quarterly*, Vol. 31, No. 3, pp. 403-421, https://doi.org/10.1111/maq.12375.

226 Hill, R. G. Jr, Sears, L. M. & Melanson, S. W. 2013, "4000 clicks: a productivity analysis of electronic medical records in a community hospital ED", *The American Journal of Emergency Medicine*, Vol. 31, No. 11, pp. 1591-1594, https://doi.org/10.1016/j.ajem.2013.06.028.

unanticipated consequences. We must appreciate the burden that measurement places on professionals to minimize it.

How, Then, to Get the Correct Care to the People Who Want It?

The above is only to alert you to the running interference, health budgets, competition for your health dollar, and problems which make accessing the best medical treatment, advice, and information progressively difficult. At the very top level, the system works brilliantly. We have never had it so good—MRIs, organ transplants, artificial limbs, artificial aortas, cochlear implants, heart valves replaced, and normal rhythm restored "while you wait".

Meanwhile, preventive medicine has languished and never realized its potential; and given this interference, it most likely never will. So, "What can a poor fella do?"

The following is ruthlessly honest, without the hype of fads. It provides the latest independent evidence, proven by the best-referenced trials. These trials have a huge sample of people (some over 100,000) and cover many years; and the results are blinded and interpreted by independent persons.

Bottom of the Cliff "Salvage" Medicine

Doctors Only Attend the Ill

Historically, medical practitioners were only sought if and when people were ill. Thus, health schemes, whether introduced by governments or insurance companies, were based on remunerating the doctor for treating these recognized illnesses. Doctors were not reimbursed for preventing illnesses and, thus. moved into areas of medicine where they could see immediate results and would get paid. Not only has prevention languished but doctors have become de-skilled in this area.

Because clinicians can only treat individuals after illnesses are established, they simply do not practice prevention or evidenced good health advice. This has created a vacuum and allowed the zealots, charlatans, beauty therapists, athletes, influencers, loonies, and gym, health food, and vitamin industries to swoop in and "round up the usual suspects"—the people, like you, desperate to be healthy while largely being given wrong and mostly exploitive, advice.

Prevention has not progressed because people only go to doctors when they are sick—which had accurately been identified as "Bottom of the Cliff Medicine" nearly 130 years ago in a poem by Joseph Malins.

"The Ambulance Down In The Valley"
by Joseph Malins, 1895

'Twas a dangerous cliff, as they freely confessed,
Though to walk near its crest was so pleasant;
But over its terrible edge there had slipped
A duke, and full many a peasant;
So the people said something would have to be done,
But their projects did not at all tally.
Some said: "Put a fence around the edge of the cliff";
Some, "An ambulance down in the valley."

[Final verse of seven]

Better guide well the young than reclaim them when old,
For the voice of true wisdom is calling;
To rescue the fallen is good, but 'tis best
To prevent other people from falling;
Better close up the source of temptation and crime
Than deliver from dungeon or galley;
Better put a strong fence 'round the top of the cliff,
Than an ambulance down in the valley.

And while it is pure Victorian melodrama, Malins was ahead of his time. In fact, he was 129 years ahead of his time, as prevention has never realized its promise or potential, until now—but only if you want it.

Healthcare is episodic, but health itself is continuous. Health is what happens between doctor visits.

Few doctors specialize in prevention, especially at a clinical level; and so there has been no apparent interest in an overview to "put it all together". Rather than Bottom of the Cliff Medicine, this Live Longer System is analogous to putting up a roadblock and warning lights to stop you from plummeting over the cliff—and what is more, constructing a new, alternate route. Stay on the new Super-Highway to Health and don't plummet over the cliff where, at best, all we can do is pick up and put on a patch. Don't get ill; prevent it by predicting what is most likely to afflict you and taking evidenced steps to avoid it. *Get it seen; Get it diagnosed; Get it fixed.*

Medicine has become progressively diverse and specialized. There are two main groups: one is the clinicians who see, diagnose, and treat patients; the other is the non-clinicians, who range from those who actively support clinicians (such as radiologists and pathologists, who occasionally see patients) to those who have abandoned any contact with patients to become researchers (such as epidemiologists). This division has led, in my observation and experience, to an unbalanced dichotomy.

The clinician is weighed down by the urgent and inescapable demands of patients and is time-poor, while the non-clinician has to "publish or perish"—get articles into journals—to get funding or a better job. The clinician has no time to read this tsunami of (often) dubious articles, while the non-clinician and their camp followers of non-medical graduates are busy creating this tsunami. The result is that many, if not most, clinicians don't access the rare gems hidden in this tsunami. So, the clinicians continue seeing patients, and while they keep up with clinical advances, they don't read much epidemiology or statistics, let alone prevention articles.

To confirm my observations, as noted before, I asked some colleagues what illnesses they were personally most likely to suffer or die from. My colleagues ranged in age from their 20s to 80s, both sexes, and most practising specialties and primary care fields… and none of them knew (except some over 50 who did correctly pick heart disease, but thereafter didn't know). I can't see my colleagues finding the time to source and read all this data, and the medical schools don't teach it, so I have redirected my efforts to you, the motivated individual.

While "prevention" has been my passion, it does not rate a mention when I am asked to confirm my specialty for international surveys whose lists go from "A": Aviation Medicine, to "V": Vascular Surgery. They offer no Prevention in the "P" section. So, it would seem that clinicians with an interest in prevention are thin on the ground. However, as a specialist physician/internist, I have researched, thought, mulled over, and studied being healthy and preventing illnesses for 50 years, and even longer if I count listening to the observations of my father—try 100 years. And while I went on to work in some of the most advanced, high-powered medical units in the world, these overall, holistic observations were not lost to me. I have been able to scan across the widest field of medicine and provide an evidenced health plan that maximizes our chances of living longer and healthier—past 75.

SECTION E

ARE WE LIVING TOO LONG?

CHAPTER 30

Are We Living Too Long? Do You Want to Live Longer?

"All would live long, but none would be old."

– Benjamin Franklin (1706-1790)

The Approach to Life, Quality of Life, & Living Forever

The world's billionaires and super-rich are funding research into living longer—try $44 Billion in 2020, rising to $66 Billion by 2026. According to an analysis conducted by Bank of America, the longevity industry is already worth $110 billion, and with the caveat of including "future food" and other non-longevity-focused themes, the same analysis projects the industry to grow to $600 billion by 2025.

But what works?

Innumerable companies such as Amway, Solgar, GNC Holdings, and Herbalife all offer products containing, they claim, key longevity molecules. Health shops proliferate, selling supplements that do not have to prove they are beneficial, let alone work, and many are adulterated.

But now, these supplements are not only for the super-rich, as living longer has become the red-hot, new objective of celebrities, their aspirants, and wannabees. Most are full of hope and fantasy.

That is not to say that the super-funded research is not staffed by excellent researchers—it is, but there have been little if any, breakthroughs so far.

Again, what, if anything, works?

Stopping, let alone reversing and extending, aging is obviously terribly complex—try reversing the 200,000 years of human evolution and the six million years before that of our ancestors and the billions of years before that developing a unicellular binary microbe, which could only hit and reverse, into the human brain. These pathways are incredibly complex… from that to 100 billion neurones, 3,313 different brain cells and trillions of connections.[227]

Good luck, guys. But they hope, and there seems to be evidence that in this incredibly slow and complex evolution, there may be a common genetic path shared by most if not all, animals. If so, this may well be manipulated, modified, and controlled.

The history of longevity is littered with the prematurely demised corpses of their protagonists and gurus. And is it worth all the time, money, risks, and incredibly disciplined lifestyles some of these supplicants devote themselves to in the promised, but not proven, hope of a carefree, increased lifespan—if not immortality?

Those already embarking on unproven regimes are convinced they will see them retain their youth, such as Tony Pemberton,

227 Weninger, A. & Arlotta, P. 2023, "A family portrait of human brain cells", *Science,* Vol. 382, No. 6667, pp. 168-169, https://doi.org/10.1126/science.adk4857.

who takes an astounding 25 different supplements a day. Don't forget middle-aged tech centimillionaire Bryan Johnson, who spends $2 million a year, fasting for 23 hours a day with his team of 30 doctors who say they have a plan to reboot his body. While others want to prolong their lives and live at least 120 years, some aspire to longer than that. Some are even freezing their corpses in hopes of a revival.

There is nothing very new here. In the 1960s, Roy Walford, a professor of pathology and medical researcher in California, is credited with significantly furthering aging research, first done in the 30s. Laboratory mice, when fed a diet that restricted their caloric intake by 50% yet maintained nutritional requirements, almost doubled their expected life span, so he wrote a series of books. One was titled *The 120 Year Diet.* He then wrote *Beyond the 120 Year Diet* and chronically underfed himself.

Sadly, he died aged 79 from amyotrophic lateral sclerosis (ALS), commonly known as Lou Gehrig's disease.

So, Walford fell some 40 years short of his 120-year ambition. In photos of him, he looked skeletal, like a survivor of Belsen or Changi POW camps. He was also the doctor for the biosphere, where, according to reports, it wasn't much different, and so I wonder if Roy's incredible discipline and miserable dietary restriction were worth it.

By contrast, a dear friend, George Melly, who, from 1965 to 1973, was the film and television critic for The London Observer, a lecturer, author on art, jazz singer, and a writer (he even wrote a profile about me in a famous English magazine) died a year older than Walford and, according to his obituary in a major UK Newspaper, "nailed the art of growing old disgracefully with style." George was an inveterate smoker and died of lung cancer, refusing all treatment. He was also, as he told me, a "hedonistic anarchist", which I then thought was an exaggeration... but, indeed, he was.

George, believe me, lived life to the fullest, and the question I now pose is: Which life would you have preferred: Roy's or George's?

The incredible regimes of others who want to live longer, such as Johnson and Pemberton, are detailed later, but most are in their 40s and 50s. Well, good luck to them! I couldn't perform 200 push-ups every morning as some do, even when I was playing first-class rugby, or swim 20-mile events (even when I was selected for an Olympic Squad), let alone eat a very dull diet and have blood samples taken every day. I hasten to add I was really a rugby 'tragic', and it was at school that the Olympic coach spotted me when I fluked a win.

I am a foodie. I have owned a restaurant and visited, reviewed, and written about "the Best Restaurants in the World." My wife is a fantastic cook, and I don't really like my veins punctured daily (once a year will do). All of this should have seen me bite the dust some years ago, but here I am, aged 83, still working and operating in my medical practice up to 10 hours a day with a 250km drive.

So, what worked for me, and what can work for you?

Quality of Life (QOL): Are You Havin' Any Fun?

QOL is a relatively new concept, and there is a lack of agreement of what it means, with over a hundred definitions. As society becomes more complex, so do expectations, and hence the criteria change. It is important to consider the broader concerns of the individual. This is a changing concept that takes into account the general well-being of individuals and societies, outlining negative and positive features of life and observing life satisfaction, including physical health, family, education, employment, wealth, religious beliefs, finance, and environment.

This would clearly be where to start. In other words, what makes us happy?

Many studies, even equations, attempt to determine what constitutes happiness, but in essence, life is a compromise between what we wish for and what we can reasonably attain.

It is proposed we should strive to live longer, healthier, and happier as well.

The incredible discipline and lifestyles of Roy Walford, Bryan Johnson, *et al.* may well have made them happy, but that wouldn't work for most of us.

The most sensible and evidence-based approach for most of us to improve our long-term health to maximize our longevity and happiness is to incorporate proven modifications that we find acceptable that can be gradually incorporated into our present lifestyles.

Therefore, the first thing to do is go away and decide what you want out of life—and what you can realistically achieve. Not all of us can win an Olympic gold medal or the Nobel Prize, but what would you do if you were told you had only a year to live… stay back at the office?

On that note a Palliative Carer asked her patients their Top Five Regrets of the Dying and wrote a book with this title.[228] Her list is:

1. I wish I'd had the courage to live a life true to myself, not the life others expected of me.
2. I wish I hadn't worked so hard.
3. I wish I'd had the courage to express my feelings.
4. I wish I had stayed in touch with my friends.
5. I wish that I had let myself be happier.

---

228 Ware, B. 2019, *The Top Five Regrets of the Dying: A Life Transformed by the Dearly Departing*, Hay House.

Be Careful What You Wish for

In 1948, The creation of the UK's National Health Service (NHS) was described, (by its instigator, Aneurin "Nye" Bevan) as "the most civilised step any country has ever taken" and was regarded as the envy of the world.[229]

75 years later, it is in shambles. Patients have seen cancer survival rates drop below the European average for nine out of 10 cancers, record waiting lists of 7.4 million people, and average waiting times for treatment that can be 16 times as long as in countries like France.[230]

When the NHS was formed, average life expectancy was 69. By 2021, it was 81. No one anticipated the effect of longer life expectancy developing complex, age-related conditions or the expensive advances in medical technology. In 1948, the old-age dependency ratio—the population over 65, relative to the working age population—was 16.5%. By 2021, it was 28%, which means Britain's pensioners are being supported by what is an ever-shrinking taxpayer base.

Along with the aging population, the obesity crisis was never foreseen in 1948, and the free safety net that the NHS provided may even have helped create it. In 1975, just 10% of adults were clinically obese. Today, more than 31% of adults are clinically obese (a staggering 64% of adults are overweight, meaning they have a BMI of 25 or over).[231]

---

229 This statement was distributed to UK households as a leaflet in May 1948, as part of a public information campaign to introduce the new National Health Service.

230 Donnelly, L. 2023, "Nine in 10 cancer survival rates worse than in Europe", *The Telegraph,* 17 January 2023.

231 NCD Risk Factor Collaboration (NCD-RisC), 2017, "Worldwide trends in body-mass index, underweight, overweight, and obesity from 1975 to 2016: a pooled analysis of 2416 population-based measurement studies in 128·9 million children, adolescents, and adults", *Lancet,* Vol. 390, No. 10113, pp. 2627-2642, https://doi.org/10.1016/S0140-6736(17)321293.

It would seem unsustainable in its present form—as, indeed, would any free health system be if we are to live much longer. The elephant in the room question no one dares ask is: "Are we living too long?"

Moral and ethical questions arise: Are longevity and health only for those who can afford it? Should we continue developing vaccines and cures, as with malaria, that will see populations increase far beyond the ability to afford even basic health care, with the real possibility that the health and longevity of far more of that population will be compromised and degraded?

COVID reminded us that nature has its way of controlling things, and, as with this example of the NHS, there are downstream complications to what is obviously ethically desrable.

Don't get too depressed: The virus wants to live, too, so it will only kill enough of us until it mutates. While it will still invade us in cycles, like the flu, it will no longer kill us—until the next new virus evolves.

Be that as it may, the pursuit for 'eternal youth' proceeds unabated with some six or so new drugs, specifically formulated for delaying aging, beginning human trials in 2024. It is reckoned that the first longevity pill is only a decade away.

Who will take it?

A Time to Think

There is a firm in Arizona that will freeze your body—or just your head—in the prospect that it can be thawed and successfully rejuvenated sometime in the future. This has led even the most enthusiastic longevity seekers, while dubious as to the success, to question what it would be like to wake up, say, in 20, 50, or 100 years—with no friends, no one you'd know, no familiarity or concept of new technology.

While that is a far-fetched scenario, how long do you seriously want to live?

The suggested optimal span is the time you can live without any major illness(es), impediments, or handicaps while being financially secure, socially mobile, happy, enjoying life, and having fun. Of course, our goals and aspirations may have to be tweaked and attenuated, but if you are secure, well, and happy, these aspirations would seem the age limit.

No one yet can predict this age for you, but it may be time to think about it. There may well be pills that prolong life, but do you seriously want to live much beyond 100? Whereas 85 would seem to be the obtainable age at present, and anything beyond that is a bonus.

As noted earlier, the Norwegian survey of 2023 found that 91 was the number of years most people wanted to live if they were healthy and had a good quality of life. Even the 'Say Forever' Immortalists couldn't convince people worldwide to want to live past 122 years (the present record).

CHAPTER 31

"Why I Hope to Die at 75." Doctors Disagree

"All the world is queer save thee and me, and even thou art a little queer."

– Robert Owen(1771-1858)

In October 2014, Dr. Ezekiel Emanuel, one of the chief architects of US President Obama's Affordable Care Act, unleashed controversy after he published an article in the respected *Atlantic* magazine entitled, "Why I hope to die at 75."[232] He wrote about the problems of aging beyond 75, including a sharp drop-off in creativity, functional declines, reduced mental capacity, and burdens placed on family members. He wrote that while death is a loss, "living too long is also a loss," and concluded, "Seventy-five. That's all I want to live."

His comments triggered an outpouring of mostly anger at the *Atlantic* website, where over 4000 responses were posted.

232 Emanuel, E. J. 2014, "Explore Why I Hope To Die at 75. An argument that society and families—and you—will be better off if nature takes its course swiftly and promptly", *Atlantic magazine*, Ootober.

Many echoed Archer R. Gravely, who wrote, inter alia, "I certainly have no desire to 'live' at an advanced age in a nursing home, but I know a number of 80+ folks who have a pretty good time going fishing and shooting at the range."

Emanuel said that once he is 75, he will not actively end his life, but he won't try to prolong it, either. He said that the default position of doctors is "almost invariably" to order tests and treatments. But Emanuel prefers to "flip… this default on its head," writing that he takes guidance from William Osler, who wrote in his textbook, *The Principles and Practice of Medicine*: "Pneumonia may well be called the friend of the aged" and that by dying of "an acute, short, not often painful illness, the old man escapes those 'cold gradations of decay' so distressing to himself and to his friends."

Emanuel, a bioethicist and oncologist (cancer specialist), described his "Osler-inspired philosophy" by saying that at 75 and beyond, he will "stop getting any regular preventive tests, screenings or interventions. I will accept only palliative—not curative—treatments if I am suffering pain or other disability."

I, too, have devoured Sir William Osler's principles and put them into practice. Osler died in 1919 and didn't have antibiotics, which would have cured his patients' "friend" pneumonia, and you simply can't tell me Osler would have withheld this treatment had he had it. Further, I simply can't agree that Osler would withhold other curative treatments to those mentally intact and otherwise physically able. I must say that I find Emanuel's reported assertion that he will not accept "curative treatments" rather odd. Run that past me again.

I have diagnosed and excised otherwise fatal cancers in over-75-year-old patients who are now cured, living, and functioning well more than 10 years later. If one of these were Dr. Emanuel, is he saying he would not want me to excise the cancer but would prefer to let it go on to metastasize to his liver and brain, leading him to die a horrible death?

Would he want me to endure incredible pain and lose the use of my legs while only taking palliation in the form of soporific, addictive pain killers, when an elegant operation would prove curative, restoring full, pain-free function?

75 and Still Going Strong

By unfortunate coincidence or serendipity, when I started the formal writing of this book in 2015 (though the actual research goes back over 50 years), I wrote how I was "rapidly approaching my 75th birthday, still find my wife disturbingly attractive, and work 10 hours a day, by choice, in my busy solo medical clinic doing quite delicate facial operations. I am in good health with normal blood pressure and cholesterol, take no medication (except an occasional paracetamol/acetaminophen for a hangover), have just completed two internationally commended medical textbooks of some 1,000 pages, and have intensively studied, for many years, how to prevent premature death and disabilities. As such, I seem to have personally demonstrated that it actually is possible to live longer, be healthy, even productive, and with an excellent quality of life past 75."

And how to do this is now available to everyone. You don't really need money, just the right information and the motivation, which, if you've read this far, you have.

A year later, I wrote: "I am now 75, and while a few things have changed, most haven't. I have no intention, nor do I hope, to die this year. I could say "fingers crossed", but instead, I prefer to access the latest medical information, techniques, and improvements. As to not accepting curative treatments, as Dr. Emanuel says he will not do at 75, I had to face some inevitable consequences of getting old, and back surgery was one of them.

While it was not life-threatening, it certainly was Quality of Life threatening.

I had a low opinion of back surgery, which was reinforced when I examined an American orthopaedic surgeon just a few months prior, who most strongly advised me to avoid it. His operation had been a wretched failure, and when my own surgeon asked bemusedly "why I had waited so long", I answered that it was "because I knew a lot about back surgery." He laughed and assured me things had changed. And they had. I have lived long enough to see back surgery emerge from the primeval swamp of barbaric butchery to elegant microsurgery.

It was unavoidable in my case (spinal stenosis—a narrowing of the spinal canal with compression of the spinal cord and spondylolisthesis—where one vertebra moves forward to further compress the spinal cord). The operation was curative, and I returned to work in less than four weeks. I am not boasting or being brave; the surgeon did a great job! The newly designed titanium screws also bring more improvements. I only cite this event as a firsthand experience that would seem to contradict Dr. Emanuel's disdain for such curative interventions completely.

But More

I am now 83, and after a year off, hiding from COVID-19, I was summonsed back to help at my old clinic, where, to boast, I think I did 'the world record' for excising a melanoma on a scalp without a graft (others, of course, have done the same, but it sure was some operation... the patient says his phone now doesn't facially recognize him!).

I also don't seem to have Emanuel's alleged "sharp drop-off in creativity, functional declines, reduced mental capacity and burdens on family members."

Morbid Personalities and Prophets of Doom

Dr. Emanuel was only 57 years old in 2014 when he hoped to die at 75. I saw a photo of him in 2016; he was a good-looking man radiating confidence and health. In his specialty of treating cancer, he would mostly see patients with established, incurable diseases, already too late to effect a cure. Treating the incurable is a laudable but morbid specialty, which surely must influence one's outlook.

I then wrote that I would like to get his later opinion, based on his own longer experience and personal realizations or insights, if and when he is 75 years old. In 2023, Helen Rumbelow interviewed him, now aged 65.

In this interview, according to Emanuel, every time he mentions his plan to refuse treatment at 75, almost everyone says 75 is too young, citing "SuperAgers" ranging from their 90-year-old grandmother who surfs to current President Joe Biden, who is 80.

"We can't all be outliers," Emanuel said.

When asked if he wants a quick illness to decide his end since it would take bravery to withstand a long treatment or take his own life, Emanuel responded, "Well, I think it's bravery to say no to interventions where the majority of people would say yes."

Emanuel also said he is sceptical of the "immortals" investing so much energy into the dream of living forever, and he wants to be realistic about when his own "consumption" exceeds his "contribution". He believes he will likely stick to his plan.

We will see.

But I not only refute his death wish ultimatum but also now provide the information that allows us to live well past 75.

Nevertheless

Dr. Emanuel's choice of 75 is not altogether curious, or even totally wrong (even though I offer what I feel is a viable alternative), because while today's 75 "is the new 65", our health symptoms seem to suddenly deteriorate at age 75. The chapter "Life Begins at 40" shows how our asymptomatic parameters of health (changes we mostly don't notice, which are just biochemical or only visible via x-rays) at age 75 become symptomatic, and we "suddenly" deteriorate.

Joints give out, blood pressure and heart troubles intervene, eyesight and hearing deteriorate, and yes, even our recollection of words may suggest we are not as sharp. The indignities, let alone the horrors, of old age now confront us. Most of us certainly do not want to then live as a progressively debilitated nursing home resident undergoing Osler's "cold gradations of decay".[233]

This finite 75-year lifespan obviously does not fit all. Given the right information, there are now ways to predict and avoid those most critical illnesses and live (and work and play) much longer. There is also evidence indicating how to stay healthier; not smoking is the best known, but there are now many other evidenced lifestyles which are not onerous nor will make us into health nuts. And while Dr. Emanuel states he doesn't want any interventions, there are many advances in modern medicine, such as cataract surgery, artificial hips, and catheter heart ablation, that return a near-blind, hobbling invalid or a potential stroke victim to being effectively normal rather than languishing and deteriorating, waiting for a premature and avoidable death.

But some are so ubiquitous that we take them for granted. This was driven home to me in the film The Name of the Rose, starring Sean Connery. It was based on the novel written by the great Italian writer Umberto Eco. In it, Connery plays an Italian priest investigating murders in the priesthood. He is only able to

233 Niburski, K. 2023, "The principles and practice of death: The Oslerian conflicted conception of dying", *Journal of Medical Biography*, Vol. 31, No. 1, https://doi.org/10.1177/09677720211018974.

do so because of a new invention—magnifying spectacles. When they fall and break, he can no longer investigate.

And so, it was with me in the 1980s as I started to push the newspaper away due to aging of my eye lenses called presbyopia, wherein a colleague eye specialist, after examining me, told me just to go to the local garage and buy a pair of magnifiers for $7.50. Now, 40 years later, I still wear them, and the price hasn't gone up much, but it has allowed me to do exquisitely fine facial surgery. I mean, think about it—40 more years of productive work for $7.50! Of course, they have cost me a deal more as I have them in every room and in my car, but do we think how wonderful it is that we can retain visual acuity, even if we need prescription glasses or laser surgery?

Still, I do agree with Shannon Brownlee, senior vice president of the Lown Institute (which I presume is named after Nobel Prize winner Bernard Lown, MD, inventor of the defibrillator and introducer of lidocaine into medical practice), in her effort to reform healthcare for the aging: "The pressure to undergo more tests, more treatments, and more invasive procedures as one gets older and frailer comes from all sides—from friends, from the hospital, from well-meaning clinicians... We need to make it easier for people to resist futile or unwanted treatments—to say no."

It is hard to disagree with Emanuel and Brownlee that interfering, intrusive, and invasive tests should not be done when old patients are ill and there is no real hope of improving their quality of life.

And if struck down with some serious or terminal illness consigning us to a nursing home with the aforementioned indignities, then, I agree, Dr. Emanuel may well have a point. In fact, just this week, I examined a vivacious young lawyer who worked for a large law firm and whose job was litigating aged care. She was a very pretty girl, but her face clouded over when discussing this subject. She vehemently advised me a number of times to "never go into a nursing home" and sketched out for me just the superficial horrors she saw as a lawyer—let alone the medical horrors. She appeared so affected by her experience that I doubt very much if she will, or can, continue in this branch of the law. And if I were an oncologist (cancer specialist) or a nursing home doctor, I think I, too, would like to bow out at 75 rather than endure the seemingly unavoidable progressive indignities and degradation.

Suicide and Older White Men[234]

Older white men have higher suicide rates, yet fewer burdens associated with aging. For example, they are less likely to experience death of a spouse and have better physical health and fewer disabilities than older women. They have more economic resources than ethnic minority older men and women.

White older men, however, may be less psychologically equipped to deal with the normal challenges of aging because of their privilege up until late adulthood. It is thought that an important factor in white men's psychological brittleness and vulnerability to suicide once they reach late life may be the belief that suicide is a masculine response to the "indignities" of aging. This is a script that implicitly justifies, and even glorifies, suicide among men as a rational, courageous, and powerful choice.

Two such famous cases were Eastman Kodak founder George Eastman, who died of suicide in 1932 at age 77—it was said he was "unprepared and unwilling to face the indignities of old age"—and Gonzo-writer Hunter S. Thompson, who killed

234 Canetto, S. S. 2015, "Suicide: Why Are Older Men So Vulnerable?", *Men and Masculinities*, Vol. 20, No. 1, https://doi.org/10.1177/1097184X15613832.

himself in 2005 at age 67, having thus triumphed over "the indignities of aging".

But older men are not the most suicide-prone group everywhere. For example, in China, women of reproductive age are the group with the highest suicide mortality. The "indignities of aging" suicide script, as well as the belief that suicide is a white man's powerful response to aging, can and should be challenged and changed.

Suicides in the United States increased 24% from 1999 to 2014, according to data from the CDC.[235] This rate increased from 1% to 2% annually from 2006 through 2014, a timespan that included the Great Recession. The female suicide rate increased 45% since 1999 and the male suicide rate increased 16%. Nonetheless, in 2014, the age-adjusted suicide rate among males was still three times that in females (20.7 vs. 5.8 per 100,000).

Suicide rates were highest in men aged 75 and older and in women aged 45–64. In children aged 10–14, suicide rates were low, but this age group had a large percentage increase in suicides (200% in females, 37% in males). About a quarter of suicides are attributed to suffocation, an increase since 1999. For men, the most frequent method involved firearms. For women, poisoning was the most common method.

235 Curtin, S. C., Warner, M. & Hedegaard, H. 2016, "Increase in Suicide in the United States, 1999-2014", *NCHS Data Brief*, No. 241, pp. 1-8.

CHAPTER 32

SuperAgers

"I'm very pleased to be here. Let's face it, at my age I'm very pleased to be anywhere."

– George Burns (who died aged 100)

"SuperAging" was coined as a research term at Northwestern University. The university defined SuperAgers as adults over age 80 who have the memory capacity of individuals who are at least three decades younger, whereas cognitive abilities, particularly memory, normally decline with age.

The prevalence and incidence have not yet been determined, but researchers regard it as a rare phenotype. Apparently, only 10% of those who apply to be included in the Northwestern study qualify or are accepted.

SuperAgers qualify by having a good memory, but there are no requirements as to physical performance; some might need a wheelchair or a walker but still have a great memory.

Unfortunately, despite many research projects, these opinions are all observational, and while SuperAgers do seem to have traits in common, no causes have been found. Be that as it may, we have certainly nothing to lose emulating their lifestyles.

They are at lower risk of developing dementia and would seem to have added protective factors, be they genetic, lifestyle, or a greater positive emotional outlook, against risk factors. Hence, the research is to hopefully uncover the mechanisms that act on known dementia risk factors to lessen age-related cognitive decline and brain changes.

Personally, and without any scientific basis, I am struck by their learning of music and their actively challenging their brains. While obsessive physical fitness or diets do not seem to have played a part, I suspect they have not been obese or junk food addicts.

Interestingly, some SuperAgers were just as likely to have the same levels of APOE genes, including APOE4, a risk for Alzheimer's disease, while others displayed splodges of amyloid and tau the same as AD sufferers.

SuperAgers were also found to have a lower frequency of the ε4 allele of apolipoprotein E than the general population.[236] Some SuperAgers had unusually low densities of age-related Alzheimer pathology and unusually high numbers of von Economo neurons in the anterior cingulate gyrus.

It is thought that memory declines on average over the lifespan and that decline or peak in our memory really might hit in our thirties. It starts going down from there.

SuperAgers have to be over age 80, and that's a time when, again, the likelihood of having memory decline increases (individuals who are at age 80 are at greater risk for memory decline than individuals in their 70s or 60s).

---

236 Rogalski, E. J., Gefen, T., Shi, J. *et al.* 2013, "Youthful memory capacity in old brains: anatomic and genetic clues from the Northwestern SuperAging Project", *Journal of Cognitive Neuroscience*, Vol. 25, No. 1, pp. 29-36, https://doi.org/10.1162/jocn_a_00300.

An average 80-year-old's brain versus that of a SuperAger, reveals that the average 80-year-olds are thinning at a rate of more than two, nearly two and a half times that of the SuperAgers.[237]

Research suggests that, although Alzheimer's disease-related changes and vascular changes are common in their brains, these individuals are less vulnerable to other forms of neurodegenerative changes like Lewy body disease.[238]

SuperAgers performed better for memory, physical condition, speed, and mental health irrespective of the levels of blood biomarkers of Alzheimer's disease and were able to withstand the negative effects of Alzheimer's disease-related brain changes and low levels of damage from vascular problems. They were also resistant to other types of brain changes that are not related to Alzheimer's disease.

It appears that individuals who live to be 90 and older with excellent memory and thinking abilities tend to have similar levels of Alzheimer's disease pathology in their brains but have lower levels of pathologies from other diseases that cause memory and thinking problems.

Researchers believe that a positive attitude and resilience are crucial to keeping mind and memory sharp in old age.

SuperAgers come from many different backgrounds and education levels and have encountered a variety of ups and downs throughout their lives. Some have experienced great traumas, and many seem to have incredible resilience in the face of stress.

---

237 Burke, S. N., Mormino, E. C., Rogalski, E. J. *et al.* 2019, "What are the later life contributions to reserve, resilience, and compensation?", *Neurobiology of Aging*, Vol. 83, pp. 140-144, https://doi.org/10.1016/j.neurobiolaging.2019.03.023.

238 Biswas, R., Kawas, C., Montine, T. J. *et al.* 2023, "Superior Global Cognition in Oldest-Old Is Associated with Resistance to Neurodegenerative Pathologies: Results from The 90+ Study", *Journal of Alzheimer's Disease*, Vol. 93, No. 2, pp. 561-575, https://doi.org/10.3233/JAD-221062.

Despite hardships in their life, they appeared to "bounce back". Many were even able to maintain their physical and mental health despite drinking and smoking.

SuperAgers share similar traits, say experts who study them. They challenge their brains every day by reading or learning something new. It does not seem to matter what the challenge is as long as the person likes it and doesn't feel they 'have' to do something they don't like, such as a crossword. Many continue to work into their 80s and remain actively engaged in life. They were also found to be more extroverted, valuing social interaction and friendships more highly than people of a similar age who had aged normally.

As people age, the cerebral cortex atrophies—becomes thinner—but not in SuperAgers, whose brains seem to shrink at a much slower rate.

MRI, or structural magnetic resonance imaging, allows very detailed measuring of the cerebral cortex outer layer, the grey-white junction, and measuring of its thickness, which gives a proxy measure of the health of the brain—i.e., the cortical thickness reflects the brain health.

When SuperAger brains (over 80) were compared to 50- to 60-year-olds, there was no significant cortical thinning. Their brains looked more like 50- to 60-year-old brains. SuperAgers also had a thicker anterior cingulate, which is important for attention,[239] and, thus, better memory, which is thought to contribute to superaging and has up to five times more "von Economo" neurons (giant brain cells that are thought to boost social behaviour, and which are often missing in people with

239 Rogalski, E. J., Gefen, T., Shi, J. *et al.* 2013, "Youthful memory capacity in old brains: anatomic and genetic clues from the Northwestern SuperAging Project", *Journal of Cognitive Neuroscience*, Vol. 25, No. 1, pp. 29-36, https://doi.org/10.1162/jocn_a_00300.

autism or bi-polar disorder). So far, the corkscrew-like von Economo neuron has only been found in humans, great apes, elephants, whales, dolphins, and songbirds.

The Vallecas Project[240] longitudinal cohort recruited between Oct 10, 2011, and Jan 14, 2014, aged 79.5 years or older, found in the data acquired as per protocol from up to six yearly follow-ups were used for longitudinal analyses. As with any observational study, they caution that causality of the factors reported, and super aging cannot be inferred.

SuperAgers Demonstrate Less Atrophy in Certain Areas of the Brain

The Lancet Healthy Longevity study[241] showed that, in SuperAgers, age-related deterioration of grey matter, especially in the areas responsible for memory, atrophies much more slowly than in normal older adults. However, the study also emphasized the importance of physical and mental fitness for a healthy aging process.

These results indicate that SuperAgers are resistant to age-related memory loss rather than having coping mechanisms that allow them to better offset this memory loss.

The MRI examinations confirmed that in SuperAgers, grey matter atrophy in the regions responsible for memory (such as the medial temporal lobe and cholinergic forebrain) and in regions important for movement (such as the motor thalamus)

240 Garo-Pascual, M., Gaser, C., Zhang, L. *et al.* 2023, "Brain structure and phenotypic profile of superagers compared with age-matched older adults: a longitudinal analysis from the Vallecas", *The Lancet Healthy Longevity*, Vol. 4, No. 8, https://doi.org/10.1016/S2666-7568(23)00079-X.

241 Touroutoglou, A., Wong, B. & Andreano, J. M. 2023, "What is so super about ageing?", *The Lancet Healthy Longevity*, Vol. 4, No. 8, https://doi.org/10.1016/S2666-7568(23)00103-4.

was less pronounced. In addition, the volume of grey matter in these regions, especially in the medial temporal lobe, decreased much more slowly in the SuperAgers than in the control subjects over the study period.

Activity at 40, 50 or Even 60 Years Old is Important

Clinical tests such as the Timed Up-and-Go Test and the Finger Tapping Test, which are easily accessed for those interested, revealed that SuperAgers can be distinguished from the normally aging control subjects with regard to their mobility and fine motor skills. Their physical condition was better, although they, by their own admission, did not move any more than the control subjects in day-to-day life. But this finding confirms that physical activity is paramount for cognitive function. These people were over 80 years old—the fact that there was not much difference between their levels of activity is not surprising. Much more relevant is the question of how you get there—i.e., how active you are at the ages of 40, 50 or even 60 years old was stressed.

In fact, the SuperAgers indicated that they had generally been more active than the control subjects during their middle years. Attempting to stay physically fit is essential, even if it just means going for a walk or taking the stairs.

On average, the SuperAgers also fared much better in tests on physical health than the control subjects. They suffered significantly less from depression or anxiety disorders. Earlier studies suggest that depression and anxiety disorders may influence performance in memory tests across all ages and that they are risk factors for developing dementia.

Blood sample analyses demonstrated that the SuperAgers exhibited lower concentrations of biomarkers for neurodegenerative diseases than the control group did. In contrast, there was no difference between the two groups in the prevalence of the APOE e4 allele, one of the most important genetic risk factors for Alzheimer's disease but the researchers assume that genetics also play a role. They found that, despite 89 variables employed, the algorithm used could only distinguish SuperAgers from normal older adults 66% of the time. This suggests that additional factors must be in play, such as genetic differences.

In brief, it was found that SuperAgers show resistance to age-related memory decline. They were faster in both gait speed and finger tapping than a control group with similar concentrations of blood biomarkers for neurodegenerative disease, suggesting that movement speed is associated with better memory, even in the absence of an evident dementia process. Although SuperAgers' self-reported exercise frequencies are similar to that reported by typical older adults, their faster movement speed could reflect a greater engagement in non-exercise physical activity (e.g., climbing stairs or gardening).

SuperAgers showed better mental health than typical older adults and complained less frequently about not getting enough sleep. They were more likely to have either a formal or amateur musical background than typical older adults. This finding is in keeping with reports that early-life to midlife formal musical training is associated with improved late-life episodic and semantic memory and with larger grey matter volume.

The research found an association between satisfaction in social relationships and super-aging, with SuperAgers reporting satisfying, high-quality relationships. However, they were more likely than typical older adults to be separated or divorced.

Years of education did not reach significant importance in classifying SuperAgers.

Aerobic exercise interventions in healthy older adults do not appear to yield cognitive benefits, even when the intervention leads to improved cardiorespiratory fitness, and psychiatric symptoms can accelerate aging from early midlife.

Research, published in the *Journal of Alzheimer's Disease*,[242] shows that, although the "oldest old" individuals, those who live to be 90 years or older, may possess superior cognitive abilities and still maintain good memory and thinking abilities. They may have Alzheimer's disease-related changes and vascular brain changes similar to levels of Alzheimer's patients but are less vulnerable to other forms of neurodegenerative changes like Lewy body disease, fewer co-existing brain pathologies, and low levels of damage from vascular problems. They also appeared resistant to other types of brain changes that are not related to Alzheimer's disease (AD) and multiple additional brain health problems. This 90+ Study was started in 2003, investigating aging and dementia.

See also the chapter on Alzheimer's Disease.

---

242 Biswas, R., Kawas, C., Montine, T. J. *et al.* 2023, "Superior Global Cognition in Oldest-Old Is Associated with Resistance to Neurodegenerative Pathologies: Results from The 90+ Study", *Journal of Alzheimer's Disease*, Vol. 93, No. 2, pp. 561-575, https://doi.org/10.3233/JAD-221062.

CHAPTER 33

The Evidence

"A hundred suspicions don't make a proof."

– Fyodor Dostoevsky (1821-1881)

What Works and How

Our health, including longevity, demands evidence as to what works. This idea was initially set down in 1890 by Dr. Koch as his 'postulates', which are now out of date as newer organisms, such as viruses and prions, have been discovered, along with other advances.[243]

Then, in the 1990s, evidence-based medicine developed, and better investigations and tests gradually developed along with statistical analyses such that a priority order or hierarchy has developed. This order gives us a clue as to the quality of the evidence.

243 Cohen, J. 2017, "The Evolution of Koch's Postulates", *Infectious Diseases*, Fourth Edition.

Trials and Studies

The priority order is:

1. *Observation:* Observational studies can only document associations; they cannot demonstrate causation.
2. *Case Reports:* Records of patients' illness stimulate a hypothesis, but this cannot be tested, as there is no comparison group.
3. *Clinical Trial:* A trial where administration of a drug to participants is analysed.
4. *Cohort Study:* Cohorts are groups of similar people, but studies compare one half exposed to the drug, diet, or such, to the other half not exposed.
5. *Cross-sectional Study:* A retrospective observational study where participants are assessed as to the effect of an exposure.
6. *Randomized Controlled Trial (RCT):* Participants are selected by random chance to an exposure.
7. *Double Blind RCT:* The gold standard. Here, all involved are 'blinded': participants, selectors, the drug with an identical placebo, and the assessors/analysists. Nobody knows who or which is what, so the results are a completely independent, un-interfered, unbiased 'surprise'.

The best trials are submitted for expert peer review to make it, or not, into the best medical journals, where there is also an acknowledged hierarchy.

Unfortunately, most longevity studies are only observational.

Statistics

All studies now have to show statistics, but unfortunately, statistics can be manipulated to support what the researchers want.

Values

P signifies probability, or the threshold of significance.

$P < 0.05$ confirms the result is significant.

Confidence Intervals, set at 95% by convention, suggest the true population value is represented.

Confounders are other (often outside) factors that may intrude to mask, influence, and alter the results.

Bradford Hill Criteria[244]

The Bradford Hill criteria, otherwise known as Hill's criteria for causation, are a group of nine principles that can be useful in establishing epidemiologic evidence of a causal relationship between a presumed cause and an observed effect. They have been widely used in public health research.

The list of the criteria is as follows:

- *Strength* (effect size): A small association does not mean that there is not a causal effect, though the larger the association, the more likely that it is causal.
- *Consistency* (reproducibility): Consistent findings observed by different persons in different places with different samples strengthens the likelihood of an effect.
- *Specificity:* Causation is likely if there is a very specific population at a specific site and disease with no other likely explanation. The more specific an association between a factor and an effect is, the bigger the probability of a causal relationship.
- *Temporality:* The effect has to occur after the cause (and if there is an expected delay between the cause and

244 Hill, A. B. 1965, "The Environment and Disease: Association or Causation?", *Journal of the Royal Society of Medicine*, Vol. 58, No. 5, pp. 295-300, https://doi.org/10.1177/003591576505800503.

expected effect, then the effect must occur after that delay).

- *Biological gradient* (dose–response relationship): Greater exposure should generally lead to greater incidence of the effect. However, in some cases, the mere presence of the factor can trigger the effect. In other cases, an inverse proportion is observed: greater exposure leads to lower incidence.
- *Plausibility:* A plausible mechanism between cause and effect is helpful (but Hill noted that knowledge of the mechanism is limited by current knowledge).
- *Coherence:* Coherence between epidemiological and laboratory findings increases the likelihood of an effect. However, Hill noted that "lack of such [laboratory] evidence cannot nullify the epidemiological effect on associations."
- *Experiment:* "Occasionally it is possible to appeal to experimental evidence."
- *Analogy:* The use of analogies or similarities between the observed association and any other associations.
- *Reversibility:* If the cause is deleted, then the effect should disappear as well.

Debate in Epidemiology

All scientific work is incomplete and liable to be upset or modified by advancing knowledge. However, that does not confer upon us the freedom to ignore the knowledge we already have or to postpone the action that it appears to demand at a given time.

CHAPTER 34

Sarcopenia

"It Could Happen to You."

– Music by Jimmy Van Heusen
and lyrics by Johnny Burke

Definition

Sarcopenia is the loss of muscle strength, mass, and function.

Everyone loses muscle mass over time, but people with sarcopenia lose it more quickly. Sarcopenia, from the Greek word meaning 'poverty of flesh', was only first proposed in 1989 by Irwin Rosenberg as a term to describe the loss of muscle mass with age. The definition of sarcopenia has evolved since that time to incorporate our understanding of the importance of muscle function alongside muscle mass.[245]

In 2016, the Center for Disease Control and Prevention (CDC) declared sarcopenia a specific disease by creating an International Classification of Disease (ICD) 10 code, which makes sarcopenia a reportable disease.

245 Offord, N. J. & Witham, M. D. 2017, "The emergence of sarcopenia as an important entity in older people", *Clinical Medicine*, Vol. 17, No. 4, pp. 363-366, https://doi.org/10.7861/clinmedicine.17-4-363.

It affects the musculoskeletal system and is a major factor in increased frailty, falls, and fractures involving a decrease in the size and number of your muscle fibers.

Muscle atrophy involves a reduction in the size of the fibers, but the number of fibers stays the same.

The most common cause of sarcopenia is the natural aging process. Other possible risk factors may include:

- Physical inactivity
- Obesity
- Chronic diseases such as chronic obstructive pulmonary disease (COPD), kidney disease, Diabetes, cancer and HIV
- Rheumatoid arthritis
- Insulin resistance
- Reduction in hormone levels
- Malnutrition or inadequate protein intake
- Decrease in ability to convert protein to energy.
- Decline in the number of nerve cells that send messages from your brain to your muscles telling them to move.

Muscle mass and, hence, strength begin to be lost at an estimated 1% a year from age 30, but this loss accelerates between the ages of 65 and 80.

Sarcopenia can also affect people with a high body mass index (BMI), called sarcopenic obesity.

Sarcopenia most commonly affects people ages 60 and older. The rates increase with age, and the disease affects both sexes equally. The rates increase in people with chronic disease.

It is important, as we age, to be aware of what sarcopenia is and how it affects us so it can be identified, as it can be prevented or treated and reverted to a normal state with early intervention.

It has is a range of adverse outcomes, including increased falls and exacerbations of chronic comorbidities including cardiovascular diseases, chronic kidney disease, and cancer. Sarcopenia is also associated with faster progression of cardiovascular diseases and higher risk of mortality, reduced quality of life, increased hospitalisations, and loss of independence among older adults. Obviously, it compromises longevity.

There is an apparent overlap with frailty, and the two may be hard to differentiate.

Rates of the condition range from 5% to 13% in people ages 60 and older. The estimates increase to 11% to 50% in people ages 80 and older.[246]

To me, as above, one of the earliest signs is difficulty rising up from a low chair, and I well remember my father who had been a champion athlete, rugby player, and gardener having to push himself up using the arms of the chair while his thighs quivered. But it is treatable and the earlier it is diagnosed, the better.

I was, however, taken aback when some skilled musculo-skeletal physio/physical therapists had not heard of it, so I assume many of my colleagues may also not be aware. Hence, this chapter.

The muscle loss is accelerated by a sedentary lifestyle, prolonged bed rest, smoking and alcohol intake, malnutrition, and any anorexia of aging. Midlife obesity has been found to be associated with an increased incidence of sarcopenia later in life.

Symptoms

The most common symptom of sarcopenia is muscle weakness. Other symptoms may include:

246 von Haehling, S., Morley, J. E. & Anker, S. D. 2010, "An overview of sarcopenia: facts and numbers on prevalence and clinical impact", *Journal of Cachexia, Sarcopenia and Muscle*, Vol. 1, No. 2, pp. 129-133, https://doi.org/10.1007/s13539-010-0014-2.

- Loss of stamina
- Difficulty performing daily activities.
- Walking slowly
- Trouble climbing stairs.
- Poor balance and falls.
- Decrease in muscle size.

Diagnosis

Diagnosis is clinical, as there are no blood or biochemical tests. For me, the best clinical sign is difficulty rising from a low chair.

There is a questionnaire based on self-reported symptoms called the SARC-F.

SARC-F stands for:

- S — Strength
- A — Assistance with walking
- R — Rising from a chair
- C — Climbing stairs
- F — Falls

You score each factor with a number between zero and two. The highest maximum SARC-F score is 10. A SARC-F score of four or less warrants more testing.

Nose Over the Toes

While on this subject, I have been disappointed when therapists don't tell older patients they must "put their nose over their toes". This allows for maximum power lift, which helps them stand, thereby exercising their muscles and postponing sarcopenia.

Treatment

The basic treatment is resistance training and nutritional supplementation where indicated. Drugs are being developed, and possibly hormone is being considered as a possibility.

Resistance Exercise Training

Resistance and aerobic training have been shown to increase muscle mass, strength, and physical performance. An important factor in the development of sarcopenia is the lack of physical activity followed by anabolic resistance.

One regime calls for progressive resistance and duration of sessions increasing gradually, depending on individual capability and progress. The initial suggestion is for at least two to three times a week for a duration of eight to 12 weeks.

After aerobic exercise alone, mitochondrial volume and enzyme activity increase, indicating that muscle quality improves regardless of age.

The essential fact is that we have to keep moving and exercising. Joining classes is recommended, as it ensures commitment, motivation, and progress, but you might have to inform your tutor you need progressive resistance and aerobic exercises.

Muscle Strength Tests

- Handgrip test: Handgrip strength draws a parallel to the strength in your other muscles. Providers use it to identify shortages in overall muscle strength.
- Chair stand test: Providers use the chair stand test to measure your leg muscle strength, especially your quadriceps. The chair stand test measures the number of times you can stand and sit from a chair without the use of your arms in 30 seconds.
- Walking speed test: The walking (gait) speed test measures the time it takes for you to travel four meters (about 13 feet) at your usual walking pace.
- Short physical performance battery(SPPB): With the SPPB test, you take three timed tasks: chair stand test, standing balance test, and walking speed test.

- Timed-up and go test (TUG): The TUG test measures the time it takes to rise from a chair, walk three meters (about 10 feet) away from it, walk three meters back to it, and sit back down in it.

Imaging Tests for Measurement of Muscle Mass

- Dual-energy X-ray absorptiometry (DEXA or DXA): This type of imaging test uses low-energy X-rays to measure your muscle mass, fat mass, and bone density.
- Bioelectrical impedance analysis (BIA): The BIA test is less expensive and more widely available than DEXA. It measures your body fat in relation to your lean body mass.

SECTION F

EXERCISE & PHYSICAL ACTIVITY

CHAPTER 35

Exercise & Physical Activities

"If you don t make time for exercise, you'll probably have to make time for illness."

– Robin Sharma

There is nothing else that can beneficially influence as many organ systems as can exercise/physical activity.

The latest revelations are that sub four-minute milers live longer[247] and now a new analysis indicates that physical performance, especially walking quickly, is independently associated with long-term survival in very old adults living in the community. Consistent with literature, physical performance is as a reliable metric for assessing mortality risk in octogenarians. Neither the number of diseases nor any specific disease predicted long-term survival. Our findings, together with available evidence, support the view that physical performance is a primary target for interventions to enhance longevity and extend health span.[248]

247 Rak, G. 2024, "Sub-Four-Minute Mile Runners Outlive General Population", *Medscape,* 21 May.

248 Remaly, J. 2024, "Three Keys to Longevity in Older Adults?", *Medscape,* 21 May.

Recent data suggests a correlation between a little more than four minutes of intense physical activity per day and a lower risk for cardiovascular diseases, cancer, and overall mortality in athletes and nonathletes.[249]

The following graphs say it all:

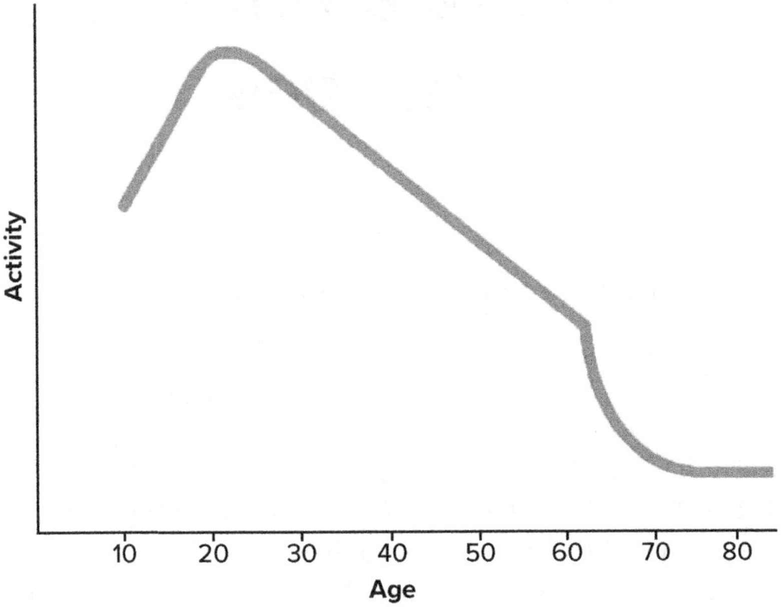

Figure 34: Exercise patterns vary with age.

From the age of 20, our exercise falls off steeply and plummets aged 60. It bottoms out aged 70. Exercise throughout life.

The more you exercise, the more health benefits.

249 Stamatakis, E., Ahmadi, M. N., Friedenreich, C. M. *et al.* 2023, "Vigorous Intermittent Lifestyle Physical Activity and Cancer Incidence Among Nonexercising Adults: The UK Biobank Accelerometry Study", *JAMA Oncology*, Vol. 9, No. 9, pp. 1255-1259, https://doi.org/10.1001/jamaoncol.2023.1830.

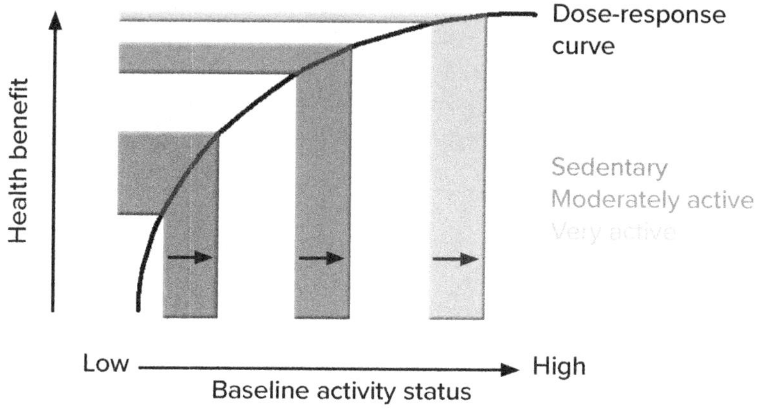

Figure 35:

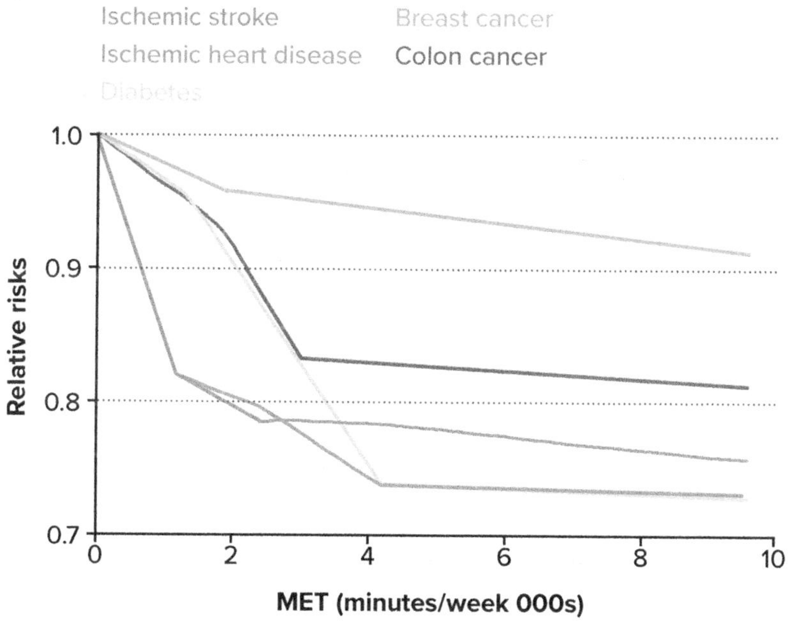

Figure 36: Continuous risk curves for association between physical activity and breast cancer, colon cancer, diabetes, ischemic heart disease and ischemic stroke.

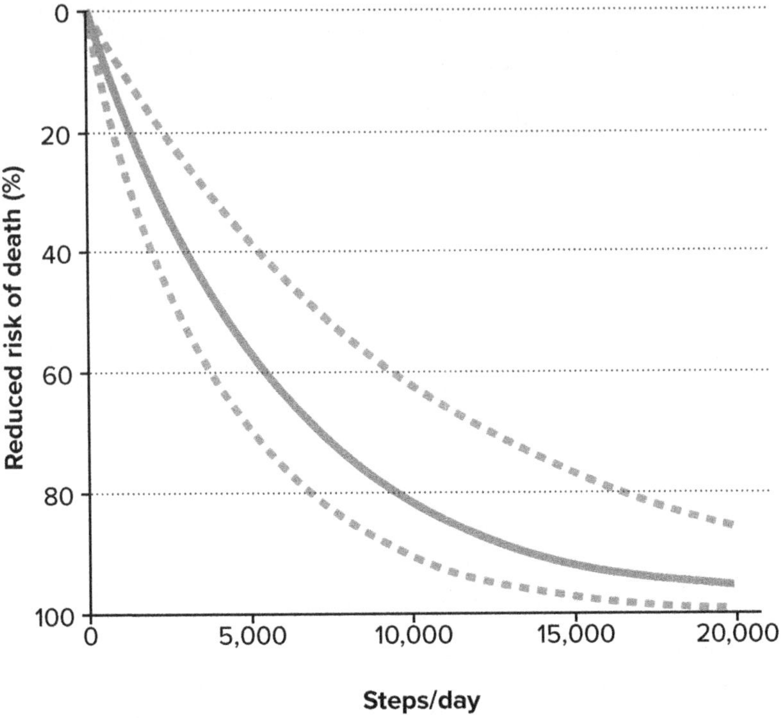

Figure 37: How walking cuts the risk of early death (*Source: ESC*).

Definitions

Physical Activity: Any movement that burns calories such as mowing lawns, walking upstairs, making the bed, walking the dog, etc.

Exercise: Structured physical activity with a series of repetitive movements designed to strengthen or develop part of your body and improve cardiovascular fitness—walking, swimming, bicycling.

Moderate activity: Gentle swimming, housework, social tennis; working hard enough to raise the heart rate and break into a sweat; able to talk but not sing the words to a song.

***Vigorous activity*:** Jogging, aerobics, or competitive tennis

Anaerobic: Not needing oxygen. Strength/weights or Resistance Training

Aerobic: Means using oxygen. Cardiovascular/Respiratory Fitness.

Maximum Heart Rate (HRmax) = 220 – your age Take it after 5 minutes of your maximum effort/exercise. Smartwatches record it and also plot your recovery.

Fitness Measurement

Your aerobic fitness is best measured by your VO_2max. VO_2max is the maximum (max) rate (V) of oxygen (O_2) your body is able to use during exercise. This is most accurately tested in a lab on an exercise bike while hooked up to a mask, but there are formulae based on heart rates, and smartwatches also give read-outs, but you usually have to exercise for > 20 minutes.

Simplest formula: $VO_2max = 15 \times (HRmax/HRrest)$

There are many charts to be found on the Internet which rate you from poor to elite. Most seem to cut out at age 60, and very few go past 80. There is also a variation as to their rating classifications. The following is the best I've found.

Your anaerobic fitness is easily measured by the increasing the amount of weight you can lift.

Recovery

It takes a day or two to recover the lactic acid build up in your muscles and to repair the minute tissue tears after exercise.

Regime

Alternating aerobic with anaerobic exercises would seem practical.

First

Find an exercise you like and can do.

Table 26: Classification of cardiorepiratory fitness by age and sex. VO_2max (estimated, VO_2peak) in mL/kg/minute of oxygen consumption. 1 MET (metabolic equivalent) equals 3.5 mL/kg/minute of oxygen consumption. Classification (percentile range) is low (< 25th percentile), below average (25th - 49th percentile), above average (50th - 74th percentile), high (75th - 97.6th percentile), and elite (≥ 97.7th percentile) (*Source: Mandsager, K., Harb, S., Cremer. P.* et al. *2018, "Association of Cardiorespiratory Fitness With Long-term Mortality Among Adults Undergoing Exercise Treadmill Testing"*, JAMA Network Open, *Vol. 1, No. 6, https://doi.org/10.1001/jamanetworkopen.2018.3605*).

	Performance group									
	Low		Below average		Above Average		High		Elite	
Age (y)	METS	VO_2max	METS	VO_2max	METS	VO_2max	METS	VO_2max	METS	VO_2max
Women										
18-19	< 10.0	< 35	10.0-11.0	35-39	11.1-12.9	40-45	13.0-14.9	46-52	≥ 15.0	≥ 53
20-29	< 8.0	< 28	8.0-9.9	28-35	10.0-11.4	63-40	11.5-14.2	41-50	≥ 14.3	≥ 51
30-39	< 7.7	< 27	7.7-9.3	27-33	9.4-10.8	34-38	10.9-13.6	39-48	≥ 13.7	≥ 49
40-49	< 7.4	< 26	7.4-8.9	26-31	9.0-10.3	32-36	10.4-13.2	37-46	≥ 13.3	≥ 47
50-59	< 7.0	< 25	7.0-8.0	25-28	8.1-9.9	29-35	10.0-12.9	36-45	≥ 13.0	≥ 46
60-69	< 6.0	< 21	6.0-6.9	21-24	7.0-8.4	25-29	8.5-11.0	30-39	≥ 11.1	≥ 10
70-79	< 5.0	< 18	5.0-5.9	18-21	6.0-6.9	22-24	7.0-9.9	25-35	≥ 10.0	≥ 36
≥ 80	< 4.4	< 15	4.4-5.4	15-19	5.5-6.2	20-22	6.3-8.3	23-29	≥ 8.4	≥ 30

Age (y)	Performance group									
	Low		Below average		Above Average		High		Elite	
	METS	VO_2max	METS	VO_2max	METS	VO_2max	METS	VO_2max	METS	VO_2max
Men										
18-19	< 10.8	< 38	10.8-12.9	38-45	13.0-13.9	46-49	14.0-16.2	50-57	≥ 16.3	≥ 58
20-29	< 10.3	< 36	10.3-11.9	36-42	12.0-13.6	43-48	13.7-15.6	49-55	≥ 15.7	≥ 56
30-39	< 10.0	< 35	10.0-11.1	35-39	11.2-12.9	40-45	13.0-14.9	46-52	≥ 15.0	≥ 53
40-49	< 9.8	< 34	9.8-10.9	34-28	11.0-12.4	39-43	12.5-14.6	44-51	≥ 14.7	≥ 52
50-59	< 8.2	< 29	8.2-9.9	29-35	10.0-11.3	36-40	11.4-13.9	41-49	≥ 14.0	≥ 50
60-69	< 7.0	< 25	7.0-8.4	25-29	8.5-9.9	30-35	10.0-12.9	36-45	≥ 13.0	≥ 46
70-79	< 6.0	< 21	6.0-6.9	21-24	7.0-8.4	25-29	8.5-11.4	30-40	≥ 11.5	≥ 41
≥ 80	< 5.1	< 18	5.1-6.2	18-22	6.3-7.2	23-25	7.3-9.9	26-35	≥ 10.0	≥ 36

I am no gym junkie, and I detest long-distance running and swimming. I think I have the brain of a dog… I have to chase something like a ball (and tennis players live longest). But my wife gets up in the middle of winter and goes swimming three times a week and loves it.

Bike riding and swimming, I have always thought the best exercises as they do not impose stress on the joints, but there are shoulder impingement injuries in elite freestyle swimmers who roll their arms over an incredible number of times.

Optimum Aging Necessitates Exercise[250]

Lack of exercise is responsible for twice as many early deaths as obesity. You have to get your VO_2max up, as there is a 50% mortality in the lowest group compared to 20% in the highest after 12 years.

High activity was associated with the following relative risk reductions:

- Diabetes: 28% lower risk
- Ischemic stroke: 26%
- Ischemic heart disease: 25%
- Colon cancer: 21%
- Breast cancer: 14%
- Whereas lack of physical activity accounts for:
- 22% of coronary heart disease
- 22% of colon cancer
- 18% of osteoporotic fractures
- 12% percent of Diabetes and hypertension
- 5% of breast cancer

250 Kyu, H. H., Bachman, V. F., Alexander, L. T. *et al.* 2013, "Physical activity and risk of breast cancer, colon cancer, Diabetes, ischemic heart disease, and ischemic stroke events: systematic review and dose-response meta-analysis for the Global Burden of Disease Study 2013", *BMJ*, https://doi.org/10.1136/bmj.i3857.

As we age, any movement is beneficial and can be broken into "fractionated" sessions, as detailed.

Intensive exercise improves the endothelium in coronary arteries, i.e., it 'smooths' the blood vessel linings. This allows better dilation and greater blood flow.

Survival of the Fittest

The more intense the activity, the better the benefit.

The relative risk of survival was four times worse for those least fit compared to those exercising most.

Greater fitness results in longer survival (all causes).

Unfit people can improve survival if fitness improves.

Table 27:

Exercise/week	Reduction CHD Risk (%)
Running 1 hr (6mph)	42
Weight training 30 min	32
Rowing 1 hr	18
Brisk walking	18
Low intensity walking	0

Longevity of Elite Athletes

Do elite athletes live longer? Apparently, they do: Those who ran a mile (1.6k) in less than four minutes – 'the epitome of extreme exercise and pushing the body to its physiological limits' – lived almost five years longer on average than their predicated life expectancy.[251]

251 Foulkes, S., Hewitt, D., Skow, R. *et al.* 2024, "Outrunning the grim reaper: longevity of the first 200 sub-4 min mile male runners", *British Journal of Sports Medicine,* Vol. 58, No. 13, https://doi.org/10.1136/bjsports-2024-108386.

Table 28: The life expectancy of elite athletes in sport (*Source: WegENT 2 July 2022*).

Sport	Life expectancy	Vs. world population life expectancy (72.6 years)
Boxing	67.7	–4.9
Football (soccer)	74.6	+2.0
Cricket	76.7	+4.1
Basketball	77.3	+4.7
Baseball	77.6	+5.0
Golf	77.8	+5.2
American Football (NFL)	78.6	+6.0
NHL Hockey	78.9	+6.3
Rugby union	79.1	+6.5
Tennis	80.4	+7.8

Methodology

100 elite athletes were identified from each of the ten selected sports to determine average life expectancy. The athlete must have competed at the elite level between 1949–1952 and been born between 1908–1931. These parameters ensured that the data collected was based on one generation of athletes only and that even the youngest of this generation had the time to live to the age of 90 by 2021.

Moderate and high physical activity led to between 1.3 and 3.7 years more in total life expectancy over those who were sedentary. Aging is not slowed, but life span increases.[252]

A graded program of regular exercise can improve fitness by 15% to 30 % in three to six months.[253]

252 Franco, O. H., de Laet, C., Peeters, A. *et al.* 2005, "Effects of physical activity on life expectancy with cardiovascular disease", *JAMA Internal Medicine*, Vol. 165, No. 20, pp. 2355-60, https://doi.org/10.1001/archinte.165.20.2355.

253 Pinckard, K., Baskin, K. K. & Stanford, K. I. 2019, "Effects of Exercise to Improve Cardiovascular Health", *Frontiers in Cardiovascular Medicine*, Vol. 6, p. 69, https://doi.org/10.3389/fcvm.2019.00069.

Women aged 75 to 93 years increased their strength by 24% to 30% with just 12 weeks of strength training (equivalent to a 'rejuvenation' of strength by 15-20 years).

Women aged 80 to 93 years produced a 15% mean increase in their aerobic power to weight ratio with 24 weeks of endurance training (equivalent to a 'rejuvenation' of endurance of 15 years).

The Women's Health Initiative Observational Study of 73,743 postmenopausal women[254] found that both walking and vigorous exercise are associated with substantial reductions in the incidence of cardiovascular events irrespective of ethnicity, age, or BMI and that prolonged sitting predicts increased cardiovascular risk.

Women aged 50 to 79 yrs. who engaged in 1.25 to 2.5 hours of brisk walking, or the equivalent had an 18% lower risk of breast cancer.[255]

A cohort of 44,452 US men enrolled in the Health Professionals' Follow-up Study were followed from 1986 through 1998, and the conclusions were that total physical activity and its intensity (running, rowing, weight training, and walking) were each associated with reduced CVS risk.[256]

In the most recent 2023 study[257] of over 500,000 cohorts, they sought the optimal combination of moderate aerobic

---

254 Manson, J. E., Greenland, P., LaCroix, A. Z. 2002, "Walking compared with vigorous exercise for the prevention of cardiovascular events in women", *New England Journal of Medicine*, Vol. 347, No. 10pp. 716-725, https://doi.org/10.1056/NEJMoa021067.

255 Mancini, M., Ordovas, J. M., Riccardi, G. *et al.* 2011, *Nutritional and Metabolic Bases of Cardiovascular Disease,* Wiley-Blackwell.

256 Lavie, C. J., Thomas, R. J., Squires, R. W. *et al.* 2009, "Exercise training and cardiac rehabilitation in primary and secondary prevention of coronary heart disease", *Mayo Clinic Proceedings*, Vol. 84, No. 4, pp. 373-83, https://doi.org/10.1016/S0025-6196(11)60548-X.

257 López-Bueno, R., Ahmadi, M. Stamatakis, E. *et al.* 2023, "Prospective Associations of Different Combinations of Aerobic and Muscle Strengthening Activity With All-Cause, Cardiovascular, and Cancer Mortality", *JAMA Internal Medicine,* Vol. 183, No. 9, pp. 982-990, https://doi.org/10.1001/jamainternmed.2023.3093.

physical activity (MPA), vigorous aerobic physical activity (VPA), and muscle-strengthening activity (MSA) to reduce the risk of all-cause, cardiovascular, and cancer mortality and concluded, "that balanced levels of MPA, VPA, and MSA combined may be associated with optimal reductions of mortality risk. Higher-than-recommended levels of MPA and VPA may further lower the risk of cancer and all-cause mortality, respectively.

A hazard ratio (HR) is the probability of an event in a treatment group relative to the control group probability over a unit of time. This ratio is an effect size measure for time-to-event data.

The category associated with the lowest hazard ratio (HR) for all-cause mortality was more than zero to 75 minutes of MPA combined with more than 150 minutes of VPA and two or more MSA sessions per week. The optimal combinations for CVD and cancer mortality risk reduction were more than 150 to 225 minutes of MPA, more than zero to 75 minutes of VPA, and two or more MSA sessions per week (and more than 300 minutes of MPA, more than 0 to 75 minutes of VPA, and 2 or more MSA sessions per week, respectively). Adjusted mortality rates represented an approximately 50% lower mortality rate for all-cause and cancer mortality and an approximately three-fold lower mortality rate for CVD mortality.

Fit & Not Fat

In 2015, as a further example of this new preventive evidence, one of the most extensive studies ever undertaken was published: 334,161 European men and women were followed for some 12.4 years, which, apparently, corresponded to over four million person-years. By any standards, this was a study of great worth and significance as, of course, were their findings. It called upon leading universities such as Cambridge and its equivalent universities of Europe to analyse the connection, if any, between physical activity and all-cause mortality for abdominal obesity. In layman's terms, it questioned whether being fat and sedentary led to premature death and if being active, and by what amount, allowed us live longer. Of course, their conclusions provided the best recommendations possible to date.[258]

Compared with people, 'Fit - Not Fat' taken as 0% reference, the risk of death is

Table 29: Fit and not fat.

	Risk of Death	
	Women	**Men**
Fit – Not Fat	0%	0%
Fit – Fat	32%	25%
Unfit – Not Fat	30%	44%
Unfit – Fat	57%	49%

Compression of Morbidity

Exercise plummets with age. For successful aging, the main aim is to compress or shorten any years of illness or disability, which invariably accompany our final years. At present, we spend as much as our last 20 years with such impositions. Keeping fit and mobile is a major contributor to successful aging and compression of morbidity.

258 Ekelund, U., Ward, H. A., Norat, T. *et al.* 2015, "Physical activity and all-cause mortality across levels of overall and abdominal adiposity in European men and women: the European Prospective Investigation into Cancer and Nutrition Study (EPIC)", *The American Journal of Clinical Nutrition*, Vol. 101, No. 3, pp. 613-21, https://doi.org/10.3945/ajcn.114.100065.

Table 30: Benefits of physical activity.

Reduced	**Increased**
All causes of death 30%	CVS - slowing of arterial aging
Osteoporosis	Post Infarct survival
Insomnia	Mobility
Stress - Depression	Wellbeing
Fat	Fitness
CAD	Disease prevention
Strokes/ cerebral haemorrhage	Balance
Diabetes 2	Health awareness
Osteoarthritis	Cognition. Lower dementia risk.
Lipids/cholesterol	Functional status
BP	Independence
Colon cancer	Social integration
Breast Ca-postmenopausal	Quality Of Life, Mood
Ovarian cancer	Disability free years
Gallstones	Total Life Expectancy
Constipation	Better sleep (not vigorous)
COPD	Better work efficiency (12.5%)
Chronic Fatigue Syndrome	Better sex (30% less ED. >female response)
Falls/ injuries	success to quit smoking doubles
	HDL cholesterol (good)

EuroPRevent 2016 Meeting

Compared to those who were inactive, older adults with low, medium and high activity levels had a 22%, 28%, and 35% lower risk of death, respectively.[259]

The more physical activity older adults do, the greater the health benefit. The biggest incremental jump in benefit was achieved at the low level of exercise, with the medium and high

259 European Society of Cardiology, 2016, "15 minutes daily exercise may be reasonable target in older adults", *ScienceDaily*, 14 June, www.sciencedaily.com/releases/2016/06/160614083104.htm.

levels bringing smaller increments of benefit. The low level of activity, which equates to a 15-minute brisk walk each day, which is half the recommended amount, was associated with a reduced risk of death in older adults compared with those who were inactive.

15 minutes a day keeps the undertaker at bay.
30 minutes a day keeps the doctor away.

Over a ten-year period, biobank participants who met recommended levels of physical activity had a 23% lower risk of cardiovascular disease, and the protective effects were even more pronounced in individuals with depression.[260]

Even Later-Life Exercise Reduces Mortality[261]

Regular exercise reduces the risk of death even when started in middle age, according to a study that measured the link between mortality and leisure time physical activity (LTPA). The results also show an association between LTPA and cause-specific mortality for the two leading causes of death, cardiovascular disease (CVD) and cancer, and that being inactive across early adulthood but increasing LTPA later at 40 to 61 years was associated with 16% to 43% risk reduction in mortality. These mortality benefits were comparable to those associated with maintaining LTPA in all age groups from adolescence and into adulthood.

260 Zureigat, H., Osborne, M. T., Abohashem, S. *et al.* 2024, "Effect of Stress-Related Neural Pathways on the Cardiovascular Benefit of Physical Activity", *Journal of the American College of Cardiology*, Vol. 83, No. 16, pp. 1543, https://doi.org/10.1016/j.jacc.2024.02.029.

261 Arem, H., Moore, S. C., Patel, A. *et al.* 2015, "Leisure Time Physical Activity and Mortality: A Detailed Pooled Analysis of the Dose-Response Relationship", *JAMA Internal Medicine,* Vol. 175, No. 6, pp. 959-967, https://doi.org/10.1001/jamainternmed.2015.0533.

Ages 40 to 79

Middle-aged and older adults, including those with cardiovascular disease and cancer, stand to gain substantial longevity benefits by becoming more physically active, irrespective of past physical activity levels and established risk factors—including overall diet quality, body mass index, blood pressure, triglycerides, and cholesterol.

Maintaining or increasing physical activity levels from a baseline equivalent to meeting the minimum public health recommendations has the greatest population health impact, with these trajectories being responsible for preventing nearly one in two deaths associated with physical inactivity. In addition to shifting the population towards meeting the minimum physical activity recommendations, public health efforts should also focus on the maintenance of physical activity levels, specifically preventing declines over mid- to late life.

Exercise—Physical Activity, Function, and Longevity Among the Very Old

A significant survival benefit was associated with initiating physical activity (PA) between ages 70 and 78 years *and* ages 78 and 85 years. Higher levels of PA, compared with being sedentary, did not show a dose-dependent association with mortality. The PA level at age 78 was associated with remaining independent while performing activities of daily living at age 85.[262]

262 Stessman, J., Hammerman-Rozenberg, R. & Cohen, A. 2009, "Physical Activity, Function, and Longevity Among the Very Old", *JAMA Internal Medicine*, Vol. 169, No. 16, pp. 1476-83, https://doi.org/10.1001/archinternmed.2009.248.

Table 31:

Age	Physically Active	Sedentary
	8 year mortality	
70	15.2	27.2
78	26.1	40.8
	3 year mortality	
85	6.8	24.4

Start Young

Aerobic fitness in adolescent males is associated with reduced risk for early death—but with no protective effect seen at BMIs of 35 or greater. Furthermore, the risk of early death was higher in fit obese individuals than in unfit normal-weight individuals.[263]

British Cyclists Study[264]

125 male and female cyclists, aged 55 to 79, who had maintained a high level of cycling throughout most of their adult lives, were studied.

Several body systems decline with age, such as muscle and bone. At mid-life, people start losing muscle mass and strength at a rate of 1% to 2% per year. Our bones also become thinner with age, and this can eventually lead to diseases such as osteoporosis.

The cyclists did not lose muscle mass or strength as they aged, and their bones only became slightly thinner.

263 Högström, G., Nordström, A. & Nordström, P. 2016, "Aerobic fitness in late adolescence and the risk of early death: a prospective cohort study of 1.3 million Swedish men", *International Journal of Epidemiology*, Vol. 45, No. 4, pp. 1159-1168, https://doi.org/10.1093/ije/dyv321.

264 Duggal, N. A., Pollock, R. D., Lazarus, N. R. *et al.* 2018, "Major features of immunesenescence, including reduced thymic output, are ameliorated by high levels of physical activity in adulthood", *Aging Cell*, Vol. 17, No. 2, https://doi.org/10.1111/acel.12750.

The immune system declines with age, making older adults more susceptible to infections such as flu and pneumonia and respond less well to vaccines.

When the immune systems of the cyclists were compared to older adults who had not done regular exercise, and to young people in their twenties, it was found that their immune systems looked most like the young persons'.

In particular, the cyclists still made lots of new immune T-cells, produced by an organ called the thymus, which normally starts to shrink after we reach puberty. The older cyclists seemed to have a thymus that was making as many new T cells as their younger counterparts. The lifelong cycling seemed to have slowed down the aging of their immune systems.

The cyclists had high levels of a hormone called interleukin 7 in their blood, which helps to stop the thymus from shrinking. Interleukin 7 is made by many cells in the body, including muscle cells, so it is thought that active muscles will make more of this hormone and keep the immune system, and especially the thymus, young.

Cholesterol and Exercise

Regular aerobic exercise modestly increases HDL levels.[265]

Cognitive Function

A clear dose-response relationship exists between exercise and cardiovascular fitness. Cardiorespiratory *fitness* response was a better predictor of cognitive gains than exercise duration.

265 Fogoros, R. N. 2022, "Exercise and HDL Cholesterol Levels", *Verywell Health*, 26 March.

Cardiovascular fitness may be the therapeutic target for achieving cognitive benefits.[266]

Physical activity linked to greater mental flexibility in older adults. Physically fit people tend to have larger brain volumes and more intact white matter than their less-fit peers. This variability is associated with better cognitive performance.

Key Messages

Health and functional benefits begin with any increase above lowest levels of activity; any activity is better than none. New guidelines now advise interspersing prolonged sitting with short bouts of standing and light activity. Small increases in moderate activity may enable older patients to get closer to the recommended 150 minutes per week. The new USA physical activity guidelines were updated in 2018 for the first time since 2008, and they still urge adults to do 75 minutes of vigorous (or 150 minutes of moderate) aerobic activity each week, plus muscle-strengthening sessions like weightlifting or yoga twice a week.[267]

Older women lowered their risk of dying early by 12% compared to their more sedentary peers with each 30-minute chunk of light activities. [268] Older men, each additional half hour

266 Vidoni, E. D., Johnson, D. K., Morris, J. K. *et al.* 2015, "Dose-Response of Aerobic Exercise on Cognition: A Community-Based, Pilot Randomized Controlled Trial", *PLOS One*, Vol. 10, No. 7, https://doi.org/10.1371/journal.pone.0131647.

267 Stamatakis, E., Straker, L., Hamer, M. & Gebel, K. 2019, "The 2018 Physical Activity Guidelines for Americans: What's New? Implications for Clinicians and the Public", *Journal of Orthopaedic & Sports Physical Therapy*, Vol. 49, No. 7, pp. 487-490, https://www.jospt.org/doi/10.2519/jospt.2019.0609.

268 "Light physical activity linked to lower risk of heart disease in older women", *NIH News*, 15 March 2019.

of light physical activity, such as walking or gardening, slashed their risk of early death by 17%.[269]

A study of over 334,000 European men and women found that twice as many deaths may be attributable to lack of physical activity compared with the number of deaths attributable to obesity, and just a modest increase in physical activity could have significant health benefits.[270]

Prolonged Sitting

There is now a clear need to reduce prolonged sitting. It is associated with higher mortality from all causes, as well as increased incidence of cancer, cardiovascular disease, and type 2 Diabetes, even among people who exercise regularly, according to a meta-analysis published in the January 20 issue of the *Annals of Internal Medicine*. However, the analysis of 47 previously published articles also shows that the association between all-cause mortality and sedentary behaviour is greatest among people who exercise the least.[271]

Move more and sit less.

---

269 Jefferis, B. J., Parsons, T. J., Sartini, C. *et al.* 2019, "Objectively measured physical activity, sedentary behaviour and all-cause mortality in older men: does volume of activity matter more than pattern of accumulation?", *British Journal of Sports Medicine,* Vol. 53, No. 16, pp. 1013-1020, https://doi.org/10.1136/bjsports-2017-098733.

270 Ekelund, U., Ward, H. A., Norat, T. *et al.* 2015, "Physical activity and all-cause mortality across levels of overall and abdominal adiposity in European men and women: the European Prospective Investigation into Cancer and Nutrition Study (EPIC)", *The American Journal of Clinical Nutrition*, Vol. 101, No. 3, pp. 613-21, https://doi.org/10.3945/ajcn.114.100065.

271 Biswas, A., Oh, P. I., Faulkner, G. E. *et al.* 2015, "Sedentary Time and Its Association With Risk for Disease Incidence, Mortality, and Hospitalization in Adults", *Annals Internal Medicine*, Vol. 162, No. 2, https://doi.org/10.7326/M14-1651.

Cancer Prevention

High vs. low levels of physical activity engagement are associated with reduced risk of 13 cancer types (including three of the top four leading cancers among men and women worldwide). The widespread generalizability of these findings is reinforced by the suggestion that the associations persist regardless of BMI or smoking status.[272]

My Personal Preferences (At My Age)

HIIPA: High Intensity Incidental Physical Activity and Walking Faster

These activities are where you can start immediately, and you can continue them every day from now on.

HIIPA uses normal lifestyle practices, without disrupting your daily schedule, to get fit. The idea is to optimize and maximise routines, e.g., walk faster, walk longer distances, take the stairs, get up and down from your desk or TV more frequently, use shopping as an opportunity to lift weights, but, above all, don't resent any of these activites. Rather, embrace them and seek other ways you can incorporate exercise into your daily life.

The Italian Study cited at the start of this chapter encourages me to walk faster.

Daily activities/necessities you can crank-up:

- Walk to work—or even 2 blocks. Walk fast.
- Walk briskly, everywhere, every time.
- Always walk if < 1 km.

---

272 Moore, S. C., Lee, I. M., Weiderpass, E. *et al.* 2016, "Association of Leisure-Time Physical Activity With Risk of 26 Types of Cancer in 1.44 Million Adults", *JAMA Internal Medicine*, Vol. 176, No. 6, pp. 816-825, https://doi.org/10.1001/jamainternmed.2016.1548.

- Walk the dog—you lead!
- Gardening—do more
- Participate in sports you love. No drive-thrus.
- No remotes.
- Have walking breaks.
- Taking 2,000 steps/day (15 min) controls weight.
- Take several trips to unload your groceries. Use them as weights ("curls").
- Regular exercise in men aged 45–75 (or even 83).
- Exercise reduced waist and body fat while weight remained the same.
- Insulin response to glucose improved by 16%.[273]

This may help prevent Diabetes 2/metabolic syndrome.

Kids who cycle to school are 8% fitter than those who walk.[274]

Ten to 15 minutes of cycling twice a day is enough to increase kid's aerobic fitness.

Take the Stairs

Climbing more than five flights of stairs daily is associated with a reduced risk of atherosclerotic cardiovascular disease (ASCVD) of about 20%, observational data suggest.[275] (A flight was regarded as 10 steps, and the more the effort required, probably the better the result).

273 Bird, S. R. & Hawley, J. A. 2017, "Update on the effects of physical activity on insulin sensitivity in humans", *BMJ Open Sport & Exercise Medicine*, Vol. 2, No. 1, https://doi.org/10.1136/bmjsem-2016-000143.

274 Andersen, L. B. 2007, "Physical activity and health", *BMJ*, Vol. 334, No. 7605, p. 1173. https://doi.org/10.1136/bmj.39225.414537.80.

275 Song, Z., Wan, L., Wang, W. *et al.* 2023, "Daily stair climbing, disease susceptibility, and risk of atherosclerotic cardiovascular disease: A prospective cohort study", *Atherosclerosis*, Vol. 386, No. 117300, https://doi.org/10.1016/j.atherosclerosis.2023.117300.

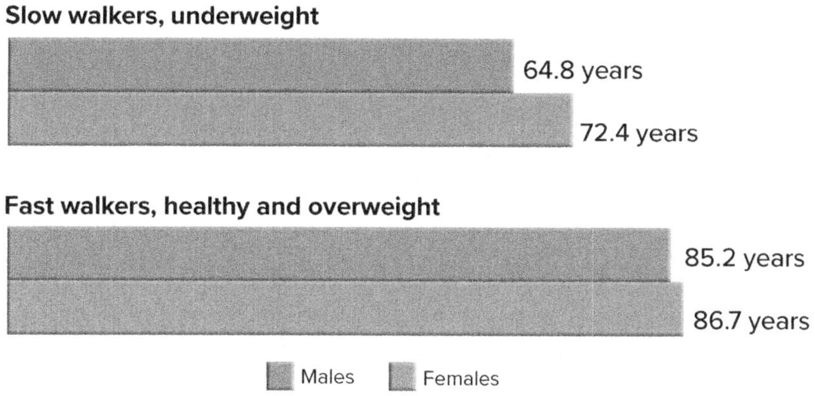

Figure 38: How walking can help you live longer. A brisk walking speed has been linked to a longer life span – even for people who are overweight. 2,337 daily steps are enough to cut the risk of premature death. 3,967 steps a day reduce the risk of dying from any cause (*Source: Tom Yates, University of Leicester*).

Timing

Moderate to vigorous physical activity timing, particularly in the evening, was consistently associated with the lowest risk of mortality relative to other timing windows.[276]

Risks

There are significant risks with sudden, unaccustomed exercise, so start slowly and have a graded plan.

Cease if distressed in any way.

There is also the risk of getting 'hooked' on the endomorphine high, as with compulsive trainers.

276 Sabag, A., Ahmadi, M. N., Francois, M. E. *et al.* 2024, "Timing of Moderate to Vigorous Physical Activity, Mortality, Cardiovascular Disease, and Microvascular Disease in Adults With Obesity", *Diabetes Care,* Vol. 47, No. 5, pp. 890-897, https://doi.org/10.2337/dc23-2448.

Scams

10,000 steps a day

The origin of clocking up 10,000 steps every day comes from Japan, back in 1965, when a device called Manpo-kei was sold. It was a pedometer – an instrument designed to measure how many steps you take – and its name literally translates to "10,000 steps meter".

It's likely that this number was entirely arbitrary. Nobody has been able to ascertain that this number was based on any kind of science, especially since even now, the science around how many steps we need to take in a day is up for debate.

The Water Bottle and two litres/eight glasses a day

Prior to the ubiquitous water bottle, you must have seen the bodies of all those people beside the road where they died from dehydration?

No?

That is because selling water and water bottles is a scam. Our body is an incredibly sophisticated piece of engineering that maintains 'homeostasis' or keeps everything in balance. Part of this system is controlling our body water, and to that end, we have our own in-built, exquisitely sensitive meter. It's called 'thirst'.

Drink only when you are thirsty.

Or you can over-guzzle water from a plastic bottle. Researchers from Columbia University and Rutgers University found roughly 240,000 detectable plastic fragments in a typical litre of bottled water. About 10% of the detected plastic particles were microplastics, and the other 90% were Nanoplastics.

SECTION G

WHAT'S NEW?

Age, it has been observed, remains the biggest threat to our health. As time passes, our fertility declines, and our bodies start to fail. These natural changes are what we call aging.

In recent decades, we've come leaps and bounds in treating and preventing some of the world's leading age-related diseases, such as coronary heart disease.

But some research takes an entirely unique view on the role of science in easing the burden of aging, focusing instead of trying to slow it down, stop it, reverse it—and some even seek immortality. These may seem like ideas reserved mainly for cranks and science fiction writers, but they're not.

Aging or growth pathways are being increasingly identified, and potential alterations to influence them seem increasingly possible.

CHAPTER 36

The Hallmarks of Aging: Anti-aging, Longevity, Successful Aging & Extended Lifespan

"You are old, Father William," the young man said,
"And your hair has become very white;
And yet you incessantly stand on your head-
Do you think, at your age, it is right?"

– Lewis Carroll, *Alice in Wonderland* 1865.

Anti-Aging vs. Longevity vs. Successful Aging and the Hallmarks of Aging

Definitions

Anti-aging is trying to look younger and delay the visible changes of age.

Successful Aging is the effective coping with, and optimizing of, these changes.

The long and complete definition is: Optimization of present health and fitness to minimize any illnesses and disabilities, to stay mentally alert, active, healthy, independent and socially integrated, with the capacity to cope with change, for the whole of our predicted lifespan, with respect to personal, social, spiritual, emotional economic goals and restrictions.

Longevity is not dying prematurely.

Extended Lifespan is living longer than presently recorded limits.

2002 Statement by 51 Pre-eminent Scientists

> "Since recorded history individuals have been, and are continuing to be, victimised by promises of extended youth or increased longevity by using unproven methods that allegedly slow, stop or reverse aging.
>
> "There are no lifestyle changes, surgical procedures, vitamins, antioxidants, hormones or genetic engineering available today that do so.
>
> "What medical science can tell us is that because age and death are not programmed into our genes, health and fitness can be enhanced at any age, primarily through avoidance of behaviour (such as smoking, excess alcohol, excess sun & obesity) that accelerate aging and adopt behaviours (such as exercise & a healthy diet) that advantage of a physiology that is inherently modifiable."[277]

Update

The above Statement was made over 20 years ago in 2002.

277 Melzer, D., Pilling, L. C. & Ferrucci, L. 2020, "The genetics of human aging", *Nature Reviews Genetics*, Vol. 21, No. 2, pp. 88-101, https://doi.org/10.1038/s41576-019-0183-6.

Since then, however, at least in mice, research has found that the *aging pathways can be intervened and are malleable* such that life (in mice) can be extended by up to 29%.[278]

Research has now found there are some two diets, four (maybe six) drugs, and three mutations that slow aging. Researchers are focusing on finding if there is a common or shared mechanism by which this may happen, and a protein molecule called GPLD1, which stimulates neurogenesis and brain health in mice, is of interest. It is manufactured in the liver and in fat and is stimulated by exercise.

While anti-aging and successful aging are different, there are places they overlap. Anti-aging is the pursuit of looking younger and, if possible, slowing down the aging process, whereas successful aging is the acceptance that age changes are inevitable but remaining fit, healthy, functional, and happy without any major financial impediments can make our lives better. Longevity, and here I propose *Live Longer* offers a unique contribution and promotes maximum lifespan by identifying, prioritizing, and preventing illnesses that may kill us prematurely. But obviously, people who are determined to look young have a vested interest in optimizing their health and welfare.

Extended lifespan at this time is thought to be potentially achievable with drugs.

Anti-aging

This term implies the pro-active pursuits to delay, minimize, or disguise the changes of aging.

These may include ensuring best-evidenced health recommendations, non-invasive to invasive procedures, cosmetic

278 Miller, R. 2022, "Longevity Supplements", Interventions Testing Program, U-Tube, Live Longer World, 12 April.

procedures, and therapies in an attempt to enhance our appearance to look younger—but often, with expenditure on unproven procedures, supplements, nutraceuticals, cosmetics, and the frankly bizarre.

Nothing has, so far, been proven.

Do not be disheartened, though, as it has been pointed out that health and fitness can be enhanced at any age.

Perhaps anti-aging is best achieved by not abusing ourselves with high-risk behaviors. Sun-damage and smoking ages our skin prematurely and poor diet is consistently responsible for more disease and death than physical inactivity, smoking, and alcohol combined.

Premature Aging

Normal Aging vs. Accelerated Aging

While, at present, lifespan cannot be extended, it can be optimized and maximized. Most "age changes" are, in effect, premature aging due to abuse, damage, or neglect to our bodies. Most gains in length of life have been achieved by treating diseases that used to kill us at birth or in our youth.

Premature or Accelerated Aging

While we can see the premature skin aging of sun damage and smoking, we can't see the damage a bad diet is doing to the insides of our coronary arteries. Even a little amount of sun and smoke, even second-hand smoke, causes early damage we can see. Both the sun and smoke actually damage our cellular DNA and compromise our immune system.

Women, especially, who smoke develop fine 'papercut' vertical wrinkles or rhytids, on their top lip and deeper wrinkles, crows' feet, and pigment spots from the sun on their cheeks.

Smoking also damages the collagen structure and support for facial skin, such that the cheeks sag and they look at least a decade older than their actual age. It is not a quantum leap to translate this to the whole of our bodies. Both the sun and the smoke also have a profound immune-compromising effect on the whole body—the skin probably reflects equal damage to the coronary arteries and whole internal health.

Prevention

If we can *prevent* damage and illness, at all stages and ages, then we optimize our health and longevity.

1. Avoidance of high-risk behaviours
2. Adopting a beneficial lifestyle
3. Immediately repair even minor damage or illness
4. Identification of age-sex incidence of likely illnesses

Biological Age

It is purported that different parts of our body, different organs and tissues, age at different rates. While we may be 50 years of age, our heart may only be 40 years old, according to how well it is functioning.

Of course, this concept is intriguing, which has seen the biohackers place great emphasis on this as they strive to turn back their biological clock. But what if the test came back that our heart was 60 years old, our brain 70, and so on?

And how is it measured?

Our bodies consist of an estimated 37 trillion different cells of 200 different types.[279]

279 Roy, A. L. & Conroy, R. S. 2018, "Toward mapping the human body at a cellular resolution", *Molecular Biology of the Cell,* Vol. 29, No. 15, pp. 1779-1785, https://doi.org/10.1091/mbc.E18-04-0260.

At present there is no agreed measurements or standards but research continues apace and it is inevitable that accurate Biological Aging measurements for our different organs and tissues is inevitable,

Aging has been reduced to the cellular level and, over the last decade or so, some 12 Hallmarks of Aging have been proposed. These cellular hallmarks each have their own proponents.

Wear and Tear: Thermal Motion

It has been pointed out[280] that the internal milieu of our bodies and cells is a dynamic, violent thermal chaos with thousands of water molecules randomly crashing into these cellular structures a trillion times a second. And while this thermal motion provides energy, it also breaks bonds between molecules, which suggests 'wear and tear' as the basis of aging.

Leonard Hayflick, PhD,[281] found our DNA cells could only replicate some 50 times (the 'Hayflick Limit') before they became senescent. Further, proteins are the essential building blocks for our bodies, but studies have shown that transcription of DNA into proteins is compromised as we age.[282] Modern medicine, good nutrition, and such, as enumerated in this book, can optimise and maximise our lives, but this wear and tear means that our bodies eventually wear out and have a use-by date.

280 Fowler, S. & Roush, R. 2013, *Concepts of Biology*, OpenStax.

281 Eissenberg, J. C. 2013, "Telomeres, cancer & aging: live long & prosper?", *Missouri Medicine*, Vol. 110, No. 1, pp. 11-6.

282 Gyenis, A., Chang, J., Demmers, J. J. P. G. *et al.* 2023, "Genome-wide RNA polymerase stalling shapes the transcriptome during aging", *Nature Genetetics*, Vol. 55, No. (2), pp. 268-279, https://doi.org/10.1038/s41588-022-01279-6.

Measurements

At this time, there is no agreed-upon standard when it comes to measuring biological age. Several approaches to quantifying biological age are used, including physical or functional measures such as appearance, blood pressure, EKG stress tests, lung capacity, VO_2max, grip strength, walking speed, nerve conductance studies, bone density, waist-hip ratio, and cognition. Different aspects of mitochondrial function appear to be responsible, while the gut microbiome loses complexity in tandem with the host as biological age increases, with likely impact on host metabolism and immunity.

No Definitive Tests: What Do You Want It to Be?

While it would seem robust and accurate biological aging of different organs and systems will be developed, there are, at present, a wide variety of results from labs touting for business. It reminds me of the "Creative Accounting" joke when a businessman asks the accountant what his income must be to minimise tax and the accountant answers, "What do you want it to be?".

Then, there are biomarkers in the form of blood test-serum analytes such as epigenetic markers, telomere length, or inflammatory markers —but, as yet no definitive tests exist.

The Epigenetic Clock

In 2013, geneticist Steve Horvath, Ph.D., while at UCLA, found he could estimate someone's age by using DNA methylation. He spent over four years collecting publicly available Illumina DNA methylation data and identifying suitable statistical methods. He used saliva/spittle. However, in an interview for Insider by Hilary Brueck in October 2023, Dr. Horvath said that biological clocks are more of a novelty—a fun measurement that people shouldn't take too seriously and that accurate biological measurements 'are not there yet'.

Methylation

Methylation are the chemical modifications that occur in DNA and other molecules that may be retained as cells divide to make more cells. They are influenced by genetics, lifestyle and environment; there are 28 million locations in the human body where this can happen.

Estimates of biological age based on DNA methylation patterns, often referred to as "epigenetic age" or "DNA age", have been shown to be the most robust biomarkers of age in humans.[283]

In a newer method, scientists measure someone's age-related changes through 10,000 plasma proteins in a fraction of a drop of blood.

However, it has been found that biological age may increase over relatively short time periods in response to stress, but this increase is transient and trends back toward baseline following recovery from stress. Transient changes in biological age also occurred during major surgery, pregnancy, and severe COVID-19 in humans or mice. Trauma patients experienced a strong and rapid increase in biological age following emergency surgery. Nevertheless, this increase was reversed and biological age was restored to baseline in the days following the surgery. Similarly, pregnant subjects experienced postpartum recovery of biological age at varying rates and magnitudes, and an immunosuppressive

283 Chen, B. H., Marioni, R. E., Colicino, E. *et al.* 2016, "DNA methylation-based measures of biological age: meta-analysis predicting time to death", *Aging,* Vol. 8, No. 9, pp. 1844-1865, https://doi.org/10.18632/aging.101020.

drug called tocilizumab enhanced the biological age recovery of convalescent COVID-19 patients. The findings imply that severe stress increases mortality, at least in part, by increasing biological age.[284]

If you want to get a helpful assessment of your health status, Dr. Horvath says visiting a doctor and having a thorough exam—weight, blood pressure, full blood panel (cholesterol, blood sugar)—is still the way to go. "Tests that are commercially available should not be taken to be more meaningful than a doctor's assessment," he says. "Getting an epigenetic test may give an individual the wrong answer and cause that person to become overly worried or stressed."[285]

Matt Kaeberlein, has tried DNA methylation tests that put his biological age in a range from 36 to 59. He is 52. "These tests are for entertainment value only," he said.[286]

The online companies or calculators that offer biological age estimates, at this point, experts say their validity is shaky.

However, it would seem biological aging of various tissues and organs will become increasingly accurate and be a useful measurement in the near future.

Cellular Focus

There have been ongoing theories as to why and how we age, but today, most research has focused on our cellular metabolism and pathways. There are, as below, some twelve distinct fields of interest within a cell.

---

284 Poganik, J. R., Zhang, B., Baht, G. S. *et al.* 2023, "Biological age is increased by stress and restored upon recovery", *Cell Metabolism*, Vol. 35, No. 5, pp. 807-820, https://doi.org/10.1016/j.cmet.2023.03.015.

285 Heid, M. 2023, "What Is Biological Age?", *Everyday Health*, 28 September, https://www.everydayhealth.com/longevity/what-is-biological-age/

286 Mosbergen, D. 2023, "What is my Biological Age?", *Wall Street Journal*, 23 October.

The overarching reasoning is to stop or reverse the deterioration in some, or even all, of these.

They are listed here FYI, as their biochemistry is complex and has even won a Nobel Prize, but I do think it helpful, as in your medical consultation/appendix, if you know what your tests do, what they are for, and if they are necessary and beneficial.

I have, however, gone into a little detail for those who are interested.

Evolutionary Biology of Aging, defined aging, in 1991, as "a persistent decline in age-specific fitness components of an organism due to internal physiological deterioration."[287]

But as you will have read, there is no agreement among longevity researchers as to what aging is and what biomarkers there are to use.

The Hallmarks of Aging

The framework for the Hallmarks of Aging was proposed in 2013 and set out a list of the biological underpinnings of the aging process—the causes behind everything from wrinkles to cancer.[288]

A framework might not sound like a breakthrough, but it really is. After decades of theories and counter-theories, there's finally some scientific agreement about what causes aging, and that means, if we can learn to slow, stop, or reverse these hallmarks, we can do the same to the aging process overall.

In fact, the rest of the breakthroughs on this list follow exactly this approach: slowing or stopping the progression of one of these hallmarks and, with it, aging overall.

287 Rose, M. R., Flatt, T., Graves, J. L. *et al.* 2012, "What is Aging?", *Frontiers in Genetics*, Vol. 3, https://doi.org/10.3389/fgene.2012.00134.

288 López-Otín, C., Blasco, M. A., Partridge, L. *et al.* 2013, "The hallmarks of aging", *Cell*, Vol. 153, No. 6, pp. 1194-217, https://doi.org/10.1016/j.cell.2013.05.039.

This focussed attention on *cellular biochemical changes*, as distinct from the many other views as to aging and pointed to the directions for future longevity research.

The twelve hallmarks of aging:

1. Genomic Instability
2. Telomere Attrition
3. Cellular Senescence
4. Epigenetic Alterations
5. Loss of Proteostasis: Misfolded proteins
6. Deregulated Nutrient Sensing
7. Mitochondrial Dysfunction
8. Stem Cell Exhaustion
9. Altered Intercellular Communication
10. Disabled Macroautophagy
11. Chronic Inflammation
12. Dysbiosis

A **Genotype** is a person's unique sequence of DNA.

A **Phenotype** is the detectable expression of this genotype—a patient's clinical presentation. A person's phenotype results from the interaction between their genotype and their environment.

The connection between genotype and phenotype is not always clear-cut.

1. Genomic Instability

Genes are the instructions for making the protein building blocks of the body.

The human genome encodes approximately 20 000 proteins. Understandably enough, investigations have concentrated on genes and proteins whose function is known. However, the human "unknome", the one fifth of human genes whose purpose remains mysterious, shouldn't be ignored. In experiments with

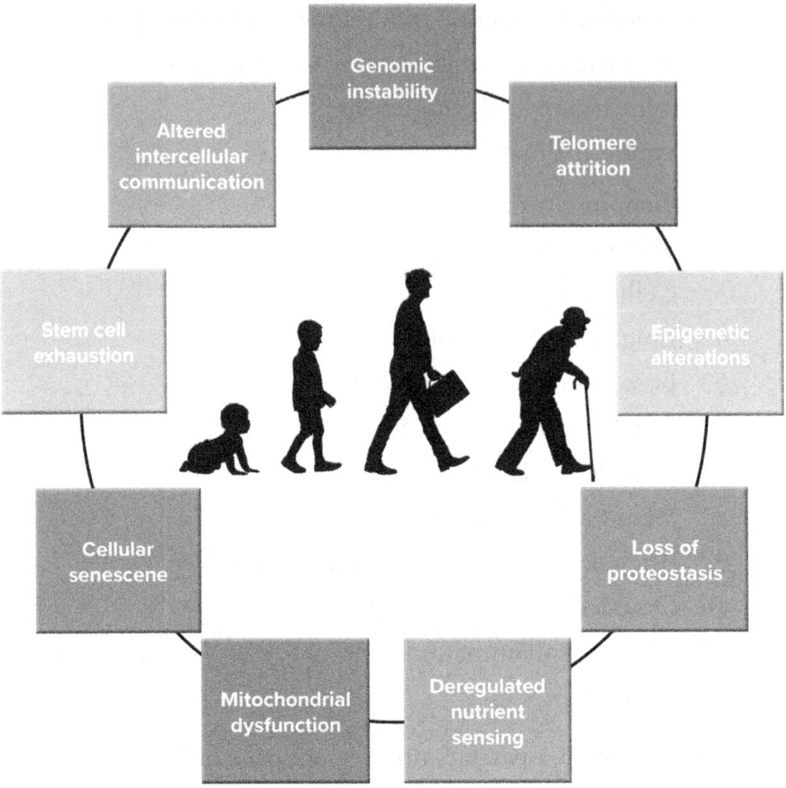

Figure 39: Hallmarks of aging (*Source: Wikipedia*).

fruit flies, removing one of these mystery genes caused the insects to die. The compilers of a new database of genes with unknown functions hope it will widen the focus of genetic research.[289]

In 2013, the Supreme Court of America ruled 9-0 that human genes were products of nature, not intellectual property, and that exclusive patent rights over genes should never be granted to anyone. This meant laboratories are not restricted by the existence of previous gene patents. Whole exome and genome

289 Rocha, J. J., Jayaram, S. A., Stevens, T. J. *et al.* 2023, "Functional unknomics: Systematic screening of conserved genes of unknown function", *PLOS Biology*, Vol. 21, No. 8, https://doi.org/10.1371/journal.pbio.3002222.

sequencing, which evaluates a large number of genes or the full genome, is an important option for paediatric genetic testing for rare diseases.

Multi-gene analysis has quickly become the standard of care and led to the choice of 286 targeted therapies in 2020, more than three times as many as were available in 2012. These advances were only made possible because information about thousands of genes and sequences in human health and disease can be incorporated into a single test. It has also opened the gate for longevity studies.

The Human Genome Project commenced in 1990, unveiled its first readout of the human DNA sequence in 2000, and was declared essentially complete in 2003. However, it took nearly 20 more years before the final, complete version was released.

This did not mark the end of humankind's genetic puzzle, however, and new study, by Matthew Freeman of the Dunn School of Pathology at the University of Oxford, a co-author, has mapped the gap between reading our genes and understanding them. Vast parts of the genome, areas the study authors have nicknamed the "unknome", are made of genes whose function are still unknown. This has important implications for medicine: Plenty of those still shrouded in darkness could have profound medical significance and may hold the keys to disorders of development, cancer, neurodegeneration, and more.

The genome is the entire set of DNA instructions found in a cell. In humans, the genome consists of 23 pairs of chromosomes located in the cell's nucleus, as well as a small chromosome in the cell's mitochondria. A genome contains all the information needed for an individual to develop and function.

Our cells protect our DNA in thick-walled cells, but even so, free radicals, pollutants, pesticides, and the sun's UV rays all attack our DNA such that it eventually breaks down.

The changes to DNA, known as somatic mutations, can impact the way blood stem cells work and are associated with blood cancers and other age-related conditions. DNA mutations throughout a person's life can significantly increase their biological age and susceptibility to heart conditions.[290]

Longevity and healthy aging are among the most complex phenotypes studied to date. The heritability of age at death in adulthood is approximately 25%. Studies of exceptionally long-lived individuals show that heritability is greatest at the oldest ages. Linkage studies of exceptionally long-lived families now support a longevity locus on chromosome 3; other putative longevity loci differ between studies. Candidate gene studies have identified variants at APOE and FOXO3A associated with longevity; other genes show inconsistent results.[291]

One finding suggests that longevity is transmitted for at least two subsequent generations only when at least 20% of all relatives are long-lived. This proves the importance of family data to avoid phenocopies in genetic studies.[292]

"Most genetic tests today are not regulated, meaning that they go to market without any independent analysis to verify the claims of the seller," according to the National Human Genome Research Institute.

290 Robertson, N. A., Hillary, R. F., McCartney, D. L. *et al.* 2019, "Age-related clonal haemopoiesis is associated with increased epigenetic age", *Current Biology*, Vol. 29, No. 16, pp. R786-R787, https://doi.org/10.1016/j.cub.2019.07.011.

291 Brooks-Wilson, A. R. 2013, "Genetics of healthy aging and longevity", *Human Genetics*, Vol. 132, No. 12, pp. 1323-38, https://doi.org/10.1007/s00439-013-1342-z.

292 van den Berg, N., Rodríguez-Girondo, M., Mandemakers, K. *et al.* 2020, "Longevity Relatives Count score identifies heritable longevity carriers and suggests case improvement in genetic studies", *Aging Cell*, Vol. 19, No. 6, https://doi.org/10.1111/acel.13139.

Scientists have successfully improved the lifespan of mice by transferring a gene from naked mole rats responsible for longevity. Researchers at the University of Rochester genetically modified mice to produce the naked mole rat version of the HAS2 gene. This led to improved health and an approximate 4.4% increase in the median lifespan of the modified mice, which were also more cancer resistant. The study provides a proof of principle that unique longevity[293] mechanisms that evolved in long-lived mammalian species can be exported to improve the lifespans of other mammals.

The Human Genome Project had spent $2.7 billion mapping our DNA by 2003, promising personalised and then precision medicine, but the gains have been small, diverting money which has recently been argued could be better spent on preventive medicine.[294]

Geneticists believed humans had some 100,000 genes and that just one or two might be responsible for the likes of Diabetes, Parkinson's, cancer, and even longevity itself (with scientists locating the Methuselah gene—a stretch of DNA that confers healthy old age in men and women). Instead, we have only about 20,000 genes, which means diseases are more likely caused by combinations of dozens or even hundreds of genes, and it is argued that most genomic studies have tiny illness effect sizes.

An exception is women with a *BRCA1* mutation have a 60%–80% risk of developing breast cancer, but most don't seem to have very much predictive power over and above what you can get in five minutes in the doctor's office, where a study suggested

293 Zhang, Z., Tian, X., Lu, J. Y. *et al.* 2023, "Increased hyaluronan by naked mole-rat Has2 improves healthspan in mice", *Nature,* Vol. 621, No. 7977, pp. 196-205, https://doi.org/10.1038/s41586-023-06463-0.

294 Tabery, J. 2023, *Tyranny of the Gene: Personalized Medicine and Its Threat to Public Health*, KNOPF US.

these scores contribute only 1% to the prediction of ischaemic heart disease.[295] Patients knowing they have a genetic risk is not a great behavioural motivator.

2. Telomere Attrition

Inside our cells, our DNA is split into 46 lengths known as chromosomes. Telomeres are protective tips at the end of each chromosome. Human cells will divide no more than 55 times in cell culture. This so-called Hayflick limit was later found to be linked to the shortening of telomeres, caps of DNA at the ends of chromosomes that prevent them from falling apart. Each time a cell copies its chromosomes and divides, its telomeres shorten slightly. Once they have worn away completely, the cell either dies or enters a twilight-zone, no longer dividing but still alive. This fate became known as cell senescence, further accelerating the aging process. This discovery won the Nobel Prize.

Research suggest that telomere length and epigenetic clock (see below) estimates are independent predictors of chronological age and mortality risk.[296]

Some people are born with longer telomeres, owing to genetic inheritance and maternal health. Environmental and lifestyle factors also significantly affect the rate at which telomeres shorten as people age. Smoking, excessive drinking, pollution, stress, social isolation, and eating processed foods, among other things, create oxidative stress, which causes telomeres to shorten faster. Oxidative stress also causes direct damage to tissue.

---

295 Salzberg, S. L. 2018, "Open questions: How many genes do we have?", *BMC Biology*, Vol. 16, https://doi.org/10.1186/s12915-018-0564-x.

296 Marioni, R. E., Harris, S. E., Shah, S. *et al.* 2018, "The epigenetic clock and telomere length are independently associated with chronological age and mortality", *International Journal of Epidemiology*, Vol. 45, No. 2, pp. 424-432, https://doi.org/10.1093/ije/dyw041, erratum in *International Journal of Epidemiology*, Vol. 47, No. 1, p. 356.

Physical activity, high levels of social support, and healthy diets rich in antioxidants can slow the rate at which telomeres shorten and reduce oxidative stress.

Numerous studies have found an association between telomere length and heart disease, cancer, cognitive decline, and other aging-related diseases. A JAMA study published in July 2023 found shorter telomeres were associated with symptoms of depression, cognitive problems, and higher levels of the inflammatory cytokine IL-6—secreted by senescent cells—among physically healthy seniors between 60 and 79.[297]

One longevity strategy is to elongate telomeres, but some scientists worry this could cause cancer. Whereas preventing telomeres from shortening and dying (telomerase) could also produce cancerous cells that can replicate indefinitely.

Telomere shortening[298] research findings can only allow a rough estimate of aging rate and can hardly be regarded as a clinically important risk marker for age-related pathologies and mortality.

3. Cellular Senescence

Humans' risk of death doubles every eight years. However, some animals live for very long times, and one is regarded as immortal.

Longer Living Animals

The oldest living land animal is a 191-year-old Seychelles giant tortoise (Aldabrachelys gigantea hololissa) named Jonathan, who

297 Han, M. H., Lee, E. H., Park, H. H. *et al.* 2023, "Relationship between telomere shortening and early subjective depressive symptoms and cognitive complaints in older adults", *Aging*, Vol. 15, No. 4, pp. 914-931, https://doi.org/10.18632/aging.204533.

298 Vaiserman, A. & Krasnienkov, D. 2021, "Telomere Length as a Marker of Biological Age: State-of-the-Art, Open Issues, and Future Perspectives", *Frontiers Genetics*, Vol. 11, https://doi.org/10.3389/fgene.2020.630186.

lives on St. Helena island, has no sense of smell, and is almost blind but has acute hearing and was brought back from the brink of death by the island vet, Jonathan Hollins[299], fed the tortoise a diet of fresh fruit and vegetables, which supplied him with all the vitamins, minerals, and micronutrients needed. Both Jonathons then combined, with the elder donating his DNA saliva for longevity/anti-cancer DNA tests via the USAF to Vanderbilt University Medical Center in Nashville, USA.

Most long living animals, however, are marine animals, often at great depths where conditions are stable and constant.

Greenland sharks (Somniosus microcephalus): researchers suggested that the sharks could be up to 512 years old.

The Bowhead Whale lives up to 200 years.

Freshwater pearl mussels (Margaritifera margaritifera): the oldest was 280 years old.

Ocean quahog clams (Arctica islandica): one found in 2006 was 507 years old.

The red sea urchins probably live more than 100 years, and the longest living may be around 200 years old,

Escarpia laminata, a cold-seep species of tube worm, regularly lives up to 200 years—and some for more than 300 years.

Hexactinellid Sponges are in deep (>1000 m) oceans and can live to be at least 220 years old. The current thinking and research is that DNA degradation has caused humans to lose the repair ability of these long-living animals.

Cellular senescence is a normal process. When a cell endures irreparable DNA damage or telomere dysfunction in response to endogenous and exogenous stresses, it no longer has the ability to divide, leading to its death, which prevents those damaged traits from proliferating further. As such, this process is, initially, a protective mechanism.

---

299 Hollins, J. 2023, *Vet at the End of the Earth*, Duckworth Books Ltd.

However, when senescent cells outnumber new replacement cells, it has a causative role in conditions associated with aging with a loss of tissue-repair capacity and proinflammatory molecules. Drugs to get rid of these excessive senescent cells are 'senolytics', stimulating much research.

A Further Note on Senescence

Over time, large numbers of old (or senescent) cells can build up in tissues throughout the body. These cells remain active and can release a complex cocktail of signalling molecules, which mobilise nearby immune cells and promote inflammation. This potent stew is called the senescence-associated secretory phenotype (SASP).

Senescence may play a role in the development of cancer and other diseases and is a leading cause of numerous age-related conditions. Senescent cells are present in living humans and become more abundant with age and have been linked with various age-related conditions, including Alzheimer's disease, osteoporosis, Diabetes, liver cirrhosis, and renal and cardiovascular disease.

Senescence initially evolved as an intrinsic defence against cancer: if old or damaged cells can no longer replicate, they can't proliferate uncontrollably. But it was a mystery why they didn't just activate apoptosis or programmed cell death. The answer was that, in people roughly under 50, at least, senescent cells play a key role in the repair of damaged tissues. They then enter this zombie-like state, inducing an immune response that kills them and cleans up wider damage to the tissue, clearing the way for replacement by new cells. As we get older, however, this process gradually diminishes and eventually backfires. As more and more cells reach the Hayflick limit or get damaged and enter senescence—including the immune cells that perform the clean-up—the sheer quantity of senescent cells overwhelms the body's ability to clear them out, and they accumulate.

Senescence was also found to be triggered by external insults, too, such as DNA damage from UV radiation or chemicals, physical injuries, and attacks by viruses or bacteria.

Unfortunately, these cells don't just sit there, benignly not dividing. We all accumulate these cells throughout our lives: they're cells that have divided too many times, accrued unacceptable levels of damage to their DNA or are just under too high a level of stress. And so, to be on the safe side, these cells stop dividing. But they secrete molecules that basically conspire to accelerate the aging process. As we age, these cells increase in number in a vicious cycle of degeneration.

Accumulation of senescent cells is associated with frailty, cardiovascular disease, obesity, Diabetes, cognitive decline, and other age- and/or chronic disease-related disorders, suggesting that senescent cells are a target for intervention and rejuvenation.

They proved very resistant to dying, so, in an attempt to clear them out of the body, researchers at the Mayo Clinic set out to discover compounds that could reactivate apoptosis, focusing on safe, natural compounds and drugs already approved for human use. In 2015, they reported a double success with a cancer drug called dasatinib (D) and a plant compound called quercetin (Q).[300] Both killed senescent cells in cell cultures, and a combination of the two was more powerful than either alone. When old mice were given D+Q, it significantly rejuvenated them. Two years later, the researchers found similar success with the combination of another cancer drug, navitoclax, and a plant compound, fisetin. Together, these treatments were dubbed senolytics.

300 Zhu, Y., Tchkonia, T., Pirtskhalava, T. *et al*, 2015, "The Achilles' heel of senescent cells: From transcriptome to senolytic drugs", *Aging Cell*, Vol. 14, No. 4, pp. 644–658. https://doi.org/10.1111/acel.12344.

In animals, senolytics were found to be effective at extending both healthspan and lifespan. They also slowed the progression of numerous age-related conditions or reversed the damage caused by them, including dementia, frailty, and cardiovascular disease, among others. Scientists have identified a number of drugs and other treatments that get rid of these errant cells in mice. They extend healthy life, defer cancer and heart problems, and even give these mice better fur.

Senescent cells are thus a target for efforts to slow, halt, or even reverse aging. Numerous drugs being researched. These senolytic drugs are agents that selectively induce apoptosis of senescent cells.

The first senolytics are beginning trials in humans. If everything goes to plan, it might only be a few years before the first senolytic treatments are approved for diseases from arthritis to cancer.

And, if those trials show that these drugs are safe and effective, it might not be many more years before we're all taking senolytic drugs to remove these cells before the problems they cause have arisen. This should be the endgame of medicines inspired by aging biology: preventative medicine that, rather than fighting a disease we've already developed, stops us getting ill in the first place.

Barring a surprise entrant from left field, senolytics are hotly tipped to win the race to be the first true anti-aging medicine.

In 2016, senolytics moved into clinical trials in humans using a combination of Dasatinib and Quercetin, which indicated reduced senescent cell burden in adipose tissue of diabetic kidney disease patients and improved physical function in patients with idiopathic pulmonary fibrosis. Clinical trials with other senolytics, including the flavonoid Fisetin and BCL-xL inhibitors, are underway.

Although studies have provided evidence that senolytics are effective at decreasing the number of senescent cells in humans, the short-term and long-term side-effects of these therapies are largely unknown. Despite the potential of senotherapeutics to transform anti-aging medicine, a cautionary approach regarding unwanted dose-dependent side-effects should be adopted.

Several of the experimental drugs designed to eliminate toxic senescent cells are available to buy over the counter or online. Quercetin, for instance, is a common supplement in health food shops in the UK, US, and elsewhere. It is also present in many dietary sources, including citrus fruits, apples, onions, green tea, and dark berries.

While eating more fruit and vegetables is good for your health in many ways, taking quercetin as a supplement in the hope of reversing aging processes in the body is a bad idea according to James Kirkland at the Mayo Clinic, who researches senescent cells and the drugs designed to destroy them. He advises not to take them, as the only place for them at the moment is in clinical trials that are carefully controlled.[301]

Despite these warnings, there is a community of biohackers who take these drugs on a regular basis. They are very cheap, readily available, and easily used.

But these compounds can be toxic, warns Linda Partridge at the Max Planck Institute for Biology of Aging in Cologne, Germany.

Another possible solution is to give up on culling senescent cells and just tame them instead. Another class of drugs called senomorphics (also known as senostatics or senomodulators) is in the offing. These medications suppress the SASP rather than push senescent cells into self-destruction.

---

301 Lawton, G. 2023, "A new class of anti-aging drugs has arrived – which ones really work?", *New Scientist*, 17 May.

The two most promising drugs, *metformin* and *rapamycin*, (see next), are already on the radar.

While we wait on senolytic drugs, other options already exist. Exercise has been shown to reduce the burden of senescent cells in skeletal muscle and fat tissue, though a recent study found that the benefits only accrue from a gruelling session of high-intensity exercise. Caloric restriction is also a senolytic.

A strategy is to clear senescent cells. A 2016 study found that clearing senescent cells in a mouse born on the same day, from the same litter, and raised in the same conditions as his brother made him look younger and delayed onset of cataracts and bent spine. Removing senescent cells also extended mouse lifespans by as much as a third.[302]

Getting closer: In a new study, Japanese researchers have identified a unique "natural senolytic" involving serotonin metabolism and the INK4a-RB signalling axis in longer-living naked mole rats. While a species-specific senescent cell-removal mechanism, it may open doors to further research paths.[303] It would be quite nice if we all had our own natural senolytic.

Hyperbaric Oxygen Therapy

A study[304] indicated that HBOT may induce significant senolytic effects, including significantly increasing telomere length and clearance of senescent cells in the aging populations.

302 Wein, H. 2016, "Senescent cells tied to health and longevity in mice", *NIH Research Matters*, 23 February.

303 Kawamura, Y., Oka, K., Semba, T. *et al.* 2023, "Cellular senescence induction leads to progressive cell death via the INK4a-RB pathway in naked mole-rats", *The EMBO Journal*, https://doi.org/10.15252/embj.2022111133.

304 Hachmo, Y., Hadanny, A., Abu Hamed, R. *et al.* 2020, "Hyperbaric oxygen therapy increases telomere length and decreases immunosenescence in isolated blood cells: a prospective trial", *Aging*, Vol. 12, No. 22, pp. 22445-22456, https://doi.org/10.18632/aging.202188.

4. *Epigenetic Alterations*

The Epigenetic Clock

How do you measure biological age? There are a number of ways to do this, but one of the most accurate is through the use of "epigenetic clocks".

Discovered in 2011 by Steve Horvath[305] and regarded as the gold standard, such epigenetic clocks are based on a process known as DNA methylation. Even though our genetic code itself—our DNA—does not change over the course of our lifetime, the way in which it is expressed does. This is called epigenetics.

DNA methylation is a key mechanism of epigenetics; molecules called methyl groups are added along the length of DNA, turning certain genes "off" or "on". Horvath's prescient contribution was the recognition that the way DNA is methylated follows a pattern, one that can be traced over time and correlates with age. Knowing the pattern allows us to read DNA methylation like a clock.

Epigenetics is the effect environment has on our genes. An epigenome is a multitude of chemical compounds that instructs our DNA what to do, such as allocating them to form different tissue cells in organs like our brain or heart. This is also known as gene expression. DNA methylation, which ages us, can be modified by a person's environment including environmental chemicals, obesity, exercise, diet, and illnesses, which can change how our epigenome operates gene expression, affecting our DNA. Epigenetic alterations such as mutations, deletions, and translocations are among the leading causes of genomic instability.

305 Palmer, R. D. 2022, "Aging clocks & mortality timers, methylation, glycomic, telomeric and more. A window to measuring biological age", *Aging Medicine*, Vol. 5, No. 2, pp. 120-125, https://doi.org/10.1002/agm2.12197.

Epigenetic age can be older or younger than our chronological age, and epigenetics can give us incredibly precise estimates of how old we are.

The 'epigenetic clock' can predict how old someone is to within a few years. If their 'epigenetic age' is higher than their chronological age, they die sooner than someone whose epigenetic age is lower.

An epigenetic clock is a biochemical test that can be used to measure age. The test is based on DNA methylation levels, measuring the accumulation of methyl groups to one's DNA molecules.

This allows for quicker experiments on anti-aging treatments with a before-and-after epigenetic age measurement a few months later.

5. *Loss of Proteostasis: Misfolded proteins*

Proteostasis, or stabilisation, of proteins is vital for all the major chemical reactions for our body and growth, but various external and endogenous stresses accumulate during aging which lead to the decline of proteostasis network capacity and proteome integrity. Periods of oxidative stress cause these protein-production mishaps to occur more frequently. There has to be a balance in protein production and protein degradation, with the tipping point occurring when replenishing good proteins no longer keeps up with depletion from *misfolding,* aggregation, and damage.

6. *Deregulated nutrient sensing*

Cells need nutrients from food, and our cells have sensors that can respond to the fluctuations of nutrient levels in our bodies. These nutrient sensors provide the molecular basis for the association between lifestyle habits and aging. The need is to absorb the correct amount because damaging by-products like free radicals are also produced in this energy production process. Over time, as our cells accumulate damage from oxidative stress, these sensors have trouble regulating this nutrient intake. This is the basis of calorific restriction, well-documented as a method of prolonging life.

7. Mitochondrial Dysfunction

Mitochondria

As we age, mitochondrial efficiency progressively declines. Mitochondria are subcellular organelles in the cells of higher organisms that convert nutrients into biochemically usable energy. They also possess their own genome, and mutations in mitochondrial DNA have been linked to a reduction in lifespan.

Paradoxically, however, several studies have shown that reducing levels of mitochondrial activity—by restricting food intake, for instance—can actually extend lifespan. These findings imply that the primary cause of aging cannot simply lie in a reduction in overall metabolic activity, so the whole issue must be more complicated.

Mitochondria produce 90% of our body's energy, but a by-product of this is that they make most of the cell's free radicals, which then damage the mitochondria's efficiency, overworking their systems and creating more free radicals in the process.

Fewer mitochondria are produced as we age, making those left work that much harder.

Loss of function in your mitochondria can result in excess fatigue, a common symptom associated with aging.

However, mitochondria are very responsive to the body's energy demand, and if power demand declines, some power plants will shut down for greater efficiency.

Sedentary lifestyles lead to further mitochondrial decline as the body responds to a lower energy need, but exercise can promote mitochondrial biogenesis, the process where the body creates more mitochondria to meet the new energy demand. The corollary is that exercise stimulates mitochondria, and the smartphone VO_2max has been recommended as a free monitor and motivator.

8. Stem Cell Exhaustion

Stem Cells at their earliest stage are also called 'pleuri-potential' cells, a more descriptive naming in that they are the basic foundation cell with the unlimited potential to turn into any cell—and hence any tissue and any organ whatsoever. As such, they present the obvious potential to repair such damaged tissues There is an active process of normal cell replenishment vital for tissue homeostasis and regeneration. Stem cell exhaustion occurs when this new, budding workforce cannot replace the retiring cells fast enough to maintain peak tissue function. Much good research has been, and is being, done, but advances so far have been limited.

Stem cell exhaustion is closely tied with the other hallmarks of aging. The imbalance between stem cells and retiring cells can occur from the proliferation of senescent cells, caused mainly by DNA damage.

Pluripotential cells were harvested from six-day-old embryos until this was banned. But in 2006, Japanese research was able to take a person's own skin or blood cells and regress them back to this stem cell state, which allowed for an autologist transfusion back into that patient without any rejection issues. These were known as induced pluripotent stem cells (iPSCs).[306]

---

306 Charitos, I. A., Ballini, A., Cantore, S. *et al.* 2021, "Stem Cells: A Historical Review about Biological, Religious, and Ethical Issues", *Stem Cells International*, https://doi.org/10.1155/2021/9978837.

They guaranteed an unlimited supply of the human-like stem cells and became the foundation for new research methods in regenerative medicine. But these cells retained some of the genetic memory of being human cells.

Now, this genetic memory of the induced stem cells can be wiped, producing reprogrammed cells that are molecularly and functionally more similar to human stem cells.

Research has developed a method using four genes to induce their production, which have already been used to treat macular degeneration, the most common cause of blindness in old people.

Their potential for treating damaged organs is obviously very exciting, but unfortunately, is also attracting much hype and offering false hope.

9. Altered Intercellular Communication

Cells have a network of chemical signalling molecules to communicate with each other, but this degrades with age—mainly due to inflammation, most often triggered by senescent cells which then further corrupt healthy adjoining cells with aging as a consequence.

10. Dysbiosis

Dysbiosis is characterized by a decrease in microbial gut diversity and an increase in proinflammatory species. This imbalanced microbiota is unable to protect from pathogenic organisms that can trigger inflammation and produce genotoxins or carcinogenic metabolites. Moreover, with obesity and its associated comorbidities, the composition of gut microbiota and intestinal epithelial barrier function are altered. Dysbiosis has been associated with colorectal, gastric, and oesophageal cancer. Antibiotics are implicated in altering this balance and probiotics restoring it.

Germline

Classical evolutionary theories propose tradeoffs between reproduction, damage repair, and lifespan. However, the specific role of the germline in shaping vertebrate aging remains largely unknown. Experiments (in fish) have shown the germline regulates longevity and somatic repair in a sex-specific manner which may add new lines of research for human longevity.[307]

Other Potential Longevity Treatments

Telomerase

Telomeres get shorter over our lifetime, and people with shorter telomeres for their age are at increased risk of diseases of old age and die sooner than people with longer ones.

Telomerase is an enzyme which can elongate our telomeres and helps provide genomic stability in highly proliferative normal, immortal, and tumour cells by maintaining the integrity of the chromosome ends—the telomeres.

Telomerase counteracts the telomere shrinking process that uniquely holds the key to delaying or even reversing the cellular aging process with the ability to synthesize DNA "repeats" (specific DNA segments of six nucleotides) onto chromosome ends, and so affords immortality in cells.

Hence the intense interest and research.

Telomerase is associated with most human cancers. There was interest and excitement in the 1990s that telomerase had life-extending potential until it was found that dosed mice had a substantially increased risk of cancer.

---

307 Moses, E., Atlan, T., Sun, X. *et al.* 2024, "The killifish germline regulates longevity and somatic repair in a sex-specific manner", *Nature Aging,* Vol. 4, pp. 791-813, https://doi.org/10.1038/s43587-024-00632-0.

Under normal growth conditions, inhibition of telomerase activity in tumour-derived cells results in continued cell division coupled with telomere shortening, eventually followed by cellular senescence or death. Thus, repression of telomerase activity may be a novel adjuvant therapy for the treatment of human cancer, and detection of telomerase activity may be important for cancer diagnostics.[308]

However, research in the last few years has shown us that as long as you turn on telomerase temporarily, you can top up telomeres seemingly without increasing cancer risk. Mice given this treatment live longer and have higher bone density and better control of their blood sugar.

Alternative Lengthening of Telomeres (also known as "ALT") is a telomerase-independent mechanism by which cancer cells avoid the degradation of telomeres.

Thymus Rejuvenation

Our thymus involutes (retrograde changes, loss of function) early around age 20, but is important for our immune system as it produces lymphocytes (T-cells), the white blood cells which help our immune system fight germs and protect us from disease. However, it involutes (functional decline) when humans reach around 20 years, and we then become more susceptible to infections.

The Amish Gene: SERPINE1

It has been found that the Amish with one copy of mutated SERPINE1 had better heart health, less Diabetes, and lived a full

308 Holt, S. E. & Shay, J. W. 1999, "Role of telomerase in cellular proliferation and cancer", *Journal of Cellular Physiology*, Vol. 180, No. 1, pp. 10-18, https://doi.org/10.1002/(SICI)1097-4652(199907)180:1<10::AID-JCP2>3.0.CO;2-D.

10 years longer than those without, which alerted researchers that a single gene, let alone a few, were a probable longevity focus.

Intermittent Reprogramming

We could one day be able to turn back the clock on our body's cells, keeping us younger for longer.

An unexpected side-effect of iPSC research is that those same four genes that can allow a cell to turn into any other kind of cell also turn back its epigenetic clock. The process, known as cellular reprogramming, seems to make cells biologically younger.

It also works in whole animals, as long as it's only done intermittently. Continuous reprogramming turns cells back to iPSCs, and this is bad news because iPSCs aren't much use in themselves, only for what they can turn into. For example, an iPSC in your heart doesn't have the skillset to pump blood, so replacing a large number of your cells with iPSCs would result in a hasty demise. However, if you just do a little bit of reprogramming—enough to shave years off of cells' biological clocks without turning them all the way back to being stem cells—you can rejuvenate the body as a whole.

Calorie Restriction (CR)

While Roy Walford became the best-known advocate for calorie restriction, it was a scientist, Clive McCay, in the 1930s, who found that rats fed less, lived longer. As mentioned, however, such CR is unsustainable for humans. In answer, drugs such as rapamycin or metformin, which mimic CR, are being trialled.

Parabiosis

Young blood plasma is known to confer beneficial effects on various organs in mice and rats. However, it was not known whether plasma from young adult pigs would rejuvenate old rat tissues at the epigenetic level. A recent study, published late 2023, recorded a remarkable near 50% reduction in biological age when pigs' plasma was transfused into rats.[309]

309 Tripathi, S. S., Kumar, R., Arya, J. K. & Rizvi, S. I. 2021, "Plasma from Young Rats Injected into Old Rats Induce Antiaging Effects", *Rejuvenation Research*, Vol. 24, No. 3, pp. 206-212, https://doi.org/10.1089/rej.2020.2354.

CHAPTER 37

Drugs, Supplements and Behaviours

"A little knowledge is a dangerous thing,
Drink deep or taste not the Pierian spring."

– Alexander Pope, 1711

"If you want a guarantee, buy a toaster."

– Clint Eastwood

Supplements are spared the rigorous regulatory approval process that legitimate medicines must submit to. So, there is no incentive for these companies that are marketing the supplements to actually demonstrate that they work. And if they did do a clinical trial, they might find out that the supplement doesn't work. In fact, there's a disincentive for these companies to prove their efficacy.

There really is, at present, no knowing what many of these supplements really do, nor any 'correct' doses, let alone what happens when they are combined into some cocktail.

Most are scams backed by incredibly convincing but pseudo-scientific claims.

Getting Closer

In late 2023, a research paper titled "Reversal of Biological Age in Multiple Rat Organs by Young Porcine Plasma Fraction" unveiled what would seem a remarkable breakthrough in the field of aging biology. A therapeutic serum called E5, developed by Harold Katcher, PhD, and his colleagues, was injected into old rats, making them significantly younger within days. E5 consists of nanoparticles of complex structure, including exosomes from young plasma sourced from another species.[310]

Steve Horvath, PhD, remarked, "Initially, I could hardly believe the profound epigenetic rejuvenation effects of E5. However, our findings are robustly supported by parallel rodent studies from different labs." Upon final analysis by Horvath and his team, there was a remarkable 67.4% average reversal in the epigenetic age of treated elderly rats. If these results translate similarly to humans, it could equate to an 80-year-old reverting to the age of 26.

ITP

The National Institute on Aging (NIA) supports the Interventions Testing Program (ITP), a multi-institutional study investigating diets and dietary supplements purported to extend lifespan and delay disease and dysfunction.

ITP allows investigators to submit proposals for interventions to be tested for their ability to decelerate aging and extend lifespan in mice, and I have downloaded some of their conclusions.

Longevity is the latest focus for research, attracting incredible scientists, but from my standpoint as a practising clinician, they are akin to Big Pharma, pursuing and developing incredible

310 Horvath, S., Singh, K., Raj, K. *et al.* 2024, "Reversal of Biological Age in Multiple Rat Organs by Young Porcine Plasma Fraction", *Geoscience*, Vol. 46, pp. 367-394, https://doi.org/10.1007/s11357-023-00980-6.

drugs but without patients or the responsibility which goes with prescribing. I have lived through enough pharmaceutical disasters and, indeed, very nearly prescribed Thalidomide, but a sixth sense stopped me. I was also responsible for getting one horrible 'tranquillizer' banned, but the process was so bureaucratic and time wasting I am frustrated that some such drugs are still allowed and are being prescribed.

And so, I watch these longevity researchers with the same healthy scepticism and wish them all the best. But what I am trying to say is that there is a hell of a gulf between research and clinical medicine, and, with the increasing complexities, it's getting wider.

I found my father's old pharmacy notes from when he was a medical student, wherein he had to extract digitalis from foxglove and then roll it into pills circa 1922. Since then, Big Pharma has exploded and taken over such that one Danish drug company, Novo Nordisk has earned more than the whole of Denmark's GDP and reputedly saved the nation from recession.

My analogy is that the longevity research is in its very early stage and has a long way to go. Practising doctors know very little about it, while the enthusiasts and scammers are touting unproven benefits.

Metformin, however, is a medicine that has been approved and beneficially used for diabetics for decades. It would seem to have other beneficial effects.

Rapamycin is the new wonder-drug and has attracted very enthusiastic and knowledgeable medical advocates. As such, I have gone into details.

1. Metformin

It has been observed that Type 2 Diabetics (T2D) taking metformin live longer. It has also been observed that people without T2D, who take metformin, do not live longer.

Retrospective data and trials in populations with Type 2 Diabetes mellitus (T2DM) have shown improved overall survival with metformin[311] as well as decreased risk of cardiovascular disease,[312] cancer incidence,[313] and cognitive decline.[314] Although these studies support the use of metformin as a potential healthspan extending treatment, these findings were largely in subjects with T2DM, and none were in adults absent of disease.

Metformin and exercise independently improve insulin sensitivity and decrease the risk of Diabetes. Metformin has thus been proposed as a potential therapy to slow aging. However, recent evidence indicates that adding metformin to exercise antagonizes the exercise-induced improvement in insulin sensitivity and cardiorespiratory fitness, and this study indicates that further research is needed before broadly prescribing metformin as a treatment to slow aging.[315]

---

311 Bannister, C. A., Holden, S. E., Jenkins-Jones, S. *et al.* 2014, "Can people with type 2 Diabetes live longer than those without? A comparison of mortality in people initiated with metformin or sulphonylurea monotherapy and matched, non-diabetic controls", *Diabetes, Obesity and Metabolism*, Vol. 16, No. 11, pp. 1165-73, https://doi.org/10.1111/dom.12354.

312 UK Prospective Diabetes Study (UKPDS) Group, 1998, "Effect of intensive blood-glucose control with metformin on complications in overweight patients with type 2 Diabetes (UKPDS 34)", *Lancet*, Vol. 352, No. 9131, pp. 854-865, erratum in *Lancet*, Vol. 352, No. 9139, p. 1558.

313 Wu, J. W., Boudreau, D. M., Park, Y. *et al.* 2014, "Commonly used Diabetes and cardiovascular medications and cancer recurrence and cancer-specific mortality: a review of the literature", *Expert Opinion on Drug Safety*, Vol. 13, No. 8, pp. 1071-1099, https://doi.org/10.1517/14740338.2014.926887.

314 Lin, Y., Wang, K., Ma, C. *et al.* 2018, "Evaluation of metformin on cognitive improvement in patients with non-dementia vascular cognitive impairment and abnormal glucose metabolism", *Frontiers in Aging Neuroscience*, Vol. 10, https://doi.org/10.3389/fnagi.2018.00227.

315 Konopka, A. R., Laurin, J. L., Schoenberg, H. M. *et al.* 2019, "Metformin inhibits mitochondrial adaptations to aerobic exercise training in older adults", *Aging Cell*, Vol. 18, No. 1, https://doi.org/10.1111/acel.12880.

Metformin is one of the most crucial first-line therapeutic agents for Type 2 Diabetes mellitus. Primarily being an antihyperglycemic agent, metformin also has a plethora of pleiotropic effects, i.e., producing more than one effect on various systems and processes. It acts majorly by activating AMPK (Adenosine Monophosphate-Activated Protein Kinase) in the cells and reducing glucose output from the liver. It also decreases advanced glycation end products and reactive oxygen species (ROS) production in the endothelium apart from regulating the glucose and lipid metabolism in the cardiomyocytes, hence minimizing the cardiovascular risks.

Its anti-cancer, anti-proliferative, and apoptosis-inducing effects on malignant cells might prove instrumental in the malignancy of organs like the breast, kidney, brain, ovary, lung, and endometrium. Pre-clinical studies have also shown some evidence of metformin's neuroprotective role in Parkinson's Disease, Alzheimer's Disease, multiple sclerosis, and Huntington's Disease.

Metformin exerts its effects through varied pathways, and the exact mechanism in the majority of them remains yet to be clearly defined.

Nir Barzilai, director of the Institute for Aging Research at the Albert Einstein College of Medicine in New York City, is seeking approval from the US Food and Drug Administration for the first clinical trial of metformin to combat aging.

The American Federation for Aging Research is currently preparing a series of six-year clinical trials to test whether metformin can delay the onset of further age-related conditions in people who already have one. Its TAME (Targeting Aging with Metformin) trial is the first large clinical trial in modern medicine to test if human aging can be treated with a drug.

One of the goals of the TAME trial is to persuade the FDA to recognise aging as a disease in its own right, which could change the landscape of the entire field. If the FDA accepts TAME results (if they are positive), they will open the door to treating aging as something that can be "cured".

But other researchers are concerned, as metformin intake has been associated with a higher risk of B vitamin deficiencies. Some studies suggest this can result in cognitive dysfunction.

Taking metformin for Type 2 Diabetes may offer protection against developing osteoarthritis compared with taking a sulfonylurea (such as glyburide, glipizide, or glimepiride), according to a 2023 study. Researchers found that, compared with participants who took a sulfonylurea, those who took metformin were 24% less likely to develop osteoarthritis. They were also 20% less likely to undergo joint replacement, but this second difference was not statistically significant.[316]

Don't Stop Metformin[317]

A study corroborated the largely consistent evidence from other observational studies showing an association between metformin use and lower dementia incidence but also found that then ceasing the drug was associated with increased dementia incidence in a diverse cohort of older adults.

It is recommended that other ways are pursued such that metformin use can continue.

Finally, check your B_{12}, as metformin interferes with its absorption.

---

316 Baker, M. C., Sheth, K., Liu, Y. *et al.* 2023, "Development of Osteoarthritis in Adults With Type 2 Diabetes Treated With Metformin vs a Sulfonylurea", *JAMA Network Open,* Vol. 6, No. 3, https://doi.org/10.1001/jamanetworkopen.2023.3646.

317 Zimmerman, S. C., Ferguson, E. L., Choudhary, V. *et al.* 2023, "Metformin Cessation and Dementia Incidence", *JAMA Network Open*, Vol. 6, No. 10, https://doi.org/10.1001/jamanetworkopen.2023.39723.

2. Rapamycin

Rapamycin has attracted the attention of excellent medical and scientific brains. As such, their opinions should be paid due attention, and I provide their opinions and some references of articles to read should you seek more information.

I am attracted to their lateral thinking and scientific approach, and I got caught up in their enthusiasm and cautiously tried it. But I developed annoying, and somewhat alarming, sub-cutaneous nodules—an unrecorded side effect to my reading—and ceased it.

Given more time to consider, I have resorted to my first principles that it has not yet been proven. The rub is that it can't be, by any double blind random controlled tests, so I will have to wait to see if those taking it do, indeed, live a longer, cancer-free life. Unfortunately, as they are in their 50s and I'm 83, I don't think I can wait around that long.

Rapamycin has been prescribed to counter organ rejection in transplant patients. In lower doses, it would seem to prolong life.

In 1991, biochemist Michael N. Hall, as a young professor at the Biozentrum of the University of Basel, was studying the control mechanism of growth in yeast and discovered that an obscure anti-fungal agent called rapamycin stopped growth.[318] Hall concluded that there is something in the yeast cell that is blocked by rapamycin. He calls that substance in the yeast cell, Target of Rapamycin or TOR or mTOR in mammals (Mammalian Target of Rapamycin).

The TOR growth pathway is universal from yeast and worms to humans and plants. TOR is activated by nutrients, insulin, and

318 Williams, C. L. 2018, "Talking TOR: a conversation with Joe Heitman and Rao Movva", *JCI Insight*, 22 February, https://doi.org/10.1172/jci.insight.99816.

growth factors. TOR drives growth, and aging is an unintended continuation of growth. TOR is a signalling pathway that contributes to cell synthesis and metabolism.

TOR (the mTOR pathway) is a master regulator of the cell's growth and metabolic state, and its dysregulation contributes to a variety of diseases, including Diabetes, obesity, neurodegenerative disorders, aging, and cancer, making the TOR pathway an attractive therapeutic target.

Rapamycin's action is, broadly speaking, slowing down growth and slowing down cell metabolism—hence, slowing aging. It can interrupt TOR to stop cells from growing and multiplying. Consequently, it becomes an effective drug in preventing cancer cells from spreading in the body and suppressing the immune system of kidney transplant patients in order to keep the body from rejecting the donor's kidney.

In terms of longevity, rapamycin is found to enhance autophagy, which is a process that removes unnecessary, abnormal, and damaged components within cells and prevents cells from stress when it inhibits mTOR. It simultaneously boosts the process and disrupts unhealthy cell growth. As a result, the body can delay the onset of the aging process and age-related diseases, giving people a longer and healthier life.

Calorie Restriction (CR) targets the exact same pathway. TOR and rapamycin may be thought of as CR in a pill.

Rapamycin has attracted a very enthusiastic group of medical practitioners and scientists who claim:[319]

1. Aging is not programmed.
2. Aging is a continuation of growth that is not turned off.
3. TOR promotes growth of cells even when cell cycle (mitosis) is blocked.

---

319 Blagosklonny, M. V. 2009, "TOR-driven aging: speeding car without brakes", *Cell Cycle*, Vol. 8, No. 24, pp. 4055-9, https://doi.org/10.4161/cc.8.24.10310.

4. TOR causes the production of senescent cells.
5. Senescent cells are hyperfunctional and damage tissues and promote diseases of aging.
6. Aging presents as hyperfunction, hyperplasia, and cell hypertrophy.
7. By analogy, aging can be viewed as a speeding car that lacks brakes and cannot slow down when the road requires going slowly and then crashes.
8. Like crashes at the end of the road, these diseases are late manifestations of aging. From the TOR perspective, death from aging and from diseases of aging has the same meaning because diseases of aging are just manifestations of aging, like smoke is a manifestation of fire.
9. According to classic gerontology, non-repaired molecular damage causes aging. In contrast, TOR-driven aging causes damage (diseases of aging).
10. From the classic perspective, nothing can be done to inhibit aging.
11. From the TOR perspective, the pharmacologic brake (rapamycin) will slow down human aging.

It is alleged Rapamycin:

1. Prolongs lifespan.
2. Prevents age-related diseases.
3. Slows production of senescent cells, and removal of senescent cells ameliorates disease.
4. Slows the epigenetic clock.

Obviously, these claims cannot be proven, but it has increased the lifespan and healthspan in animals and is currently being tested as an anti-aging drug in dogs.

Numerous studies demonstrated that inhibition of the mTOR pathways by any means (genetic, pharmacological, and dietary) extends lifespan. Currently, only two studies, as above, demonstrated that senolytics (fisetin and a combination Dasatinib plus Quercetin) extend lifespan in mice. These senolytics slightly inhibit the mTOR pathway. Thus, life extension by these senolytics can be explained by their slight rapamycin-like (gerostatic) effects.

There is an incredible list of plants with claimed senolytic properties.

Rapamycin blocks mTORC1 in the short term but not mTORC2. However, over the longer term (weeks of higher dose), eventually, there are feedback mechanisms that cause mTORC2 to be increasingly blocked.

The other issue is what else the molecule might interact with or block—other pathways that may or may not be known.

Dr. Mikhail V. Blagosklonny, MD, PhD, who has written most of the articles the above information is taken from, says that evolution doesn't explicitly program us to age. Rather, it leaves a hyperactive life script that promotes aging and age-related diseases. This process involves mTOR (Target of Rapamycin), which acts like an overzealous growth engine.

By managing mTOR, we can slow aging and combat a host of age-related conditions from heart disease and cancer to Alzheimer's and Parkinson's. Rapamycin, he claims, is our most promising weapon in this battle against aging.

He wrote this free access opinion article: "Rapamycin for longevity."[320]

Abstract

"While ruling out programmed aging, evolutionary theory predicts a quasi-program for aging, a continuation of the

320 Blagosklonny, M. V. 2019, "Rapamycin for longevity: opinion article", *Aging,* Vol. 11, No. 19, pp. 8048-8067, https://doi.org/10.18632/aging.102355.

developmental program that is not turned off, is constantly on, becoming hyper-functional and damaging, causing diseases of aging. Could it be switched off pharmacologically? This would require identification of a molecular target involved in cell senescence, organism aging and diseases of aging. Notably, cell senescence is associated with activation of the TOR (target of rapamycin) nutrient- and mitogen-sensing pathway, which promotes cell growth, even though cell cycle is blocked. Is TOR involved in organism aging? In fact, in yeast (where the cell is the organism), caloric restriction, rapamycin and mutations that inhibit TOR all slow down aging. In animals from worms to mammals' caloric restrictions, life-extending agents, and numerous mutations that increase longevity all converge on the TOR pathway. And, in humans, cell hypertrophy, hyper-function and hyperplasia, typically associated with activation of TOR, contribute to diseases of aging. Theoretical and clinical considerations suggest that rapamycin may be effective against atherosclerosis, hypertension and hyper-coagulation (thus, preventing myocardial infarction and stroke), osteoporosis, cancer, autoimmune diseases and arthritis, obesity, Diabetes, macula-degeneration, Alzheimer's and Parkinson's diseases. Finally, I discuss that extended life span will reveal new causes for aging (e.g., ROS, 'wear and tear', Hayflick limit, stem cell exhaustion) that play a limited role now, when quasi-programmed senescence kills us first".

He goes on:

"From the dawn of civilization, humanity has dreamed of immortality. So why didn't the discovery of the anti-aging properties of mTOR inhibitors change the world forever? I will discuss several reasons, including fear of the actual and fictional side effects of rapamycin, everolimus and other clinically approved drugs, arguing that no real side effects preclude their use as anti-aging drugs today. Furthermore, the alternative to the reversible (and avoidable) side effects of rapamycin/everolimus are the irreversible (and inevitable) effects of aging: cancer, stroke, infarction, blindness and premature death. I will also discuss why it is more dangerous not to use anti-aging drugs than to use them and how rapamycin-based drug combinations have already been implemented for potential life extension in humans. If you read this article from the very beginning to its end, you may realize that the time is now".

I suggest you read this whole free access article: *Aging and immortality: quasi-programmed senescence and its pharmacologic inhibition* by Mikhail V Blagosklonny .[321]

Dr. Peter Attia, author of *Outlive*, podcaster, and longevity expert, is another enthusiastic user.

Rapamycin Clinical Use

A protein (kinase) called mTOR is in every cell membrane, in many varieties of life from yeast to worms to fruit flies to mice and other mammals—probably dogs, primates, and humans. This universality is attributed because the genes for our metabolic growth path(s) would seem to be universal in all life forms and have persisted through evolution.

This commonality also provides the basis for research discoveries, but no studies have yet been conducted on humans.

mTOR is now known to be a central regulator critical to cell growth, proliferation, autophagy, apoptosis, metabolism, and survival by participating in multiple signalling pathways in the body.

321 Blagosklonny, M. V. 2006, "Aging and immortality: quasi-programmed senescence and its pharmacologic inhibition", *Cell Cycle*, Vol. 5, No. 18, pp. 2087-102, https://doi.org/10.4161/cc.5.18.3288.

There are two mTORS: mTOR 1 regulates protein synthesis and cell growth through downstream molecules and is sensitive to rapamycin. mTORC2 is sensitive to growth factors, not nutrients, and is insensitive to rapamycin.

mTOR is sensitive to nutrients, mostly in the form of amino acids, and it may stimulate anabolism or growth and, therefore, may provoke tumor formation and angiogenesis; or it may be catabolic and deregulate growth in diseases including cancer and insulin resistance/Type 2 Diabetes. It is also associated with arthritis, osteoporosis, and other diseases.

Inhibition of mTOR improves and boosts autophagy and simultaneously disrupts unhealthy cell growth. As a result, the body can delay the onset of the aging process and age-related diseases, *potentially giving people a longer and healthier life.*

The discovery and development of rapamycin is a 50+ year saga, but briefly, in 1964, a Canadian medical expedition to Easter Island, Rapa Nui, where Dr. Georges Nógrády took soil samples looking for tetanus spores. Few were found, but the samples ended up in laboratories in the USA and Switzerland.

In 1972, the scientist Dr. Surendra (Suren) Sehgal defied his USA laboratory's order to shut his research down, and in 1988, he sent a memo about rapamycin that allowed for the animal testing of the compound. While he was initially developing rapamycin as an antifungal drug, he also believed that rapamycin possessed novel properties as well as immunosuppressive activities and sent samples to the U.S. National Cancer Institute (NCI) so they could isolate rapamycin for screening. Indeed, rapamycin demonstrated incredible anti-tumor activity against many of the solid tumors tested, leading to it being designated as a priority drug by NCI for immunosuppression in transplant patients.

In 1991, Michael Hall, a senior investigator in Switzerland, discovered this *'target of rapamycin'*, which was a protein in yeast cells and proposed the name TOR, German for 'door'. In 1994, David Sebatini then isolated it in mammals while still a doctoral student and gave it the name mTOR (for mammalian target of).

Sabatini has continued his research to this day and, in 1994, named Rapamycin after its origin in the island of Rapa Nui. It would seem he knows as much or more than anyone about rapamycin, but there are many other, highly qualified researchers, such as Matt Kaeberlein, who support the claims for rapamycin, going so far as to say that, "As a potential long-term therapeutic that it always works and is, without question, the most robust and reproducible drug, at least from pre-clinical studies, that we know about today for impacting not only longevity but, to the extent that we can measure various metrics of healthspan in complex animals rapamycin also seems to impact pretty well every aspect of healthspan that we measured".[322]

Kaeberlein and Peter Attia take rapamycin, but David Sabatini does not. They are awaiting Kaeberlein's study on supplementing middle-aged heavier dogs due in 2026 to see if their lifespan is increased.

Initially, rapamycin was used in high doses as an immunosuppressant but in low doses would seem to have both health and lifespan benefits with few side effects and is used off-label by many, especially the biohackers, with the most usual dosage of 6mg once per week.

In the UK, Professor João Pedro de Magalhães at Birmingham University has studied the DNA of our longest-living animals and, citing cancer resistance genes and enhanced repair of DNA damage, rejuvenating the thymus and thus our immune system, thinks drugs will be developed to extend human lifespan.[323]

322 Kaeberlein, M. 2023, "Rapamycin: potential longevity benefits", *The Drive Broadcast*, 25 September.

323 de Magalhães, J. P. 2023, "Aging: is it driven by our genetic coding?", *University of Birmingham News*, 28 March.

My conclusion, as a physician/internist: I am conservative and want to wait and see, and I can't help being a little wary of any unbridled enthusiasm and claims. As the old observation goes, "if it sounds too good to be true, it probably is." It would seem, however, that such drugs will be developed, and I may change my mind.

Other Potential Supplements

Acarbose

Acarbose is a drug prescribed for diabetics and similar to metformin.

In mice studies, it extended life and worked best in younger mice, being only half as effective at middle age.

It reduces glucose absorption from the gut and blunts peak levels of glucose but causes flatulence—especially with wheat.

However, it had the most significant life extension when combined with rapamycin, viz:

Rapamycin + Acarbose = 29% lifespan extension in male mice (not female).[324]

AKG

AKG (alpha-ketoglutarate), is an antioxidant which inhibits protein degradation in muscles.[325]

---

324 Strong, R., Miller, R. A., Cheng, C. J. *et al.* 2022, "Lifespan benefits for the combination of rapamycin plus acarbose and for captopril in genetically heterogeneous mice", *Aging Cell*, Vol. 21, No. 12, https://doi.org/10.1111/acel.13724.

325 Wu, N., Yang, M., Gaur, U. *et al.* 2016, "Alpha-Ketoglutarate: Physiological Functions and Applications", *Biomolules & Therapeutics*, Vol. 24, No. 1, pp. 1-8, https://doi.org/10.4062/biomolther.2015.078.

17 Alpha Estradiol

17-α Estradiol is a weak estrogen and a potent 5-α reductase inhibitor that has been shown to improve metabolic function, enhance insulin sensitivity, and reduce fat and inflammation in old male mice without causing feminization (Stout et al., 2017). It increased AMPK levels and reduced mTOR activity in visceral adipose tissue. It worked in male mice only, increasing life extension by some 12%.[326]

Astaxanthin

This compound improves lifespan in male (not female) mice.The Astaxanthin compound CDX-085 (developed by Cardax) showed the ability to significantly increase the expression of the FOXO3 gene, which plays a proven role in longevity.[327]

Canacaflozin

This is a human diabetic drug which stops resorption of glucose in the kidneys. It may have subsidiary effects in reducing cancer and heart disease, and male mice lifespan was extended by 15%.[328]

326 Stout, M. B., Steyn, F. J., Jurczak, M. J. *et al.* 2017, "17α-Estradiol Alleviates Age-related Metabolic and Inflammatory Dysfunction in Male Mice Without Inducing Feminization", *The Journals of Gerontology: Series A*, Vol. 72, No. 1, pp. 3-15, https://doi.org/10.1093/gerona/glv309.

327 University of Hawaii Cancer Center, 2017, "Astaxanthin compound found to switch on the FOX03 'Longevity Gene' in mice", *ScienceDaily*, 28 March, www.sciencedaily.com/releases/2017/03/170328092428.htm.

328 Korfhage, J., Skinner, M. E., Basu, J. *et al.* 2022, "Canagliflozin Increases Intestinal Adenoma Burden in Female ApcMin/+ Mice", *The Journals of Gerontology: Series A*, Vol. 77, No. 2, pp. 215-220. https://doi.org/10.1093/gerona/glab254.

Captopril

Captopril is an anti-hypertensive drug prescribed for humans, It gave a 5% life extension to female mice but had no effect in males.[329]

DHEA

Some research has found that the synthetic hormone DHEA (dehydroepiandrosterone) slows aging in both cells and skin.[330]

Fisetin

Fisetin is one of the most potent senolytics yet discovered among plant-derived polyphenols, destroying dysfunctional senescent cells and, in one study, extending lifespan by approximately 10% in animals but not in the mice studies of ITP. In mice, it not only had no effect on lifespan, but it had no effect on decreasing senescent cells.[331]

Glycine

Glycine is a non-essential (can be produced by the body) amino acid that is involved in many important cellular processes. During aging, glycine levels decline. Recent findings claim that glycine may reverse some aspects of the aging process and may even

---

329 Strong, R., Miller, R. A., Cheng, C. J. *et al*, 2022, "Lifespan benefits for the combination of rapamycin plus acarbose and for captopril in genetically heterogeneous mice", *Aging Cell*, Vol. 21, No. 12, https://doi.org/10.1111/acel.13724.

330 *Ibid.*

331 Yousefzadeh, M. J., Zhu, Y., McGowan, S. J. 2018, "Fisetin is a senotherapeutic that extends health and lifespan", *eBioMedicine*, Vol. 36, pp. 18-28, https://doi.org/10.1016/j.ebiom.2018.09.015.

provide value in lifespan extension by some 5% in both mice sexes.[332]

GPLD1

A study published July 9, 2020, in Science showed that after mice exercise, their livers secrete a protein called GPLD1 into the blood. Levels of this protein in the blood correspond to improved cognitive function in aged mice, and it is also elevated in the blood of elderly humans who exercise regularly. Simply increasing the amount of GPLD1 produced by the mouse liver could confer many of the same brain benefits as regular exercise.[333]

Meclizine

Meclizine improves lifespan in male mice and appears to be a fairly potent mTORC1 inhibitor.[334]

NAC (N-Acetylcysteine)

The primary role of NAC as an antioxidant stems from its ability to increase the intracellular concentration of glutathione (GSH). NAC acts as a precursor to intracellular cysteine, increasing the

332 Razak, M. A., Begum, P. S., Viswanath, B. & Rajagopal, S. 2017, "Multifarious Beneficial Effect of Nonessential Amino Acid, Glycine: A Review", *Oxidative Medicine and Cellular Longevity*, https://doi.org/10.1155/2017/1716701.

333 Horowitz, A. M., Fan, X., Bieri, G. *et al.* 2020, "Blood factors transfer beneficial effects of exercise on neurogenesis and cognition to the aged brain", *Science*, Vol. 369, No. 6500, pp. 167-173. https://doi.org/10.1126/science.aaw2622.

334 Harrison, D. E., Strong, R., Reifsnyder, P. *et al.* 2023, "Astaxanthin and meclizine extend lifespan in UM-HET3 male mice; fisetin, SG1002 (hydrogen sulfide donor), dimethyl fumarate, mycophenolic acid, and 4-phenylbutyrate do not significantly affect lifespan in either sex at the doses and schedules used", *GeroScience*, Vol. 46, pp. 795-816, https://doi.org/10.1007/s11357-023-01011-0

pool of GSH, which in turn is essential in several diseases linked to oxidative stress as a consequence of glutathione depletion. Thus, although NAC is used in a range of diseases, further studies are needed.

Cysteine is found in most high protein foods such as chicken, turkey, yogurt, cheese, eggs, sunflower seeds, and legumes. Consuming adequate cysteine and NAC is important. While NAC may improve brain health, more human research is needed to make firm conclusions.[335]

NMRA

No effect on (mice) longevity.[336]

NMN

NMN is a naturally occurring molecule.

It has been popularised by David Sinclair, a Harvard professor, whose claims about its benefits have earned him cult status. He argues it has been shown to increase NAD+ (nicotinamide adenine dinucleotide) levels, which play a critical role in DNA repair, energy production, and cellular signalling. That includes reversing mitochondrial dysfunction, one of those primary hallmarks of cellular aging.

But there is no proof.

NMN joins an ever-growing list of health trends, although this one has some evidence to it. NMN, or Nicotinamide Mononucleotide, is derived from vitamin B3 (niacin) and is found in human cells. It has a critical role to play in how the

335 Tenório, M. C. D. S., Graciliano, N. G., Moura, F. A. *et al.* 2021, "N-Acetylcysteine (NAC): Impacts on Human Health", *Antioxidants*, Vol. 10, No. 6, p. 967, https://doi.org/10.3390/antiox10060967.

336 Mitchell, S. J., Bernier, M., Aon, M. A. *et al.* 2018, Nicotinamide Improves Aspects of Healthspan, but Not Lifespan, in Mice", *Cell Metabolism*, Vol. 27, No. 3, pp. 667-676, https://doi.org/10.1016/j.cmet.2018.02.001.

body uses cellular energy. Natural NMN is present in various food sources such as raw beef, fruits, and vegetables, including broccoli, cabbage, edamame, cucumber, avocado, and tomato.[337]

NAD (nicotinamide adenine dinucleotide)

NAD levels appear to decline as we age, hence the interest.[338]

NDGA

12% life extension in male mice only. It is an antioxidant and anti-inflammatory.

Peptides

Peptides are short-chain amino acids. There are thousands in the human body, such as insulin. Now, lab-produced versions that mimic it and others have been approved for treating diseases such as multiple sclerosis, Type 2 Diabetes, and obesity. The term "peptides" has entered the consumer vernacular, some providers have come to market them not as drugs but as rejuvenation treatments, and people are increasingly open to injecting themselves with peptides at home. Proponents say that peptides help them build lean muscle, shed weight, increase energy, and get a dewy glow along with physiological transformations that go beyond diet and exercise.

They are being prescribed to patients by doctors as well as paramedical providers, even though several in-demand peptides are not approved by regulators. This lack of control raises concerns about the purity of ingredients, improper dosing, and

337 Shade, C. 2020, "The Science Behind NMN-A Stable, Reliable NAD+Activator and Anti-Aging Molecule", *Integrative Medicine*, Vol. 19, No. 1, pp. 12-14.

338 McReynolds, M. R., Chellappa, K. & Baur, J. A. 2020, "Age-related NAD+ decline", *Experimental Gerontology*, Vol. 134, https://doi.org/110888.https://doi.org/10.1016/j.exger.2020.110888.

unknown side effects. But advocates say they're comfortable with any risks.

For years, peptides such as BPC-157, CJC-1295, and ipamorelin have been popular among bodybuilders and athletes who are seeking to speed up healing or build muscle, but regulators have cracked down on their sales, and the World Anti-Doping Agency has expressly banned their use. However, that hasn't stopped interest (and experimental versions) with peptide spas popping up across the USA.[339]

Procyanidin C1

In 2021 Chinese researchers found this compound in grape seeds and that it prolonged the lifespan of old mice by 9%. It acts as a senolytic.

Quercetin

Polyphenol quercetin removes harmful older cells before they accumulate, i.e., it is a senolytic.[340]

Rilmenidine

Treating the nematode worm, *C. elegans*, with rilmenidine, an anti-hypertensive drug in humans, at young and older ages increases lifespan. Further, transcriptional changes similar to Caloric Restriction were observed in liver and kidney tissues in mice treated with rilmenidine. Together, these results reveal a geroprotective and potential caloric restriction mimetic effect

339 Yang, H., Zhang, Q., Zhang, B. *et al.* 2023, "Potential Active Marine Peptides as Anti-Aging Drugs or Drug Candidates", *Marine Drugs*, Vol. 21, No. 3, https://doi.org/10.3390/md21030144.

340 Kirkland, J. L. & Tchkonia, T. 2020, "Senolytic drugs: from discovery to translation", *Journal of Internal Medicine*, Vol. 288, No. 5, pp. 518-536, https://doi.org/10.1111/joim.13141.

by rilmenidine.[341] The longevity effects of rilmenidine likely involve inhibition of mTOR activity and upregulation of autophagy pathways, both of which are also associated with Caloric Restriction (CR).

Taurine

Taurine is an amino sulfonic acid. It occurs naturally in the body. The best food sources of taurine are meat, fish, and eggs. It has important functions in the heart and brain. It helps support nerve growth. Taurine abundance decreases during aging. A reversal of this decline through taurine supplementation increases healthspan and lifespan in mice and worms and healthspan in monkeys. This identifies taurine deficiency as a driver of aging in these species. To test whether taurine deficiency is a driver of aging in humans as well, long-term, well-controlled taurine supplementation trials that measure healthspan and lifespan as outcomes are required.[342]

This study, of course, stimulated a run-on taurine which the supplement manufacturers were only too happy to supply. But there is no reliable indication that supplementation with this amino acid would result in any improvement in any health claims or longevity in humans or even that supplementation would be effective in raising serum taurine levels.

Taurine is found in biological effective doses in shellfish, especially scallops, mussels, and clams and the dark meat of turkey and chicken.

---

341 Bennett, D. F., Goyala, A., Statzer, C. *et al.* 2023, "Rilmenidine extends lifespan and healthspan in Caenorhabditis elegans via a nischarin I1-imidazoline receptor", *Aging Cell,* Vol. 22, No. 2), https://doi.org/10.1111/acel.13774.

342 Singh, P., Gollapalli, K., Mangiola, S. *et al.* 2023, "Taurine deficiency as a driver of aging", *Science*, Vol. 380, No. 6649, https://doi.org/10.1126/science.abn9257.

L-theanine

Theanine is an amino acid found in tea and some mushrooms. People use L-theanine to improve mental function. It is also used for anxiety, mental impairment, stress, and other conditions, but there is no good scientific evidence to support these uses.[343]

Urolithin A

Urolithin A is a natural gut microbiome-derived food metabolite that has been shown to stimulate mitophagy and improve muscle function in older animals and to induce mitochondrial gene expression in older humans.

It has been shown to re-energise cells. The health benefits attributed to pomegranate have been associated with its high content in polyphenols, particularly ellagitannins. This is also the case for other ellagitannin-containing fruits and nuts including strawberry, raspberry, blackberry, walnuts, and muscadine grapes. The bioavailability of ellagitannins and ellagic acid is, however, very low.

These molecules suffer extensive metabolism by the gut microbiota to produce urolithins that are much better absorbed. Research, mostly based on in vitro testing, has shown preliminary evidence of the anti-inflammatory, anticarcinogenic, antiglycative, antioxidant, and antimicrobial effects of urolithins, supporting their potential contribution to the health effects attributed to pomegranate and ellagitannin-rich foods. The number of in vivo studies is still limited.[344]

---

343 Baba, Y., Inagaki, S., Nakagawa, S. *et al.* 2020, "Effects of l-Theanine on Cognitive Function in Middle-Aged and Older Subjects: A Randomized Placebo-Controlled Study", *Journal of Medicinal Food*, Vol. 24, No. 4, pp. 333-341, https://doi.org/10.1089/jmf.2020.4803.

344 Singh, A., Andreux, P. A., Fouassier, A. M. *et al.* 2022, "Urolithin A improves muscle strength, exercise performance, and biomarkers of mitochondrial health in a randomized trial in middle-aged adults", *Cell Reports Medicine*, Vol. 3, No. 5, https://doi.org/10.1016/j.xcrm.2022.100633.

The following had no effect on life extension in mice:

- Resveratrol
- Spermidine
- Curcumin
- Green tea extract (less early deaths in female mice)
- MCT oil
- Fish oil.

Presence and Quantity of Botanical Ingredients with Purported Performance-Enhancing Properties in Sports Supplements[345]

Eighty-nine percent of dietary supplement labels did not accurately declare the ingredients found in the products, and 12% of products contained FDA-prohibited ingredients.

Diets

Calorie Restriction

Calorie restriction without malnutrition, commonly referred to as dietary restriction (CR), results in a well-documented extension of life span. CR also produces significant, long-lasting improvements in biomarkers of metabolic health that begin to accrue soon after its introduction. The improvements are attributable in part to the effects of CR on energy balance, which limit fat accumulation of excess body fat that occurs when energy intake chronically exceeds the energy costs for growth and maintenance of existing tissue.

The resulting obesity promotes the development of insulin resistance, disordered lipid metabolism, and increased expression

345 Cohen, P. A., Avula, B., Katragunta, K. 2023, "Presence and Quantity of Botanical Ingredients With Purported Performance-Enhancing Properties in Sports Supplements", *JAMA Network Open*, Vol. 6, No. 7, https://doi.org/10.1001/jamanetworkopen.2023.23879.

of inflammatory markers in peripheral tissues. The link between the life-extending effects of CR and adiposity is the subject of an ongoing debate, but it is clear that decreased fat accumulation improves insulin sensitivity and produces beneficial effects on overall metabolic health.

Methionine Restriction (MR)[346]

Over the last 30 years, dietary methionine restriction (MR) has emerged as a promising CR mimetic because it produces a comparable extension in lifespan but, surprisingly, does not require food restriction. Dietary MR also reduces adiposity but does so through a paradoxical increase in both energy intake and expenditure. The increase in energy expenditure fully compensates for increased energy intake and effectively limits fat deposition. Perhaps more importantly, the diet increases metabolic flexibility and overall insulin sensitivity and improves lipid metabolism while decreasing systemic inflammation.

Behaviours

Exercise is recognised as the most important 'investment' in health and, therefore, longevity and deserves its own chapter, which it received earlier in this book.

Diet is incredibly important, with over 5,000 micronutrients as well as 13 vitamins. The key is variety, and I based the Newtrition-Mediterranean diet (see end chapter) on this.

Regarding active behaviours, saunas and hot baths seem to reduce heart attacks while at the opposite end there is the ice therapy, which also seem to reduce inflammation. Wim Hof

346 Orgeron, M. L., Stone, K. P., Wanders, D. *et al.* 2014, "The impact of dietary methionine restriction on biomarkers of metabolic health", *Progress in Molecular Biology and Translational Science*, Vol. 121, pp. 351-376. https://doi.org/10.1016/B978-0-12-800101-1.00011-9.

is known as the Iceman and can hold himself in ice water for nearly two hours with an elevated body temperature. He climbed to a great height on Mount Everest, in shorts and no shirt, and attributes much to his breathing technique.

Sleep is restorative while our brain goes on learning in its deep, slow-wave phase. It would seem light is detrimental, even to marine life like oysters from street light spillage, and so complete black out curtains or a mask should be considered mandatory.

Challenging the mind by multiple and varied novel learning disciplines such as a language, painting, and computers has seen a 200% improvement in cognition after a year in elderly participants.

Meditation reduces stress with beneficial downstream effects.

The Thymus gland produces our 'Killer T-Cells' but is allowed to atrophy, whereas increasing our muscle mass releases a chemical which reactivates it.

The cytokine Interleukin 7 increases in the sedentary, so again, aerobic exercise is recommended.

Tai Chi has remarkably reproduced and even improved the benefits of exercise.

Hyperbaric Oxygen Therapy experiments have lengthened participant's telomeres.

Biohacking

It is impossible to keep up with the biohackers who now buy whole houses with both good and useless wellness gadgets. The Wall Street Journal had a good article for those interested.[347]

I can only conclude, "Show me the proof."

347 Flint, J. 2023, The Biohacking Devotees Spending Hundreds of Thousands—Even Millions—to Enhance Their Homes", *The Wall Street Journal*, 9 August.

CHAPTER 38

Experts, Individuals, Players, & Investors

"Having the data is not the same as having the expertise to look through the data—if it were, everybody with a smartphone would be a doctor or a scientist."

– Abhijit Naskar (1991-)

"People who think they know everything are a great annoyance to those of us who do."

– Isaac Azimov (1920-1992).

At the outset, I apologize profusely to all those eminent medical practitioners and scientists I have missed. This is not an almanac for such distinguished people, so the ones listed are those I have just happened upon without the diligent research necessitated for such an undertaking. I ask forgiveness for any such omissions and for any misinformation.

As to Longevity, no one has all the answers, but there are some fundamental agreements and also many unproven theories and practices.

Investors are investors, but it is my impression that many are incredibly rich, have great trouble spending their fortunes, and are getting older. What better way for them to invest?

My own bias is that, for advice on longevity, I favour clinicians—and old clinicians at that. It's a case of having decades of observation as well as the *clinical responsibility* of having to deal with patients and not being carried away by the drug companies' latest spiel, the researchers' enthusiasms, and the desperate need for funds. It is also a case of them having achieved extreme old age—and it's not all genetics, so they must know something.

The great clinicians have what we call 'clinical acumen', which I translate as having a sixth sense that there is 'something else'. This, I equate to the machine learning of AI in that they have seen so many other similar cases they recognise the odd one out. But it makes them pursue a case like Sherlock Holmes (who was based on an Edinburgh Doctor and where I 'walked' the same wards and was inculcated with the same methods of observation), and I find their conclusions somewhat more gentle, perhaps thoughtful and less didactic, based on their ultra-long clinical experience.

That said, Ancel Keys died aged 100, and he was not a medical practitioner, but I agree with what he said.

I have added their age, as best I can, as it helps me place their interests and theories in a temporal context.

My recommendation is to read widely, check the qualifications of the author, and be circumspect if they are super-keen enthusiasts, let alone zealots, and if they are selling anything (other than fresh produce) or promoting the unproven.

Practitioners

As promised, I hereby identify those experts who have detailed their regimes or programs and tests by an asterisk before their names if you wish to access their websites.

I draw your attention to the following disclaimer that accompanies most longevity commentaries. As such, I have identified those who are not medical practitioners.

As I stated elsewhere, my preference is for clinicians who actually consult and treat patients and not medical graduates who have gone into research, such as epidemiology, or who don't see patients face to face, such as pathologists and radiologists. As to the scientists, I liken them to pharmaceutical chemists researching new drugs. Some of them are quite brilliant, but feeding monkeys or mice, new drugs is simply not the same as treating human patients. Whereas any new drug has to go through years of testing to get approved, these supplements don't, and I sometimes feel these scientists get carried away by their own field of minutiae.

But I try to have an open mind and try to follow their achievements.

In the USA, the usual medical practitioner qualification is MD, whereas scientists are mostly PhDs and, as such, entitled to be called 'Doctor' but not to advise medically.

I was recently approached by a young medical graduate interested in opening a longevity clinic. He was most disarming and honest, saying how he 'wanted to make money'.

I replied as follows:

"As I see it, there are three approaches to longevity clinics, and I don't hold any holier-than-thou attitudes in as much that, while a doctor can advise what is regarded as ethical and needed, there will always be patients who want more…I don't think the plastic surgeons refuse women boob jobs.

1. As a specialist physician, my approach is based on Evidence-Based Preventive Medicine. This prioritises and investigates what kills or ills us and offers prevention/ treatment. Today's biohackers may criticise this as not being proactive, but I refute this.

Cardiovascular Disease is our greatest killer, so I test for it (and the other killer illnesses) and then proactively take steps to prevent it and them. However, some tests may reveal an unfixable potential disorder. I discuss these with the patient if they want them.

2. Dr Attia (see below) offers extended testing and enthuses longevity via rapamycin and such. This may be regarded as being proactive, but as yet, it is not proven, which is not really being proactive.
3. ETK (my abbreviation for 'Every Test Known') is the practice the biohackers demand, such as six-monthly full-body MRIs and up to some 50(+) blood tests. This practice has no known benefits as of yet."

What I didn't add was that the pendulum has swung such that, when I was young, I accepted all responsibility for the patient, even withholding fatal diagnoses. Before anyone becomes judgemental, I saw many patients who "felt" something was wrong but didn't want to know what (nor did their loved ones want them to know). Those patients sailed off blissfully. Consider the example of an ex-veteran who begged me to tell him his diagnosis, as he "could take it". But when I told him his 'lung shadow' was, in fact, cancer, he simply folded and went into a steep, deep depression from which he never recovered. And today, the 'loved ones' would sue the doctor for 'non-full disclosure'.

In this brave new world, there are no longer 'patients' but 'consumers and customers', and they are always right and get what they want and demand.

In addition, I have an open mind but some reservations as to extended testing, extended exercise, and extended dependence on laboratory tests, which I sometimes feel border on obsessive, introspective behaviour by both consumer-demanding 'clients' and the doctor.

I well remember a jaundiced patient (yellow eye sclera) who my fellow medical student was presenting to the Consultant Surgeon, giving a long rundown of all the laboratory tests, but missing this essential clinical sign. Finally, the Surgeon exploded 'Look! Look at the patient! *There* is your laboratory!'

In the same way today's biohackers want a laboratory to estimate their 'biological age' but the astute clinician would immediately note many more accurate signs of aging. But there I go on my Sherlock Holmes bent again. There would seem no doubt, however, that accurate biological aging of individual tissues and organs will eventuate.

Dr. Gladys McGarey MD (102-year-old)

Residing in Scottsdale, Arizona, Gladys is still a practising doctor and was one of the first physicians in the United States to adopt a holistic approach to medicine. She has now written *The Well Lived Life*—a tome advising the six secrets to long-lasting health and happiness.

"In essence, the secret is to live in every moment," she explains. "As I've gotten older, I've become more content, and I have my rich bank of memories to thank for that."

Gladys is disparaging of the stricter regimes the 1% swear by to reverse aging. "Laughter and joy aids healing," she argues. Her secret for living a long and fulfilled life is having a purpose to keep us going.[348]

---

348 McGarey, G. 2023, *The Well-Lived Life: A 102-Year-Old Doctor's Six Secrets to Health and Happiness at Every Age*, Atria Books.

Dr. Howard Tucker, MD (101-year-old)

The World's 'Oldest Practicing Doctor'[349] (what about Dr. McGarey above?)

While genetics and luck are a good head start, he says, stimulating your mind (at all ages) is crucial for staying mentally sharp and keeping your brain healthy as you age.

Here are his best tips for brain health.

1. Engage in something thought-provoking and enjoyable
2. Interact with other people
3. Adjust your mindset
   "I recognize that I am 101 years old, but I don't dwell on it," he says. Instead, he focuses more on being grateful for how many years he's lived. Research backs up how gratitude can help people live longer.
4. 4. Create sustainable habits
   "I don't believe in any fad diets, miracle cures, or specific exercise routines that promise you'll live to 100," he says.

Rather, he encourages health-promoting behaviours and moderation. Loving what you do is the ultimate key, according to Dr. Tucker. "Enthusiasm about your work, personal life, and having a sense of purpose, will naturally lead to motivation."

Ancel Keys Physiologist (100, deceased)

Keys popularised and promoted the Mediterranean diet. He died aged 100 and his wife, Margaret, aged 97.

Keys always believed in the benefits of regular exercise—he walked and swam a lot in Italy and found time for safe, useful

349 Guinness Book of World Records verifies record of neurologist Dr.Howard Tucker, who still teaches medical residents at local hospital and takes on legal expert witness work in his spare time. The day after his 100th birthday on 10 July 2022.

exercise such as working in his yard. But he had no intention of joining up with the joggers. "I try to persuade people to have some pleasurable, safe exercise, preferably useful, when they are older." And dieting can be dangerous, too. "Diet fads are for the birds."

Dr. George D. Lundberg, MD (92-year-old)

Professor of Pathology, Editor at Large Medscape

Dr. Lundberg has written *How to Live to a Ripe Old Age,* which is a delightful and very wise synopsis I would urge all to read.[350]

Dr. Leroy Hood MD (84-year-old)[351]

Lee is the cofounder of the Institute of Systems Biology (ISB) and is best known for inventing revolutionary biological instruments that paved the way for the Human Genome Project.

He wakes up around 5:30 a.m. He spends the first two hours of his day at his desk; then he begins a 40-minute workout routine: 200 push-ups, 100 sit-ups, and 100 deep-knee bends, followed by a series of stretches and balance exercises.

He takes 25 supplements, like vitamins C and D, zinc, and magnesium, and skips breakfast as part of an intermittent-fasting routine. After that, he walks about a mile to his office in Seattle. He reads roughly a book a week, plays folk music on his

---

350 Lundberg G. D. 2022, "Would You Like to Live to a 'Ripe Old Age'?" *Medscape*, 31 August. As President and Chair of the Board of Directors of The Lundberg Institute, Dr George D. Lundberg, MD, has more than 30 years' combined experience as Editor-in-Chief of *JAMA* (*Journal of the American Medical Association*), the 10 AMA specialty journals, *AM News*, *Medscape*, *The Medscape Journal of Medicine*, *eMedicine* from WebMD, and *MedPage Today* from Everyday Health.

351 Moens, J. 2023, "Leroy Hood Wants To Show You How To Live for a Really, Really Long Time", *Popular Mechanics*, 28 June.

recorder, and takes long, meandering hikes. At 7 p.m., he eats dinner, usually a combination of leafy greens, whole grains, and fresh fruit, then goes to sleep around 10:30. Over the past decade of living by a philosophy of disease prevention, he has lost 25 pounds.

He wears a Fitbit on his right wrist and a thick black Oura Ring on his left ring finger that monitors his sleep. At least twice a year, he gets blood tests from his physicians to monitor his levels of cholesterol, vitamin B_{12}, vitamin B9, lipid profile, and markers of inflammation. He takes drugs like NAD+, which has been shown to slow aging in animals, but is still considered unproven.

Dr Michael Mosley (67, deceased)

Dr. Mosley described himself as a medical journalist and has hosted a number of excellent BBC TV medical series and written books such as *The 5:2 Diet*, which he claims cured his Type 2 Diabetes and popularized Intermittent Fasting. He studied philosophy, Politics and Economics at New College, Oxford, before working for two years as a banker in the City of London. He then decided to move into medicine, intending to become a psychiatrist, studying at the Royal Free Hospital Medical School, now part of UCL Medical School. He was no longer a registered doctor. His BBC Series, "Trust Me, I'm a Doctor", is well worthwhile. He even had a longevity series. Tragically, he died from heat exhaustion hiking alone while on holiday on a Greek Island in June 2024.

Dr Peter Attia, MD (50-year-old)

Peter Attia is a Canadian-American author, physician, and researcher. He earned his Bachelor of Science in mechanical engineering and applied mathematics from Queen's University in 1996, then attended Stanford University School of Medicine, graduating in 2001 with a Doctor of Medicine degree. From 2001 to 2006, Attia embarked on a residency in general surgery at Johns Hopkins Hospital in Baltimore, Maryland. However, he did not complete his residency, nor did he pursue a fellowship or become board-certified in surgery. During this period, he also conducted research at the National Institutes of Health (NIH), focusing on cancer immunotherapy for melanoma. After leaving his residency program, Attia joined the consulting firm McKinsey & Company in Palo Alto, California. His work there spanned the Corporate Risk Practice and Healthcare Practice.

In 2012, Attia co-founded the Nutrition Science Initiative (NuSI) with Gary Taubes, focusing on promoting nutrition research and addressing health challenges related to obesity, diabetes, and metabolic diseases.

In 2014, he founded a private clinic dedicated to longevity medicine. Attia is also known for his blog, initially called "The Eating Academy," which later evolved into "War on Insulin" and is now hosted at peterattiamd.com. He launched the podcast "The Peter Attia Drive", where he interviews experts on topics related to longevity, metabolic health, and medical research.

Attia has authored a book titled "Outlive: The Science & Art of Longevity", co-authored with Bill Gifford, which was published in 2023.

The book has been a bestseller since its release and has garnered significant attention.

He is arguably the best-known pundit on longevity, with his podcast and his best-selling book. He is gratifyingly very scientifically and medically based but at the cutting edge. He is evidently very physical, having been a boxer, swum 20-mile marathons, and now lifts weights.

According to an interview in the Wall St Journal,[352] Matt Kaeberlein, a molecular biologist and longevity scientist and a regular guest on "The Drive", says Attia taps into widening frustration with modern healthcare. "There is a growing dissatisfaction with the status quo, which also is driving people to look for alternatives to try to empower themselves."

He promotes some practices and treatments outside of mainstream medicine. Attia has said he takes, and prescribes to some patients, rapamycin as well as extensive blood tests, preventive full-body scans, and continuous glucose monitoring. As alluded to before, I see this as where medicine is headed: From physician counsel to consumer demand, which is titillated by the media and, often dubious, research articles.

Dr Perry Wilson, MD, MSCE

Dr. Wilson does the 'Impact Factor' for Medscape which, thanks goodness, analyses the many, often questionable, claims made in published papers, and I highly recommend it. He attended Harvard College, where he graduated with honors in biochemistry. He then attended medical school at Columbia College of Physicians and Surgeons before completing his internship, residency, and fellowship at the University of Pennsylvania.

In 2012, he received a Master's degree in Clinical Epidemiology, which has informed his research ever since. At Yale since 2014, his goal is using patient-level data and advanced analytics to personalize medicine to each individual patient. He is the creator of the popular online course "Understanding Medical Research: Your Facebook Friend Is Wrong" on the Coursera platform and the author of *How Medicine Works and When It Doesn't—Learning Who to Trust to Get and Stay Healthy*.

352 Janin, A. 2023, "The Favorite Doctor of Bio-Hackers and the Longevity-Obsessed", *Wall Street Journal*, 10 September.

Norman Swan, AM FAHMS (born 1953)

A Scottish-born Australian physician, journalist and broadcaster, Swan moved to Australia to continue his training but transitioned from medicine when he became a producer and broadcaster with the Australian Broadcasting Corporation in 1982. He co-hosted the Radio National program *Life Matters* between 1996 and 2001, and produced and presented ABC radio program *The Health Report* from its inception in 1985, which is well worth while. From March 2020 till 2023 Swan co-hosted *Coronacast*, a podcast about pandemics and the coronavirus. This has been replaced with the *What's That Rash* podcast. He is the author of three books: *So You Think You Know What's Good for You*; *So You Want to Live Younger, Longer?*; and *So You Want to Know What's Good for Your Kids?*.

Dr Claudia Kawas, MD

Dr. Kawas attended the School of Medicine, University of California, Irvine and has spent 15 years studying people aged over 90 and advocates the following to lessen the risks of dying young:

- Exercise for 15 minutes a day: 11% less risk of dying young
- Drink two glasses wine a day: 18% less risk
- Drink two cups coffee a day: 10% less risk
- Spend at least two hours a day on hobbies: 21% less risk
- Body mass index being slightly overweight for older people: 3% less risk.[353]

353 Institute on Aging (IOA), 2022, "'Clinical and Pathological Studies of the Oldest-Old' Claudia Kawas, MD discusses 90+ Study", 2 June, https://penninstituteonaging.wordpress.com/2022/06/02/kawas.

Dr Luigi Ferrucci MD, PhD

Dr. Luigi is a geriatrician and an epidemiologist who conducts research on the causal pathways leading to progressive physical and cognitive decline in older persons. He refined the design of the Baltimore Longitudinal Study of Aging to focus on the Geroscience Hypothesis, which states the pace of biological aging is the root cause of many age-related chronic diseases, as well as physical and cognitive disability.

Dr Richard Miller, MD, PhD

Professor of Pathology at the University of Michigan and the Director of Michigan's Paul F. Glenn Center for Biology of Aging and Interventions Testing Program (ITP).

He runs one of the three laboratories for the Intervention Test Programs, which trials drugs and supplements. While these are on mice, they are the best guides available. The three labs test independently and publish their results which put off the supplement sellers and bring a refreshing validity. His "Live Longer World" interviews are well worthwhile. "One of the key things that's happened is that the evidence that you can actually slow down and interfere with the aging process in mammals … has become so overwhelming that only the willfully blind can ignore it," he has said.

Dr. Michael Lustgarten, PhD, Scientist (53-year-old)

He is part of the Nutrition, Exercise Physiology, and Sarcopenia (NEPS) Team at the Human Nutrition Research Center on Aging at Tufts University. His academic research currently focuses on the role of the gut microbiome and serum metabolome on muscle mass and function in older adults. Dr. Lustgarten has contributed to 30 publications in peer-reviewed journals that have been cited more than 3,200 times. He also has a growing YouTube channel that is focused on biohacking aging and presenting aging-related news. He supplies great amounts of data for his 9 or so biomarkers and optimises these by then modifying his diet, weighing all his food, and analysing its macro and micronutrient constituents. He also gets his blood taken for testing four to six times a year.

Dr Aubrey De Grey PhD, Scientist (Biomedical Gerontologist) (60-year-old)

The author of *Ending Aging*, *The Mitochondrial Free Radical Theory of Aging*, and *Advancing Conversations* has launched a new non-profit initiative called the Longevity Escape Velocity Foundation (LEVF), which is now close to cooling organs for transplant. His approach to aging, called Strategies for Engineered Negligible Senescence (SENS) earned him worldwide recognition, while his eccentric looks, and lifestyle are sometimes the source of controversy.

Dr Nir Barzilai, MD (68-year-old)

Nir Barzilai, the director of the Institute for Aging Research at the Albert Einstein College of Medicine, is sometimes credited with discovering the first "longevity gene," an unusual variation in DNA that is linked to exceptionally long life. He has studied the lives of hundreds of centenarians, the people they've married, and their kids, observing that the children of centenarians are "about 10 years healthier" than their peers. As a somewhat salutary check, around half the centenarians in his study have been overweight; thirty per cent of the women and sixty per cent of the men have been heavy smokers.

He is seeking approval from the US Food and Drug Administration for the first clinical trial of metformin to treat aging as a 2014 UK clinical trial involving over 150,000 people, which revealed that diabetics taking metformin live longer than non-diabetics who don't.[354] But a robust clinical trial was needed, so Barzilai began the 'Targeting Aging with Metformin' (TAME) trial over a four-year period. Instead of looking at the ability of metformin to delay a single age-related disease, as the other trials have done, this study will assess the drug's capacity to delay the onset of age-related disease in general. It will show if metformin can increase healthspan.

The evidence for metformin is impressive, but as detailed elsewhere, once you start, don't stop.

Dr Mikhail V Blagosklonny MD, PhD

Probably the greatest advocate for rapamycin (see Rapamycin previous chapter).

Dr Steve Horvath PhD, Scientist (55-year-old)

Horvath is a professor at the University of California, Los Angeles, known for developing the Horvath aging clock, which is a highly accurate molecular biomarker of aging and arguably the Gold Standard, His work on the genomic biomarkers of aging, the aging process, and many age-related diseases/conditions has earned him several research awards. Horvath is a principal investigator at the anti-aging start-up Altos Labs and co-founder of the non-profit Clock Foundation.

354 Bannister, C. A., Holden, S. E., Jenkins-Jones, S. *et al.* 2014, "Can people with type 2 Diabetes live longer than those without? A comparison of mortality in people initiated with metformin or sulphonylurea monotherapy and matched, non-diabetic controls", *Diabetes, Obesity and Metabolism*, Vol. 16, No. 11, pp. 1165-73, https://doi.org/10.1111/dom.12354.

Dr David Sinclair BSc, PhD, Scientist (53-year-old)

Sinclair studied at the University of New South Wales, Sydney, obtaining a BSc in biochemistry with honours in 1991 and a PhD in molecular genetics, focusing on gene regulation in yeast.

He lifts weights two to three times per week.

He performs "time-restricted fasting" for 20 hours per day and eats within a four-hour window. This, he believes, puts his body in a state of 'autophagy,' which means the cells begin to renew themselves as the body isn't designed to digest food constantly all day, every day.

He takes NMN, Berberine, Resveratrol, and eats a predominantly plant-based diet. particularly leafy greens and varied colourful vegetables. He gets at least eight hours of sleep every night. He promotes his supplements.

However, a long article in the Wall Street Journal (April 27, 2024) concludes, "But he has increasingly drawn criticism for hyping his own research or promoting unproven products, especially when he stood to benefit financially".

Dr Matt Kaeberlein, Scientist (52-year-old)

Biogerontologist and director of the Healthy Aging and Longevity Research Institute at the University of Washington.

One of several scientists warning of the longevity molecule industry's potential to be riddled with "snake oil". He cites resveratrol, which was the "wonder molecule" of its day 15 years ago, as a cautionary tale as it, in fact, has no effect on lifespan or healthspan, at least in mice. One main area of focus is rapamycin, a drug that has been found to extend healthy lifespan in a number of trials in mice and fruit flies; he is also involved in the University of Washington's Dog Aging Project, which, because of the speed with which dogs grow old, means "we can actually get answers in a reasonable timeframe." He foresees being able to prove the efficacy of certain interventions in the next five to 10 years.

Disappointingly, the funding for the dog project has not been renewed at this juncture.

Vadim Gladyshev, PhD (49-year-old)

Vadim N. Gladyshev is a professor of medicine at Brigham and Women's Hospital, Harvard Medical School, who specializes in antioxidant biology. He is known for his characterization of the human selenoproteome. He is also known for his work on the effects of aging in humans.

He was, apparently, a professional footballer in Russia. His colleagues esteem him for remaining independent.

Dr. Valter Longo, Scientist (55-year-old)

Professor of Gerontology and Biological Sciences and Director of the Longevity Institute at the University of Southern California, Los Angeles

Dr. Longo is also the Director of the Longevity and Cancer Program at the IFOM Institute of Molecular Oncology in Milan, Italy. He is a biogerontologist and cell biologist known for his studies on the role of fasting and nutrient response genes on cellular protection aging and diseases and for proposing that longevity is regulated by similar genes and mechanisms in many eukaryotes. He is the author of *The Fasting Mimicking Diet* and takes a multivitamin.

Prof Janet Lord CBE FMedSc

Institute of Inflammation and Aging, Professor of Immune Cell Biology, Director of the MRC-Versus Arthritis Centre for

Musculoskeletal aging Research and a theme lead in two NIHR funded centres: the NIHR Birmingham BRC and the NIHR Surgical Reconstruction and Microbiology Research Centre.

She is scathing over experimental measures some of the super-rich favour, such as cryogenics and blood plasma transfusion. "There's literally no evidence cryogenics will ever work."

Dr Oliver Zolman, MB, BS, BSc (29-year-old)

Leads the 30-plus doctor team behind Bryan Johnson's reportedly $2 million "Project Blueprint" longevity craze (see next). He studied at King's College London, graduating with a degree in Regenerative Medicine & Biology. His project encompasses over 200 longevity-related protocols to help Johnson reverse his biological age.

Patients and Experiments

The Brave New World; The Worried Well

Some of these regimes are beyond the discipline and pockets of most. But even spookier, there is little, if any, proven evidence for their regimes and supplements, although many do incredible research into their biomarkers.

The proof and evidence, of course, is in if they actually do live longer and healthier.

And I can't help but wonder if these incredible regimes don't impact them having fun or their quality of life, as alluded to elsewhere.

This explosion in science has created a new class of lifestyle, health, and longevity 'enthusiasts', for want of a better word, who describe themselves as:

- ***Biohackers*** who make purposeful tweaks to their lifestyle for a desired outcome such as weight loss, reduced anxiety, or increased libido.

- ***Spanners***, people who proactively seek to expand their own healthspan and lifespan indefinitely.
- ***Transhumanists*** believe technology can and should evolve humans beyond their physical limitations.

There are overlaps and merges.

Despite them apparently not having any medical training, some eschew and seem critical of traditional medicine, with a logic I find somewhat akin to criticising Daimler or Henry Ford for not having invented the electric car. Their evolution has been made possible by this explosion in science along with new tests and home-tests, which they analyse and recommend, allowing the money-making pop-up laboratories pander to their 'need'.

They seem obsessed with regularly testing themselves, adopting strict diets, and taking supplements.

While most of us have an interest in our health, the hypochondriac is a well-known entity. Clinicians call them 'The Worried Well'. It is, of course, a very difficult decision to refuse a patient a test. The media delights in exposing how a person's fatal diagnosis was missed. So where does it now begin and end?

A small study[355] looked into the "Perspective of Healthy Asymptomatic Patients Requesting General Blood Tests from Their Physicians: A Qualitative Study" which revealed "a substantial gap between patients' attitudes and beliefs about general blood tests and current evidence-based guidelines."

The eruption of these laboratories, who will apparently do any tests an individual is prepared to pay for, would seem to satiate these Biohackers' and Worried Wells' curiosity. Other than that, there are the 'current evidence-based guidelines'.

---

355 Shaked, M., Levkovich, I., Adar, T. *et al.* 2019, "Perspective of healthy asymptomatic patients requesting general blood tests from their physicians: a qualitative study", *BMC Family Practice*, Vol. 20, No 1, p. 51, https://doi.org/10.1186/s12875-019-0940-9.

I do not know if the following consider themselves as such, but they have been the subject of much publicity or self-promotion.

As of 2003:

Robert Nelsen, 60

Co-founded Arch Venture Partners and is the largest institutional investor in Altos Labs. He downs a daily cocktail of almost a dozen different drugs, including rapamycin, metformin, taurine, and nicotinamide mononucleotide, and has a full-body MRI every six months, sees a dermatologist every three months, and has annual blood tests to detect cancer. At his home, he works out in an "electric suit" that he says emits low-frequency impulses to build muscle and improve health.

Tony Pemberton, 37

"I fast for 14 hours a day. Upon waking up, I go to the gym. Three to four times a week, O'll use the sauna after, as it activates the FOXO3 gene, which is nicknamed the longevity gene. I'll have a low carb/sugar breakfast, and during the day I'll drink six to eight cups of green tea and eat around 10 portions of fruit and vegetables. I try to stop eating by 6pm."

"I didn't want to be decrepit and look awful when I was older," the 37-year-old tells Metro.co.uk. "I wanted to get more out of life."

He also swears by peptide therapy, using a vast range of supplements to stimulate cellular regrowth, to reverse the natural aging process. He takes an astounding 25 different supplements a day, specifically tailored to his needs.[356]

356 Bond, K. 2023, "Who Wants To Live Forever", *Metro UK*, 11 June 11.

Bryan Johnson, 46

"The Most Measured Man in Human History"

The US entrepreneur and tech company CEO made headlines with a body modification plan he hopes will see him last forever. Johnson's $2 million-a-year routine involves popping 111 pills a day, apparently including metformin, glucosamine sulfate, *N*-acetylcysteine (NAC) and rapamycin. He is a vegan. His daily workout routine, which takes between 45 to 60 minutes, consists of roughly 25 exercises specifically designed to lower his rate of biological aging,

He tracks every area of his health, from hearing to liver function, and employs a team of 30 doctors and scientists. He claims he has achieved metabolic health equal to the top 1.5 % of 18-year-olds, inflammation 66 % lower than the average 10 year old, and reduced his speed of aging by the equivalent of 31 years. While he probably has achieved some of this, as noted elsewhere, these measurements are questionable. His testing and lifestyle are extreme and the subject of many interviews, as he does not seem shy of publicity.[357] The latest article about him appears in the February 2024 Vanity Fair.

Investors & Labs

"We are drowning in information while starving for wisdom."

– E. O. Wilson (1929-2021)

The world's billionaires and entrepreneurs figured if age is a condition or an illness, it can be cured. They are pouring money into age-reversal investments.

357 Alter, C. 2023, "The Man Who Thinks He Can Live Forever", *Time Magazine*, 20 September, https://time.com/6315607/bryan-johnsons-quest-for-immortality/.

But to discover and develop a novel therapeutic agent that could pause, stop, or even reverse aging and prolong life is incredibly complex and expensive. Developing just one single drug by the usual method takes over a decade,

and Deloitte found that the average cost of developing a new drug among the top 20 global biopharmas it studied rose 15% ($298 million) in 2022, to approximately $2.3 billion. That figure includes the average cost of developing a candidate from discovery through clinical trials to the market. And such new drug developments fail 80% of the times.[358]

Understandably, their research is clouded by stealth and secrecy, with no progress reported thus far.

The global longevity and anti-senescence therapy market was valued at $25.1 billion in 2020 and is projected to reach $44.2 billion by 2030, growing at a CAGR of 6.1% from 2021 to 2030.[359]

The statistics show the estimated size of the anti-aging market worldwide in 2021 and provide a forecast for 2022 to 2027. In 2021, the global anti-aging market was estimated to be worth about USD$62.6 billion. The anti-aging market is estimated to see a compound annual growth rate (CAGR) of nearly seven percent between 2022 and 2027.[360]

A number of impressive laboratories and research institutes have started backed by a host of billionaires and institutional

---

358 Deloitte, 2023, "Deloitte pharma study: Drop-off in returns on R&D investments – sharp decline in peak sales per asset", press release, 23 January.

359 Allied Market Research, 2022, *Longevity and Anti-senescence Therapy Market Size, Share, Competitive Landscape and Trend Analysis Report by Therapy, by Application, by End user: Global Opportunity Analysis and Industry Forecast, 2020-2030,* https://www.alliedmarketresearch.com/longevity-and-anti-senescence-therapy-market-A14010.

360 Petruzzi, D. 2023, "Operating income of Givaudan worldwide from 2013 to 2023", *Stasista,* 30 January, https://www.statista.com/statistics/482559/operating-income-givaudan-worldwide/.

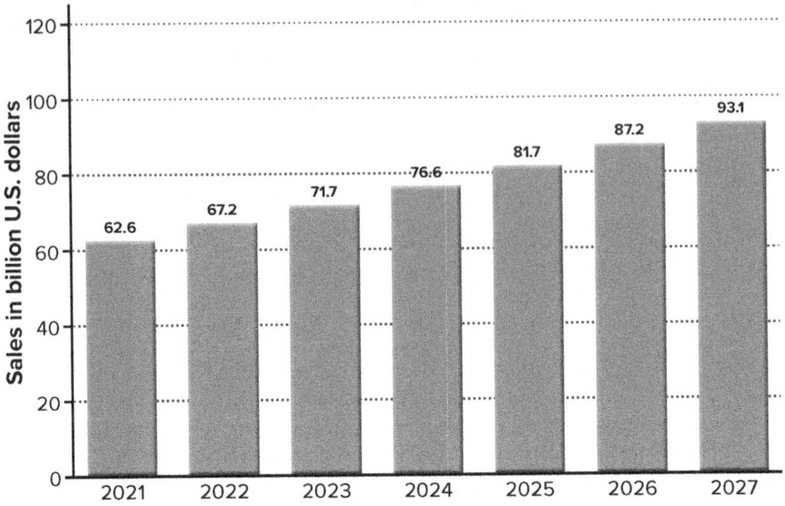

Figure 40: Size of the anti-aging market worldwide from 2021 to 2027 (in billion U.S. dollars) (*Source: Statista*).

investors such as Jeff Bezos, Peter Thiel, Larry Ellison, and Larry Page. Many employ Alphabet and Nobel laureates.

Their methodologies revealed so far are varied, including cellular reprogramming, mind uploading, body part replacement/cyborg technology, genetic editing/gene therapy, cryonics, anti-aging drugs/regenerative medicine, cloning, and parabiosis (young-blood transfusions).

The cosmetic market is distinct from the longevity market and confuses the issue by assuming the name "Anti-Aging". It, however, reflects just how interested people are in looking young(er), hence the attraction of investors to produce a therapeutic agent that actually makes us younger.

The Anti-Aging Market Trends and Forecast, which is the cosmetic anti-wrinkle appearance part of the market and not the longevity part, is expected to reach an estimated $78.2 billion by 2028, and it is forecast to grow at a CAGR of 5.2% from 2023 to 2028.[361]

361 ReportLinker, 27 April 2023

These are, by no means, all the labs and start-ups, with one database listing over 560 longevity companies, but just a sample to show what's out there and the intense interest in longevity projects. It has been suggested that such developments will take a decade, but one promises a pill sooner.

AgeX Therapeutics

Listed in the NYSE, AgeX Therapeutics develops innovative medicines and advanced therapeutics that seek to address human aging. Utilizing tissue regeneration technologies, small molecule drug delivery systems, and stem cell research, the firm aims to crack the code of cellular immortality to revitalize health and reverse the effects of degenerative diseases and aging in humans.

The firm was founded in 2017 by Michael D West, a prominent biogerontologist and pioneer in stem cell research, cellular aging, cloning, and telomerase. Both Juvenescence Chairman Jim Mellon and CEO Dr. Greg Bailey backed AgeX in its early stage.

Alcor

Alcor, based in Arizona, reportedly has around 100 dead bodies on ice. For $230,000, your body can be frozen in liquid nitrogen in the hope it can be regenerated in the future. For $90,000, just your head can be frozen, with the hope it may be attached to a new, young body in the future.

Altos Labs, $3 billion, 2022

Altos is backed by Amazon's "Reprogramming" is the scientific term for turning old cells young again. It was discovered in 2012 by Japanese scientist Shinya Yamanaka, who called it a potential "elixir of life" and was awarded the Nobel Prize in Medicine.

Altos is on a mission to restore cell health and resilience and reverse disease, injury, and disabilities. The company focuses on cellular rejuvenation programming to create a completely new approach to medicine based on the emerging concepts of cellular health.

BioSplice Therapeutics Inc

Formerly known as Samumed, BioSplice Therapeutics focuses on developing the science and the techniques for tissue-level regeneration to treat cancer, osteoarthritis, and other aging-related diseases. As its new name suggests, the company's stated mission is to restore human health via novel therapies that use alternative splicing.

BioSplice was founded in 2008 by Turkish American billionaire Osman Kibar. Kibar holds a doctorate in biophotonics and invented a cancer diagnosis system that was eventually acquired (as the emergent company Genoptix) for USD$476 million by Swiss pharmaceutical giant Novartis in 2011.

BlueRock Therapeutics

Toronto-based BlueRock Therapeutics develops authentic cellular medicines and engineered stem cell therapies to cure a range of diseases, regenerate damaged tissues, and elevate the potential of human health. In 2021, BlueRock announced that the US FDA granted Fast Track designation for DA01 for advanced Parkinson's disease. DA01 is the company's "pluripotent stem cell-derived dopaminergic neuron therapy" being evaluated in a Phase 1 study.

Brian Armstrong

Coinbase Co-founder and CEO, recently invested in a company developing epigenetic reprogramming therapies to radically extend human healthspans.

Calico Life Sciences LLC

The Google-backed company is also focused on longevity via reprogramming and Lineage Cell Therapeutics, backed by BlackRock, Raffles Capital Management, Wells Fargo, and others.

As the health research and longevity science subsidiary of Alphabet, Calico enjoys the enormous social and financial clout of being the reputedly 5th most valuable (just around US$1.54 trillion) company on the planet.

Calico was formed in 2013 by American venture capitalist and entrepreneur Bill Maris with Google's Larry Page and hired Apple Chairman Arthur D. Levinson to serve as CEO. Calico has yet to make a breakthrough announcement. In July 2021, the company extended its partnership with AbbVie to develop novel therapeutics that combat senescence and prolong human lifespan.

Elevian

Elevian develops medicines that restore youthful regenerative capacity in humans, with the potential to halt and treat a range of diseases related to aging by conducting research that demonstrates tissue and organic regeneration capabilities acquired by older animals after being transfused with the blood of young animals.

These experiments—largely conducted by Elevian's scientific founders working at the Harvard Department of Stem Cell and Regenerative Biology—enabled the company to identify its lead drug candidate: recombinant human GDF11, which shows efficacy in regenerating heart, brain, muscle, and other tissues damaged by age-related diseases such as stroke and Diabetes. The biotech start-up has exclusive global rights to the patent portfolio for GDF11 held by Harvard University.

Hevolution Foundation

This foundation was established as a non-profit in 2018 by Saudi royal decree. Hevolution doesn't conduct its own research but, instead, aims to work with established institutions to pump money into underfunded areas of study. It receives funding from the Saudi Arabian government of up to $1 billion per year to fund the science of increasing healthy human lifespans.

Human Longevity Inc.

Operating under the wellness service brand Health Nucleus, Human Longevity Inc. was founded in 2013 by author-entrepreneur Peter Diamandis and genomics pioneer Craig Venter. The company aims to build the planet's most comprehensive database on human phenotypes and genotypes then use advanced AI, machine learning, and genome sequence analysis to develop new methodologies and therapeutics to treat age-related diseases, reverse the aging process, and empower people to have full, better lives. Human Longevity raised a total of US$330 M after a Series C funding round in 2019 that included Emerging Technology Partners and Celgene among its latest investors. The company managed to command a post-money valuation of USD$1 billion to USD$10 billion in the same year, despite previously having suffered numerous setbacks, including the departure of and subsequent lawsuit against founder Craig Venter that was later dismissed.

Insilico Medicine

Formed in 2014 and domiciled in Hong Kong, Insilico Medicine develops AI technologies to accelerate drug discovery, development, and testing. As its main business model, the firm provides solutions to biotechnology and pharmaceutical companies aimed at improving efficiencies in their development of therapeutics and medicines—from discovery to clinical trial analysis.

Currently, Insilico's in-house research focuses on the treatment of cancer, fibrosis, Alzheimer's Disease, and aging. In early 2021, Insilico successfully demonstrated the transformative benefit of its AI solutions by discovering, designing, and testing a new drug for pulmonary fibrosis within just 18 months for less than USD$3 million. A few months after, the company replicated its drug development success for kidney fibrosis.

Juvenescence

A life sciences company geared towards the consumer health market, Juvenescence develops prescription drugs and consumer products for age management, disease prevention, and enhanced metabolic efficiency. A pioneer in cellular and tissue regeneration, the company also uses AI, machine learning, and data to accelerate the development and drive the effectiveness of new drugs.

With five funding rounds under its belt, Juvenescence has raised around USD$219.2 million so far and is valued at USD$500 million.

Life Biosciences

Boston-based Life Biosciences develops new medicines and advanced therapies that prevent, treat, or reverse multiple diseases related to aging and has exclusive licenses with top research and academic institutions for at least three of eight well-known factors that underly the process of senescence. The ultimate goal is to therapeutically target aging itself and prolong the human lifespan. Key people behind the start-up include Tristan Edwards (co-founder and Chief Investments Officer), top genomics researcher Dr. David Sinclair (Director), and veteran pharma executive Jerry McLaughlin (CEO).

Tel Aviv University

For the first time, scientists encoded a toxin into mRNA molecules and delivered them to cancer cells. The cells produced the toxin, which eventually killed them.

Tel Aviv University researchers have, in 2023, used a single injection into the tumor bed of animals with melanoma to cause 44% to 60% of the cancer cells to disappear completely and permanently.

Unity Biotechnology

PayPal's Peter Thiel and Amazon's Jeff Bezos are two of the big names that supported Unity Biotechnology, even before its IPO in May 2018. Now listed in the Nasdaq exchange, the company was formed in 2009 to develop advanced therapeutics and transformative medicines that address age-related diseases, focusing on senescent cells.

Prior to its IPO, Unity raised a total of USD$290.6 million from seven funding rounds. Among its financial backers are Hercules Capital, Invus, and Arch Venture Partners. In 2020, the firm laid off some staff and incurred a drop in its market valuation. In addition to senescence, the company currently focuses on ophthalmology and neurology.

SECTION H

LONGEVITY NUTRITION

CHAPTER 39

The Super-Newtrition Evolutionary Longevity Diet

"Let food be thy medicine, and let medicine be thy food."

– Hippocrates (c. 460 – c. 370 BC)

The Newtrition Micronutrient Diet: Best for both physical and brain health

This is the basic excerpt from *Live Longer's Super-Newtrition: The Micronutrient Revolution,* being revised. The following foods provide all 13 vitamins and 5,000 micronutrients. It is based on a Mediterranean diet.

At the outset it must be pointed out that many medical studies (as previously documented), but especially nutrition, depend on observational studies and observation does not prove causation.

Whilst striving for evidence medicine nevertheless has fads. The latest 'evidence' i.e., observational studies are that meat and alcohol are bad. I suspect these are inspired by the very aggressive vegan-vegetarian lobby and the prohibition lobby, both of which have significant religious inputs. However, I don't think vegetarian teetotallers live longer than omnivores who drink a little alcohol and eat a little meat. Like most things it would seem excess is the problem.

There is some truth in their claims especially as to processed meats and excess booze. We have been ingesting too much of both due to their availability. *Newtrition,* however, notes that cardiovascular disease is our greatest killer but that the cleanest coronary arteries in the world are found in meat eaters – the Tsimene of Bolivia - and that our primate ancestors have been drinking alcohol probably for some 21 million years while humans for some 3,200 years and seem to have increased their longevity. Meat provides a few nutrients than plants cannot, and a little meat would seem beneficial, and a little alcohol would not seem too detrimental. Both also add to the enjoyment of life, which is beneficial.

In addition, there are many ways to analyze a dataset. Data methodologists from McMaster University have pointed out that just one method should not be used but rather, thousands should be used, then the results combined to ascertain the real truth. This methodology is known as 'multiverse analyses'.

In doing so, they studied the relationship between red meat and early mortality and found 70 unique ways to analyze the association. Of the 48 analyses deemed statistically significant, 40 indicated that red meat consumption reduced early death, and eight indicated that eating red meat led to higher mortality.[362]

362 Wang, Y., Pitre, T., Wallach, J. D. *et al.* 2024, "Grilling the data: application of specification curve analysis to red meat and all-cause mortality", *Journal of Clinical Epidemiology,* Vol. 168, No. 111278, https://doi.org/10.1016/j.jclinepi.2024.111278.

Not many studies are this rigorous, but *Newtrition* has consulted the best information available.

That said, many medical journals restrict the use of causal language to the reporting of randomized clinical trials but methods for observational studies have advanced such that causal interpretations of the results of well-conducted observational studies may be possible when strong assumptions hold. Furthermore, observational studies may be the only practical source of information for answering some questions about the causal effects.[363]

There is an excellent article in *Scientific American*, "What Did Humans Evolve To Eat," July/August 2024, by Kate Wong. Highly recommended.

Other problems with nutritional studies are peoples' memories of what they ate, but also *what they don't eat* e.g., does olive oil reduce the risk of dementia or is it that the people who can afford olive oil have a better diet and lifestyle.

It is very hard to resist the sales spiel of the supplement and vitamin pushers, especially if they are medically or scientifically qualified, but humans evolved and prospered over the last 200,000 years or so. Our ancestors evolved for some seven or eight million years before that and did so before the first vitamin was discovered in 1913, let alone the micronutrients and supplements.

Humans are the successful peak of evolution with the best brain, and we achieved this without any synthetic vitamins or supplements. To do so, I think it is obvious, we had to find the

363 Dahabreh, I. J. & Bibbins-Domingo, K. 2024, "Causal Inference About the Effects of Interventions From Observational Studies in Medical Journals", *JAMA*, Vol. 331, No. 21, pp. 1845-1853, https://doi.org/10.1001/jama.2024.7741.

foods that made us so prosper. This was achieved by seasonal variation of fruits and vegetables and by being *opportunistic omnivores*—i.e., eating anything and everything that didn't kill us, and, in doing so, the inherent 'goodies' in these foods became desirable. They supplied, not only the macronutrients of proteins, fats, and carbohydrates but also the vitamins and, I maintain, these helpful micronutrients whose secrets are only now being revealed.

But more than this, due to humans evolving by identifying what foods we liked, aka needed, they delivered their vitamins, minerals, and micronutrients in the exquisitely optimum dose, easily absorbed and metabolised but also by enforced variety due to seasonal produce, famines and scarcity. This, of course, does not occur in the Western world today and we can become picky and faddists.

Gratifyingly and reassuringly recent research corroborates this wrt our mental health (and I would claim our physical health too). viz: "Food preferences significantly influence dietary choices, yet understanding natural dietary patterns in populations remains limited. Here we identifiy four dietary subtypes by applying data-driven approaches to food-liking data from 181,990 UK Biobank participants: 'starch-free or reduced-starch' (subtype 1), 'vegetarian' (subtype 2), 'high protein and low fiber' (subtype 3) and 'balanced' (subtype 4). These subtypes varied in diverse brain health domains. The individuals with a balanced diet demonstrated better mental health and superior cognitive functions relative to other three subtypes. Compared with subtype 4, subtype 3 displayed lower gray matter volumes in regions such as the postcentral gyrus, while subtype 2 showed higher volumes in thalamus and precuneus. Genome-wide association analyses identified 16 genes different between subtype 3 and subtype 4, enriched in biological processes related to mental health and cognition. These findings provide new insights into naturally developed dietary patterns, highlighting the importance of a balanced diet for brain health".[364]

Most certainly, there have been vitamin and nutritional deficiencies. The classic was scurvy when sailors were deprived of citrus fruits or vitamin C, but these were all abnormal situations of restrictions, famines, fetishists, or poverty.

Even today, it has been found that a multivitamin tablet a day helps cognition in the elderly. But, sadly, most old people do not eat well.

Super-Newtrition is, of course, a gimmick to catch your attention. But there would seem certain foods that donate specific benefits and, perhaps, we can call them 'super', but it is the variety of fresh foods which is the secret. If you can access and afford these, there is no need for vitamins and unproven supplements. Fresh food has had eight million years of clinical trials, which is how we are here. Sadly, our food has changed in the last 60 years more than the previous 600,000 with the progressive introduction of ultra-processed foods, which I maintain 'we cannot process'.

The *Super-Newtrition* recommendations / foods include all the ingredients of the 'Mind Diet' or the The Mediterranean-DASH Diet Intervention for Neurodegenerative Delay. The MIND diet had already been associated with preservation of cognitive function, presumably through their protective effects against cardiovascular disease, which in turn preserved brain health.[365]

---

364 Zhang, R., Zhang, B., Shen, C. *et al.* 2024, "Associations of dietary patterns with brain health from behavioral, neuroimaging, biochemical and genetic analyses", *Nature Mental Health*, Vol. 2, No. 5, pp. 535-552, https://doi.org/10.1038/s44220-024-00226-0.

365 Harvard T.H.Chan School of Public Health, 2023, "Diet Review: MIND Diet", https://nutritionsource.hsph.harvard.edu/healthy-weight/diet-reviews/mind-diet/.

US News

US News has a Best Diets Panel of nationally recognized experts in nutrition, obesity, food psychology, disease management, and has developed a survey in partnership with The Harris Poll. The survey asked the panel to carefully compare diets for their nutritional completeness, health risks and benefits, long-term sustainability, and evidence-based effectiveness.

These are the 2024 results. The Mediterranean diet has been No.1, justifiably in my opinion, for seven years in a row. For *Super-Newtrition,* I have amalgamated the best of these top diets, urging *variety* to maximize our ingestion of natural vitamins and micronutrients.

Table 32:

Rank		Overall Score
1	Mediterranean Diet	85.1%
2	DASH Diet	75.4%
3	MIND Diet	60.7%
4	Mayo Clinic Diet	55.3%
5	Flexitarian Diet	3.6%
6	Weight Watchers	46.1%
7	Volumetrics Diet	41.4%
8	Dr. Weil's Anti-Inflammatory	41.1%
9	TLC Diet	39.9%
10	Vegan Diet	17.9%
11	Ornish Diet	13.6%
12	Pritikin Diet	9.9%
13	Zone Diet	5.0%
14	Noom	1.4%
15	Plantstrong Diet	0.7%
16	South Beach Diet	-3.6%
17	Nutritarian Diet	-4.3%
18	Jenny Craig Diet	-8.7%

19	Profile Plan	-9.3%
20	Paleo Diet	-17.6%
21	HMR Program	-33.1%
22	Nutrisystem Diet	-35.7%
23	Keyto Diet	-38.3%
24	OPTAVIA	-40.0%
25	Keto Diet	-46.1%
26	Atkins Diet	-46.2%
27	SlimFast Diet	-48.6%
28	Dukan Diet	-54.3%
29	Herbalife Nutrition	-57.2%
30	Raw Food Diet	-61.4%

Super-Newtrition

Easy! Just some from each of the five groups daily:

- 20% Fruit
- 20% Vegetables
- 20% Grains, Seeds, and Nuts
- 20% Protein - mostly plants
- 20% Superfoods (Micronutrients)

No added sugar, No added salt, No Processed Foods

Salt Substitution: Flavorful salt-free spices, herbs, lemon and lime juices, and vinegars.

Fish two to three times a week. Some lean meat if desired.

20ml Extra Virgin Olive Oil (EVOO) daily.

Eating at least 7 g of olive oil daily -- about a half tablespoon -- was tied to an adjusted 28% lower risk of dementia-related death (pooled hazard ratio compared with never or rarely consuming olive oil for women but not men.[366]

366 Tessier, A., Cortese, M., Yuan, C. *et al.* 2024, "Consumption of Olive Oil and Diet Quality and Risk of Dementia-Related Death", *JAMA Network Open,* Vol. 7, No. 5, https://doi.org/10.1001/jamanetworkopen.2024.10021.

Latest News: I have maintained that humans successfully evolved and prospered, more than any other animal, on such a, plant-based with some meat, diet and, in 2024, this has now been gratifyingly corroborated by the Max Planck Institute.[367]

Slowed Brain Aging

The beneficial nutrient blood biomarkers that reflected slower brain aging were a combination of fatty acids (vaccenic, gondoic, alpha linolenic, elcosapentaenoic, eicosadienoic and lignoceric acids); antioxidants and carotenoids including cis-lutein, trans-lutein and zeaxanthin; two forms of vitamin E and choline. *This profile is correlated with nutrients found in the Mediterranean diet,* which research has previously associated with healthy brain aging.[368]

The Newtrition Micronutrient Superfoods

Some foods are richer in micronutrients, and which donate greater benefits: Apples/pears (white fruit), Apricots (dried), Beans, Beetroot, Berries, Celery, Chillies, Cocoa, Citrus, Coffee, Eggplants, Fish, Garlic/onion family, Grains, Green Leafy Vegetables (bok choy),Inulin vegetables (chicory, leeks, asparagus, Jerusalem artichokes), Legumes, Mushrooms, Nuts (all), Oats (barley) (rolled/cut), Olive oil, Peppers, Prunes, Sweet Potato (purple), Vegetables (green-yellow-cruciferous), Purple/red vegetables.

---

367 Moubtahij, Z., McCormack, J., Bourgon, N. *et al.* 2024, "Isotopic evidence of high reliance on plant food among Later Stone Age hunter-gatherers at Taforalt, Morocco", *Nature Ecology & Evolution*, Vol. 8, pp. 1035-1045, https://doi.org/10.1038/s41559-024-02382-z.

368 Zwilling, C. E., Wu, J., & Barbey, A. K. 2024, "Investigating nutrient biomarkers of healthy brain aging: A multimodal brain imaging study", *Npj Aging*, Vol. 10, No. 1, pp. 1-12, https://doi.org/10.1038/s41514-024-00150-8.

Maybe: Magnesium, Curcumin, Cinnamon, Pomegranate Juice, Dates, Rosemary, Sage, Shitake mushrooms, Vinegar, Vitamin D, Chamomile, Peppermint and Kombucha teas, Kefir (fermented milk).

Every Day—Variety is the key.

1. Fruit variety: ensure berries, apples (skin), citrus
2. Vegetable variety: especially green leafy, purple, legumes, and lentils
3. Nuts: 20g, two handfuls. Walnuts, pecans, peanuts, almonds, etc.
4. Grains
5. Berries
6. Beans: at least half a cup per day.
7. Chilies
8. Cocoa (heavy metal free)
9. Tea, coffee, red wine, water
10. Extra Virgin Olive Oil (EVOO)
11. Fish (two to three times a week)
12. Fiber
13. Leave something on your plate. Never get full.
14. Calm, pleasant meals. Happy people only at meals.
15. No distractions: Concentrate on your food.
16. Superfoods

NO

1. Processed foods or meats
2. Butter or cream (well, maybe a little every now and then!)
3. Added sugar
4. Sugar sweetened beverages (SSB)
5. Added salt

Foods that Sound Healthy but Aren't

1. "Light" products
2. Flavored yogurt
3. Veggie chips or straws
4. Meatless meats
5. Granola bars
6. Fruit leather
7. Vitamin water
8. Dairy-free cheese
9. Diet soda
10. High-protein snacks

Do not worry about the occasional lapse or treat. It is the long-term, everyday ingestion of junk food that is harmful.

Always use only cold-pressed oils.

Newtrition's World's Best Breakfast

1. Blueberries—brain health
2. Granny Smith-skin on—gut health and stroke prevention
3. Walnuts, pecans—anti-cancer, heart health
4. Oats or bran—lowers cholesterol, better microbiome
5. Grains—reduce All-Cause-Mortality, CVD, and cancer
6. Flax (ground)—richest source Omega-3, ALA
7. Inulin—reduces visceral fat
8. Dried apricots—high potassium, lowers BP
9. Green bananas—fiber speeds gut transit, Potassium
10. Biodynamic unsweetened yoghurt—(< 4g sugar / 100g)
11. Fruit, in season
12. Prunes—fiber/microbiome gut health
13. Coffee—super-food

Breakfast is not necessary unless you feel you need it to function better.

World's Worst Breakfast Foods

1. Cereals high in sugar and salt (processed)
2. Sausages
3. Bacon/ham
4. Eggs – only once a week
5. Hash browns
6. Butter
7. Crumpets
8. Waffles/pancakes/pastry
9. Golden/maple syrup
10. Muffins
11. Sugar in your tea or coffee

A whole grain contains the nutrient-vitamin rich endosperm, germ, and bran in contrast to refined grains, which retain only the endosperm. Corn flake breakfast cereals are not whole grains despite their advertising, as the nutritious, natural bran and germ have been removed such that synthetic vitamins and flavorings have to be added. They are arguably the most insidious ultra-processed of all foods as intensive advertising has given them a false 'health-halo'.

A serving of corn flakes includes about 24 grams of carbohydrates and 1 gram of fiber, a less than-

ideal ratio. Then, there is the sugar and salt content and, of course, we add sugar on top.

Bran, however, is whole grains, just crushed.

In a study published in 2023, researchers found that adherence to the Mediterranean lifestyle by middle-aged individuals living in the United Kingdom reduced all-cause and cancer-related mortality by 29% and 28%, respectively.[369]

This is the fundamental diet you should eat. If you want more (much more) detail as to why, my book, *Super-Newtrition: The Micronutrient Revolution* is being updated and will be available soon.

Increased mortality risks from ultra-processed foods[370]

Processed meats such as sausages and ham have a 13 per cent higher chance of dying.

Sugary and artificially sweetened drinks had a 9 per cent increased risk.

Packaged goods and snacks were found to have a 4 per cent higher risk of death.

Dairy desserts – such as cheesecake and fromage frais – were linked to a 6 per cent increased risk.

Breads and breakfast cereals were linked to a 4 per cent increase.

Emulsifier additives that are ubiquitous in western diets and consumed daily by millions of children and adults worldwide are associated with increased risks of cardiovascular disease (CVD) and now first epidemiological insight as to their potential involvement in the development of type 2 diabetes

369 Maroto-Rodriguez, J., Delgado-Velandia, M., Ortolá, R. *et al.* 2023, "Association of a Mediterranean Lifestyle With All-Cause and Cause-Specific Mortality: A Prospective Study from the UK Biobank", *Mayo Clinic Proceedings*, Vol. 99, No. 4, pp. 551-563, https://doi.org/10.1016/j.mayocp.2023.05.031.

370 Fang, Z., Rossato, S. L., Hang, D. *et al.* 2024, "Association of ultra-processed food consumption with all cause and cause specific mortality: population based cohort study", *BMJ*, Vol. 385, https://doi.org/10.1136/bmj-2023-078476.

have been linked. Recent experimental studies have shown that emulsifiers can directly modulate the composition and function of the intestinal microbiota, driving microbiota encroachment and chronic low-grade intestinal inflammation, thus exacerbating metabolic disorders.[371]

Among the various additives that could contribute to these associations, food emulsifiers (food additives with emulsifying properties, referred to as emulsifiers from this point onwards) are the most ubiquitous. They are extensively used by food manufacturers to enhance texture and allow a longer shelf-life in a variety of ultra-processed foods such as chocolate, ice cream, cookies, pastries, ultra-processed fruits, vegetables and cereals, dairy products, mayonnaise, edible oils, and syrups. Globally, the most commonly used emulsifiers are lecithins (E322; found in 14% of food products in the EU according to data from the European Food Safety Authority [EFSA]), monoglycerides and diglycerides of fatty acids (E471; found in 7% of foods), guar gum (E412; found in 6% of foods), xanthan gum (E415; found in 5% of foods), carrageenans (E407; found in 4% of foods), and celluloses (E460–469; found in 2% of foods).[374]

While *Super-Newtrition* provides a complete diet contributing all the macronutrients, vitamins, minerals, and micronutrients necessary, there are many people, usually as people get old, that either can't afford the fresh variety or are stuck in a nursing home with poor nutrition. Such people will benefit from a multivitamin.

In a study published in the *American Journal of Clinical Nutrition*, researchers report that taking a multivitamin that you

371 Salame, C., Javaux, G., Sellem, L. *et al.* 2024, "Food additive emulsifiers and the risk of type 2 diabetes: analysis of data from the NutriNet-Santé prospective cohort study", *Lancet Diabetes and Endocrinology*, Vol. 12, No. 5, pp. 339-349, https://doi.org/10.1016/S2213-8587(24)00086-X.

can buy at the pharmacy can slow cognitive decline associated with aging by as much as two years.[372]

Pizzas and hamburgers are widely condemned but if (home) made with all fresh ingredients, no processed meats, and no commercial sauces/emulsifiers, they can be healthy.

I am also a bit of a fan of intermittent fasting, which accords with how we humans evolved. We sure didn't sit down to three calorie-dense meals a day or eat the junk delivered through our car window 200,000 years ago. The following study would seem to add support.[373]

Multiomics (A new approach where the data sets of different omic groups are combined during analysis. The different omic strategies employed during multiomics are genome, proteome, transcriptome, epigenome, and microbiome.) analyses reveal dynamic bioenergetic pathways and functional remodelling of the heart during intermittent fasting.

Intermittent fasting (IF) has been shown to reduce cardiovascular risk factors in animals and humans and can protect the heart against ischemic injury in models of myocardial infarction. Comprehensive, system-wide analyses and transcriptome, followed by functional analysis and advanced mass spectrometry, profiled the proteome and phosphoproteome of heart tissues obtained from mice that were maintained on

---

372 Vyas C. M., Manson J. E., Sesso, H. D. 2024, "Effect of multivitamin-mineral supplementation versus placebo on cognitive function: results from the clinic subcohort of the COcoa Supplement and Multivitamin Outcomes Study (COSMOS) randomized clinical trial and meta-analysis of 3 cognitive studies within COSMOS", *The American Journal of Clinical Nutrition*, Vol. 119, No. 3, pp. 692-701, https://doi.org/10.1016/j.ajcnut.2023.12.011.

373 Arumugam, T. V., Alli-Shaik, A., Liehn, E. A. *et al.* 2023, "Multiomics analyses reveal dynamic bioenergetic pathways and functional remodeling of the heart during intermittent fasting", *elife*, Vol. 12, https://doi.org/10.7554/eLife.89214.

daily 12- or 16-hour fasting, every-other-day fasting, or ad libitum control feeding regimens for six months. Analyses revealed that IF significantly affected pathways that regulate cyclic GMP signalling, lipid and amino acid metabolism, cell adhesion, cell death, and inflammation. Additionally, functional echocardiographic analyses demonstrated that IF enhances stress-induced cardiac performance.

Proteomic technology now allows examination of global alterations in protein expression in the diseased heart and can provide new insights into cellular mechanisms involved in cardiac dysfunction.[374]

Routine, periodic fasting is associated with a lower risk of Diabetes and coronary artery disease (CAD) and may reduce weight and improve metabolic parameters. Multiple related biological pathways are acutely affected by water-only fasting, potentially leading to long-term health improvements, including lower CAD. Trimethylamine N-oxide (TMAO) is produced by intestinal bacteria and may increase CAD risk. Water-only, 24-hour fasting reduced plasma levels of TMAO, a potential risk factor for CAD.

These findings suggest that routine, periodic fasting (multiple episodes overtime on a regular basis) may have a long-term impact on TMAO levels and related CAD risk, but this requires further investigation.[375]

The latest fad for 'Super Nutritional' Drinks is nutritional fearmongering and just another unproven supplement scam.

---

374 McGregor, E. & Dunn, M. J. 2006, "Proteomics of the Heart: Unraveling Disease", *Circulation Research*, Vol. 98, No. 3, pp. 309-321, https://doi.org/10.1161/01.RES.0000201280.20709.26.

375 Horne, B. D., Cox, J. E., Muhlestein J. B. *et al.* 2014, "Abstract 13412: 24-Hour Water-Only Fasting Acutely Reduces Trimethylamine N-Oxide: the FEELGOOD Trial", *Circulation*, Vol. 130, No. Supplement 2.

SECTION I

ARTIFICIAL INTELLIGENCE AI

This would seem to be the greatest recent leap forward in medicine today. From my standpoint, of Preventive Medicine, it makes it more exciting than any other development in longevity. AI can predict or diagnose the previously undiagnosable—and up to seven years before traditional symptoms, signs, or tests.

The prestigious New England Journal of Medicine (NEJM) even now has a dedicated AI Subscription.

Much of this information was inspired by a TED presentation by cardiologist Eric Topol, whom I have admired and followed for years.

Firstly, my primitive understanding of how AI can provide medical input is how it 'learns', aka 'Supervised Learning', from scanning hundreds of thousands of records. Authors and magazines are upset that their original work has so been 'copied' and may now be used as AI reproductions.

In medicine, however, AIs have scanned hundreds of thousands of X-rays and can, in the blink of an eye, run through all these to compare them with an X-ray of a patient that was just taken. AI regularly finds spots in mammograms that even expert physicians have missed, and when AI is added to colonoscopies in real-time, significantly more polyps are found. This is pretty daunting stuff! I don't know if I'd like to compete with 100,000 other diagnostic reviews!

But that is its power. As noted, it sometimes to pick up what the radiologists may have missed and the combining, cross-referencing, and checking between the two will offer the best patient outcomes/results.

Healthcare provider Kaiser Permanente added AI in 19 of its hospitals in recent years to see whether it could predict which inpatients' conditions were dangerously worsening via regular inputs, including lab test results, vital signs, nurses' reports, medical histories, and other factors. Then, it issued alerts for any who were showing signs of decline. In more than 35,000 patients over 2.5 years, there were 16% fewer deaths in the 30 days following the alert, saving 520 lives.

From chest X-rays, observers then went on to images of the retina, and, incredibly, AI could diagnose not just eye problems but Parkinson's Disease seven years before any hitherto known clinical tests!

GPT-4, in the context of medicine.

1. Supervised Learning:
    - Definition: Supervised learning is a type of machine learning where the model learns from labelled training data. It involves mapping input features to corresponding output labels.

- Process:
  - Training: The model is exposed to input-output pairs (features-labels). It learns to predict the correct label based on the input features.
  - Loss Function: The model's performance is evaluated using a loss function that quantifies the difference between predicted and actual labels.
  - Optimization: The model adjusts its parameters (weights) to minimize the loss function.
  - Inference: Once trained, the model can predict labels for new, unseen data.
- Application in Medicine: Supervised learning is commonly used for tasks like disease diagnosis (e.g., classifying x-rays as normal or abnormal) and predicting patient outcomes (e.g., survival prediction based on clinical features).

2. Transformer Models (GPT-4):
   - Definition: GPT-4 (Generative Pre-trained Transformer) is an advanced language model based on the Transformer architecture. It was developed by OpenAI.
   - Architecture:
     - Transformer: Introduced in 2017, the Transformer architecture relies on self-attention mechanisms. It processes input sequences (such as text) in parallel, capturing contextual information effectively.
     - GPT-4: GPT-4 is a large-scale language model pre-trained on massive text data using unsupervised learning techniques. It predicts the next word in a sequence based on preceding context.
   - Capabilities:
     - Natural Language Understanding: GPT-4 can generate coherent and contextually relevant responses based on user input.

- Medical Applications: GPT-4 has the potential to assist with various medical tasks:
- Patient Discharge Notes: It can help generate concise and accurate discharge summaries.
- Clinical Trial Summaries: GPT-4 can summarize recent clinical trials, aiding healthcare professionals.
- Ethical Guidelines: It can provide information on ethical guidelines relevant to medical practice.
- Innovation: GPT-4 may drive medical innovation by assisting clinicians and researchers.

In summary, supervised learning focuses on labelled data and specific tasks, while GPT-4 leverages its language understanding capabilities to assist in various medical contexts. Both approaches contribute to advancing healthcare practices.

What is more, GPT-5 is apparently incredibly more powerful than GPT-4. It accesses so much more data that it may even be slower.

As detailed elsewhere, there are some 800,000 mis- or missed diagnoses made every year in the USA, leading to deaths or disabilities. The incidence would be the same in most developed countries.

When AI was trained using supervised learning of 100,000 images of the retina to assess if it could see what trained ophthalmologists could not, the experts picked the patients' gender correctly 50% of the time, but AI got it 97% right.

AI, through supervised learning, has then been found to be just as good, if not better, with x-rays, CT scans, and MRIs.

AI picked up colonic polyps better than the gastroenterologist performing the procedure.

These deep learning machine eyes can pick up things the human eye doesn't.

Retina Individual Models:

Just from a retinal image alone, AI could pick up:

- Diabetes and Blood Pressure Control (*Nature Biomed Engineering*, 2018)
- Kidney Disease (*Lancet Dig Health*, 2020)
- Liver and Gall Bladder Disease (*Lancet Dig H*, 2021)
- Predicting Heart Attack and Stroke (*Nature Mach Intel*, 2022)
- Hyperlipidemia (*Eye*, 2023)
- Parkinson's Disease (*Neurology*, 2023)

Now, just from the one using 1.6 images, AI could predict:

- Myopia
- Diabetic retinopathy
- Glaucoma
- Ischaemic stroke
- Parkinson's Disease
- Myocardial Infarction

It is proposed that the retina will be 'the gateway to almost every system in the body'.

ECG/EKGs

AI could pick up what experienced Cardiologists could not.

AI could propel the biggest transformation in the history of medicine, says physician-scientist Eric Topol. He explains how sophisticated AI models can interpret medical images as well or better than human experts can—and, beyond that, even pick up things that human eyes can't see. Learn all the ways AI is poised to make a difference for both patients and doctors.

- Age and Sex (*Circulation*, 2019)
- Ejection Fraction (*Nature Medicine*, 2019)

- Difficult Diagnoses (*Circulation*, 2019)
- Anaemia/Hemoglobin (*Lancet Digital Health*, 2020)
- Predicting Atrial Fibrillation/Stroke Risk (*Lancet*, 2022)
- Prediabetes and Diabetes (*BMJ*, 2022)
- Filling Pressure of Heart (*JACC*, 2022)
- Hyperthyroidism (*Lancet*, 2023)
- Kidney Disease (*Comms Med*, 2023)

Chest X-Rays

- Race (*Lancet Dig Health*, 2022)
- Diabetes and Conitaltrol (*Nature Comms*, 2023)
- Heart (*Lancet Digital H*, 2023)
    - Ejection fraction
    - IVC dilation
    - Aortic stenosis and regurgitation
    - Mitral stenosis and regurgitation
    - Tricuspid regurgitation
    - Pulmonary regurgitation

Pathology

Expert pathologists often disagree as to an exact diagnosis; one classic is between a severely dysplastic nevus and a melanoma, as the former merges into the latter.

Now, from a tissue slide:

- Driver Mutations
- Structural Genomic Changes
- Tumor vs. Normal and Origin
- Prognosis

These studies were done with supervised learning, covering up to hundreds of thousands of images.

GPT4 was also used for 70 very difficult cases at the NEJM Clinical-Pathological Conference, and the Chatbot did as well as, if not better than, the expert clinicians in making the diagnoses.

Future Projections: The projection is that AI will finally free doctors from being 'data clerks' and allow them to actually talk with and spend more time with their patients.

SECTION J

APPENDIX: YOUR MEDICAL CONSULTATION

This Appendix concentrates on the evidence-based, best, and most appropriate tests, investigations, and information you need at your age for the longest life presently possible.

Inherent in this:

- Get a full medical check as a baseline.
- Get the recommended tests for your age.

Disclaimer: The following is for your information only and can and does not take the place of a personal consultation and examination by your own doctor.

No one has all the answers, and individual doctors may differ as to what is most appropriate for you.

In addition, these recommended tests are to identify some major problem that is hopefully treatable and not to 'fine tune' if there is such a thing as a reasonably healthy body e.g., Statins are protective against a heart attack or stroke but only if the patient has demonstrable major risks and not a marginally elevated cholesterol that could be lowered by better nutrition, weight loss and exercise. Most good health and longevity are due to a healthy lifestyle, good nutrition and exercise, and the early identification and treatment of a potentially fatal illness.

This is where to start. Medications should only be prescribed when there is a proven need, and supplements are totally superfluous on a Mediterranean no ultra-processed food diet.

As cardiovascular disease (CVD) is the greatest cause of our premature demise, and as high Blood Pressure is the greatest cause of CVD, I strongly recommend getting your BP checked regularly and, when you hit 45, buying a wrist machine, some of which are only $25. Like this book, a pretty cheap investment to save your life.

This information is based on the best studies, trials, and clinical experience, but given the pace of medicine, newer tests may become available.

1. Preliminary Basic Measurements

- Height and weight
- Waist-hip ratio (BMI no longer used)
- Skin—dermoscopy
- Cardiovascular
- Central nervous system
- Respiratory system
- Gastrointestinal system
- Genito-urinary system: male/female
- Endocrine
- ENT (Ear, Nose, Throat).
- Eyes—visual acuity and fields, fundi.
- Hearing—auditory acuity
- Musculoskeletal/Locomotor

- Age grip, mobility, posture, nutrition, hydration, feet, walking speed
- Psychiatric/mental

2. Medical Symptoms & Signs

The earlier an illness can be diagnosed, the more chance of a cure. It is, therefore, important for you to know what *symptoms and signs* to look for and not to ignore them. The following is a list of the main signs and symptoms which should be reported.

General

- Undue fatigue or tiredness
- Unexplained loss of weight
- Unexplained bruising/prolonged bleeding
- Any blood transfusions
- Slowness of movement or mental process

Eyes

- Grittiness/inflammation/watering/discharge
- Pain & blurring
- Reduced or loss of vision
- Stuck lids

GIT (Gastrointestinal Tract)

- Heartburn/indigestion
- Abdominal pain
- Change of bowel habit
- PR mucus, blood, slime
- Weight loss
- Yellow whites of eyes
- Recurrent diarrhea
- Intolerance to bread

CVS (Cardiovascular System)

- Blood pressure
- Palpitations/fluttering
- SOBOE (Shortness of breath on effort)
- Chest pain
- Swollen ankles

Respiratory

- Smoking
- Persistent cough/blood in sputum
- Wheeze/asthma/difficulty breathing
- Bad snoring/choking in sleep
- Any previous exposure to asbestos

CNS (Central Nervous System)

- Head trauma (sports, etc.)
- Transient loss of vision/consciousness (TIA)
- Altered behaviour
- Fits
- Pins and needles
- Weakness of grip
- Disturbances of balance
- New headache
- Tremors
- Increasing forgetfulness/confusion

Locomotor / Muscle or Joints

- Pain
- Swelling
- Inflammation

- Joint pains—note any climbing stairs, especially hip or knee
- Increasing tendency to choke on food
- Unaccounted-for limp
- Finger nodes
- Weaker grip
- Balance problems
- Muscle wasting and weakness, especially thighs or legs

Men

- Diminished stream & cut off
- Frequency/nocturia
- Terminal dribbling
- Pink urine
- Testicular lumps

Women

- Any lump
- Mammogram/pap
- Stress incontinence
- Frequency/nocturia
- Cystitis/pink urine
- Discharge/inter-menstrual bleeding

Endocrine

- Slowing down (compared with one year ago)
- Thinning hair
- Menstrual problems
- Pop eyes
- Fast talk
- Central obesity
- Thirst, polyuria

Age

- Trouble getting out of chairs
- Increasingly fixed opinions
- Memory problems
- Feet—not cared for
- Back pain

Mental Health

- Feeling something is wrong
- Sadness/hopelessness/worthlessness
- Worried all the time
- Loss of interest
- Inappropriate guilt
- Sleep difficulties
- Suicidal thoughts
- Memory problems
- Repetition
- Isolation, loneliness
- Social activity

Work

- Exposure to asbestos, diesel, pesticides

3. Age-Specific Tests & Investigations

In my experience, most people just want to know "what to do" and don't want a laborious, complex explanation or reasons thrust down their throats.

Then, there are the others who do want to know the minutiae.

As such, I have tried to satisfy both.

Costs and cost-effectiveness are also significant to most, even though today, the super-rich, the wellness-longevity clinics, and the influencers (who often don't have to pay) are urging us to spend big.

You can just get these basic tests done and then delve deeper if any are abnormal, or, as best I can, I have tried to explain and simplify these investigations and tests. But whatever, you are not Robinson Crusoe. Many of these tests are highly complex and challenging, even for doctors to understand. They are also debatable as to need and choice.

Most of the following blood tests, I have done yearly since 1968 and refined them as better tests evolved. But I was using myself as a guinea pig, and you do not need such frequent tests unless abnormal.

These are *all, I recommend, should be needed* initially.

Symptoms and abnormal results may suggest others.

Again, I would emphasize priorities. Heart (cardiovascular) disease is our greatest killer, so get your heart tests first. To this end then, as emphasized later, I strongly recommend buying a wrist Blood Pressure machine and monitoring your BP; hypertension is arguably the greatest cause of our premature demise.

Then, as per the lists, I have prioritized your tests based on your sex and age as per official proven data.

Some tests may not need to be repeated after a baseline: Lipids should only be done every five years if normal.

For other tests, 10-year screening is otherwise suggested, reducing to five-year intervals after 45 years or as clinically assessed.

There are increasing scams, promises, and dubious tests of up to some 50 to 200 effectively useless "biomarkers".

These are flattering if you are 50, and they record your biological age as 30, hence their popularity. But different laboratories or tests seldom, if ever, agree.

Whereas *Live Longer* tests and investigations are the absolute bedrock of advanced, evidenced, legitimate medicine to provide the foundations to live longer.

Ensure you use a well credentialed laboratory that has certified checks as to standards.

Explanation of these abbreviations are detailed below these tables.

Table 33: Note: Lp(a) (if high, repeat at different laboratory to confirm).

Age	**Male**	**Female**
15-30	BP	BP
	Low-dose CT Chest scan	Low-dose CT Chest scan
	C/FBC/hsCRP	C/FBC/hsCRP
	MBA incl. Uric A. Creatinine	MBA incl. Uric A. Creatinine
	Lipids ApoB ApoA1 ApoB/ApoA-1 ratio Lp(a) (do once only – rpt if high)	Lipids ApoB ApoA1 ApoB/ApoA-1 ratio Lp(a) (do once only – rpt if high)
	Coeliac D screen	Coeliac D screen
	Cardiovascular check	Cardiovascular check
		Gynecology (cervical screen, breasts)
	Others as indicated STD/HPV hsTropinin Grip strength Balance Hearing VO_2max	Others as indicated STD/HPV hsTropinin Grip strength Balance Hearing VO_2max
30-40	BP	BP
	Low-dose CT Chest scan	Low-dose CT Chest scan
	C/FBC/hsCRP	C/FBC/hsCRP
	MBA incl. Uric A. Creatinine	MBA incl. Uric A. Creatinine

30-40	Lipids ApoB ApoA1 ApoB/ApoA-1 ratio Lp(a) (do once only)	Lipids ApoB ApoA1 ApoB/ApoA-1 ratio Lp(a) (do once only)
	Coeliac D screen	Coeliac D screen
	Cardiovascular check	Cardiovascular check
		Gynecology (cervical screen, breasts)
	Others as indicated Colon cancer hsTropinin Grip strength Balance Hearing VO_2max	Others as indicated Colon cancer hsTropinin Grip strength Balance Hearing VO_2max
40-50	BP	BP
	Low-dose CT Chest scan	Low-dose CT Chest scan
	C/FBC/hsCRP	C/FBC/hsCRP
	MBA incl. Uric A. Creatinine	MBA incl. Uric A. Creatinine
	Lipids ApoB ApoA1 ApoB/ApoA-1 ratio Lp(a) (do once only)	Lipids ApoB ApoA1 ApoB/ApoA-1 ratio Lp(a) (do once only)
	Coeliac D screen	Coeliac D screen
	Cardiovascular check	Cardiovascular check
	Prostrate check	Gynecology (cervical screen, mammogram, DEXA)
	Colon Cancer colonoscopy	Colon Cancer colonoscopy
	Others as indicated hsTropinin Grip strength Balance Hearing VO_2max	Others as indicated hsTropinin Grip strength Balance Hearing VO_2max

50–64	BP	BP
	Low-dose CT Chest scan	Low-dose CT Chest scan
	C/FBC/hsCRP	C/FBC/hsCRP
	MBA incl. Uric A. Creatinine	MBA incl. Uric A. Creatinine
	Lipids ApoB ApoA1 ApoB/ApoA-1 ratio Lp(a) (do once only)	Lipids ApoB ApoA1 ApoB/ApoA-1 ratio Lp(a) (do once only)
	Coeliac D	Coeliac D
	Cardiovascular check	Cardiovascular check
	Prostrate check	Gynecology/Hormones
	Colon Cancer	Colon Cancer
	Others as indicated Hearing test/Eyes Apo B if not done hsTropinin Grip strength Balance Hearing VO_2max	Others as indicated Hearing test/Eyes Apo B if not done hsTropinin Grip strength Balance Hearing VO_2max
65–74	BP	BP
	C/FBC/hsCRP	C/FBC/hsCRP
	MBA incl. Uric A. Creatinine	MBA incl. Uric A. Creatinine
	Lipids ApoB ApoA1 ApoB/ApoA-1 ratio Lp(a) (do once only)	Lipids ApoB ApoA1 ApoB/ApoA-1 ratio Lp(a) (do once only)
	ECG/EKG annually—to exclude AF	ECG/EKG annually—to exclude AF
	Prostrate check	Gynecology (cervical screen, mammogram, DEXA)
	Colon Cancer	Colon Cancer

65–74	Ultrasonography for Abdominal Aortic Aneurysm	
	hsTropinin	hsTropinin
	Grip strength	Grip strength
	Balance	Balance
	Hearing	Hearing
	VO_2max	VO_2max
75-85 Previously no tests recommended?!	BP	BP
	C/FBC/hsCRP	C/FBC/hsCRP
	MBA incl. Uric A. Creatinine	MBA incl. Uric A. Creatinine
	Lipids ApoB ApoA1 ApoB/ApoA-1 ratio Lp(a) (do once only)	Lipids ApoB ApoA1 ApoB/ApoA-1 ratio Lp(a) (do once only)
	ECG/EKG annually—to exclude AF	ECG/EKG annually—to exclude AF
	Prostrate check	Gynae as indicated
	Colon Cancer	Colon Cancer
	Ultrasonography for Abdominal Aortic Aneurysm	
	Apo B if not done	Apo B if not done
	hsTropinin	hsTropinin
	Grip strength	Grip strength
	Balance	Balance
	Hearing	Hearing
	VO_2max	VO_2max

Special Note

I emphasize cardiovascular disease prevention as priority one – because it is. It is gratifying, reassuring and timely to read this latest analysis and Editorial in the *JAMA*.

Cardiovascular risk assessment has become an essential part of preventive strategies and has contributed to dramatic reductions in cardiovascular disease mortality during the past 60 years in the US and other countries. Beginning in the 1960s, investigators from the Framingham Heart study identified key physiological, behavioral, and biochemical risk factors for atherosclerotic cardiovascular disease and were the first to develop multivariable risk equations using major risk factors to predict first-time fatal and nonfatal myocardial infarction and later atherosclerotic cardiovascular disease events during a period of up to 12 years. These risk equations are able to explain about 70% to 80% of the variability of cardiovascular risk in the populations in which they were derived. The generalizability of these early tools has been enhanced by using large, diverse, pooled cohorts in the US, Europe and elsewhere. Since their development, many attempts to improve the models have been pursued, yet the basic models have stood the test of time.[376]

Prognostic Value of Cardiovascular Biomarkers in the Population[377]

Measurement of high-sensitivity cardiac troponin I, high-sensitivity cardiac troponin T, N-terminal pro-B-type natriuretic peptide, B-type natriuretic peptide, or high-sensitivity C-reactive protein.

Cardiovascular biomarkers were strongly associated with fatal and nonfatal cardiovascular events and mortality.

376 Gaziano, T. A. & Gaziano, J. M. 2024, "Can Cardiovascular Risk Assessment Be Improved in the 21st Century?", *JAMA*, Vol. 331, No. 22, pp. 1891-1893, https://doi.org/10.1001/jama.2024.7644.

377 Neumann, J. T., Twerenbold, R., Weimann J, *et al.* 2024, "Prognostic Value of Cardiovascular Biomarkers in the Population", *JAMA*, Vol. 331, No. 22, pp. 1898-1909, https://doi.org/10.1001/jama.2024.5596.

The addition of biomarkers to established risk factors led to only a small improvement in risk prediction metrics for atherosclerotic cardiovascular disease, but was more favorable for heart failure and mortality.

What These Tests Are and What They Are For

1. Blood Pressure (BP)

This is arguably the most useful test but also the most under-used.

The first World Health Organization (WHO) report dedicated to hypertension indicates that four out of five patients do not receive adequate treatment.[378]

Hypertension affects one in three adults worldwide, but nearly half of people with hypertension globally are currently unaware of their condition. High blood pressure is associated with various cardiovascular problems, including stroke and heart failure, and is viewed as a "silent killer", given the absence of initial symptoms for most patients.

I highly recommend a wrist BP machine and monitoring your own BP.

In fact, after I had written this, a recent study as to the "Long-Term Effect of Home Blood Pressure Self-Monitoring Plus Medication Self-Titration for Patients with Hypertension" would suggest that this simple, inexpensive, and easy-to-implement self-management interventions have the potential to improve the long-term control of hypertension.[379]

---

378 WHO, 2023, "First WHO report details devastating impact of hypertension and ways to stop it", news release, 19 September.

379 Martínez-Ibáñez, P., Marco-Moreno, I., García-Sempere, A., *et al.* 2024, "Long-Term Effect of Home Blood Pressure Self-Monitoring Plus Medication Self-Titration for Patients With Hypertension: A Secondary Analysis of the ADAMPA Randomized Clinical Trial", *JAMA Network Open*, Vol. 7, No. 5, https://doi.org/10.1001/jamanetworkopen.2024.10063.

2. *Blood Profile: CBC/FBC/ESR/hsCRP*

Hematology:

- CBC = Complete Blood Count
- FBC = Full Blood Count—same tests

Hemoglobin/Hematocrit--indicates if you are anemic

White Cell Count—indicates infection, leukemia

Blood Film—abnormal cells as in myeloma, lead poisoning

Platelet Count—indicates bleeding problems.

ESR—indicates inflammation, now not used as much as *CRP*—C-reactive protein, indicates inflammation.

hs-CRP—high-sensitivity is more sensitive and can help show the risk of getting coronary artery disease.

3. *Biochemistry: MBA = Multiple Biochemical Analysis*

This measures the electrolytes that compose the body fluids & their balance, viz*: Sodium, potassium, chloride, bicarbonate, anion gap, and osmolality.*

Calcium/Phosphate/Alkaline phosphatase—bone disorders

Urea and creatinine—indicate kidney function.

Urate—elevated in gout & metabolic syndrome in children

Uric Acid—While related, it is not quite the same and low levels have been associated with longevity.

Glucose—elevated in Diabetes

Protein (Albumin and Globulin)—low in kidney and some liver disease and high in some metabolic disorders

Bilirubin—indicates gall bladder/liver disease.

Liver Function Tests (LFT)—The most common liver tests include liver enzymes, viz: alkaline phosphatase (ALP), alanine transaminase (ALT), aspartate aminotransferase (AST), and gamma-glutamyl transferase (GGT). Albumin and total protein, Bilirubin, L-lactate dehydrogenase (LD), and Prothrombin time (PT).

Centenarians tend to have lower levels of glucose, creatinine, and uric acid from their sixties onwards, according to the largest study of its kind[380] that may lead to a simple blood test being able to predict a person's chance of reaching 100,

**HbA1c*: This measures your glucose average over the last three months and should be done if B. glucose is elevated.

4. Cardiovascular Check

Lipids:

- ApoB
- ApoA1
- ApoB/ApoA-1 ratio
- Lp(a) (but, if high, repeat at different laboratory to confirm)

See notes on Lipids/Cholesterol below

ECG/EKG: Heart Tracing: Do annually over 65 or a smart watch/Kardia. There is an increasing prevalence of a heart arrythmia, Atrial Fibrillation, as we age.

Lipids (Cholesterol and Triglycerides)

I'm going to spend some time on cholesterol, as it may well be the greatest killer of all time. To be blunt, it's *what's going to kill you and me…* unless we take immediate preventive actions.

380 Murata, S., Ebeling, M., Meyer, A. C. *et al.* 2023, "Blood biomarker profiles and exceptional longevity: comparison of centenarians and non-centenarians in a 35-year follow-up of the Swedish AMORIS cohort", *GeroScience,* Vol. 46, pp. 1693-1702, https://doi.org/10.1007/s11357-023-00936-w.

Default

I have done my best to simplify and de-mystify it all for those of you who want it clarified.

If you do not want to grapple with this biochemistry, all you have to know is:

Get your

- ApoB level
- ApoB:ApoA ratio
- Triglycerides

done regularly and

- Lp(a) done once (but, if high, repeat at different laboratory to confirm)

Detail

Cholesterol and triglycerides are lipids, aka fats, aka fatty acids. Cholesterol is an essential substance in most cells in our body but, if elevated, is implicated in causing heart attacks and strokes when carried on a transport lipoprotein, ApoB, which then sticks to the vascular endothelium (the lining of arterial walls), forming plaques (atheroma). These plaques of cholesterol undergo damaging oxidation via free radicals, initiating atherosclerosis and blocking the coronary arteries (atherosclerosis)-a heart attack.

- The cholesterol that causes heart attacks and strokes is only bound to apolipoprotein (ApoB).
- ApoB measures each such damaging cholesterol particle.
- As such, ApoB is the most accurate measurement of damaging cholesterol (to prevent heart attacks and strokes).

Basically...

Cholesterol has been subdivided into sub-fractions.:

1. Low (LDL-C) 'Bad'
2. High Density (HDL-C) 'Good'

The "C" is often dropped, i.e. LDL and HDL

By binding to lipoproteins, five further classifications are made (see below).

LDL in plasma is a mix of *lipoproteins,* ***Cholesterol ester (CE), Triglyceride (TG), Free cholesterol (FC),*** and ***phospholipid (PL).***

Transport and Distribution

The fat we eat, such as steak fat (stearic acid), butter (butyric acid) and so on, is broken down in our gut lumen and then amalgamated into chylomicrons, particles whose function is the transport of this fat from the intestinal lumen to the liver.

Lipids (cholesterol and triglycerides) are insoluble, and to be transported in the plasma, they must be attached to specific 'transport' apoproteins.

Apoproteins

These are classified alphabetically (A, B, C, D, E).

Each type of lipid is associated with different apolipoproteins to carry out specific functions.

These Lipoproteins allow for division into five main classes based on size, lipid composition, and apolipoproteins. They have different functions and carry different substances:

1. ***Chylomicrons:*** Large, triglyceride-rich lipoproteins. Intestinal cells produce them from dietary fats.
2. ***Very low-density lipoproteins*** (VLDL): The liver later produces these triglyceride-rich particles.
3. ***Intermediate-density lipoproteins*** (IDL): These carry cholesterol and triglycerides.

4. ***Low-density lipoproteins***, LDL(-C): The main carrier of cholesterol to deliver to dependent tissues, such as the adrenal glands and the gonads.
5. ***High-density lipoproteins,*** HDL(C): These play an essential role in reverse cholesterol transport—bringing cholesterol from other tissues to the liver— and may help prevent atherosclerosis or the build-up of fat in the arteries.

Not all the contents of these Low-Density Cholesterols (LDL) cause atheroma. ApoB, as pointed out, is thought to be the only part of LDL that causes atheroma.

Each LDL particle is surrounded by one molecule of apoprotein B (apoB) to facilitate transport in the plasma.

ApoB (or apoB) is found in chylomicrons, LDL, very-low-density lipoprotein (VLDL), intermediate-density lipoprotein (IDL), and Lp(a) particles.

All contain one ApoB molecule per particle.

Hence, measurements of ApoB most accurately reflect the number of atherogenic particles. This is why ApoB is a more accurate predictor of heart disease risks than LDL levels alone, as it reflects the actual number of LDL particles, which are the atherogenic agents.[381]

On the other hand, HDL does not contain ApoB and is not atherogenic. In fact, HDL appears to play a protective role, and high numbers of HDL particles are associated with less risk of heart disease.

381 Behbodikhah, J., Ahmed, S., Elyasi, A. *et al.* 2021, "Apolipoprotein B and Cardiovascular Disease: Biomarker and Potential Therapeutic Target", *Metabolites*, Vol. 11, No. 10, p. 690, https://doi.org/10.3390/metabo11100690.

ApoB Further Evidence

In 2006, a 30 person, 10 panel stated:[382]

"There is abundant evidence that the risk of atherosclerotic vascular disease is directly related to plasma cholesterol levels. Accordingly, all of the national and transnational screening and therapeutic guidelines are based on total or LDL cholesterol. This presumes that cholesterol is the most important lipoprotein-related proatherogenic risk variable. *On the contrary, risk appears to be more directly related to the number of circulating atherogenic particles that contact and enter the arterial wall than to the measured concentration of cholesterol in these lipoprotein fractions. Each of the atherogenic lipoprotein particles contains a single molecule of apolipoprotein (apo) B, and therefore the concentration of apo B provides a direct measure of the number of circulating atherogenic lipoproteins* (my italics). Evidence from fundamental, epidemiological and clinical trial studies indicates that apo B is superior to any of the cholesterol indices to recognize those at increased risk of vascular disease and to judge the adequacy of lipid-lowering therapy. On the basis of this evidence, we believe that apo B should be included in all guidelines as an indicator of cardiovascular risk. In addition, the present target adopted by the Canadian guideline groups of an apo B <90 mg dL (1.7544 μmol/L) in high-risk patients should be reassessed in light of the new clinical trial results and a new ultra-low target of <80mgdL (1.56μmol/L) be considered. The evidence also indicates that **the apo B/apo A-I ratio** is superior to any of the conventional cholesterol ratios in patients without symptomatic vascular disease or Diabetes to evaluate the lipoprotein-related risk of vascular disease".

382 Lips, P., Hosking, D., Lippuner, K. *et al.* 2006, "The prevalence of vitamin D inadequacy amongst women with osteoporosis: an international epidemiological investigation", *Journal of Internal Medicine,* Vol. 259, No. 3, pp. 245-254, https://doi.org/10.1111/j.1365-2796.2006.01685.x.

In the FOURIER[383] and IMPROVE-IT[384] trials, each 1-SD (standard deviation) increase in ApoB and non-HDL was associated with a 19% and 16% higher risk, respectively, of myocardial infarction (MI): a heart attack. In the model adjusted for clinical risk factors plus ApoB, non-HDL and HDL cholesterol, and triglycerides, only ApoB was significantly associated with the risk of MI.

(Standard deviation (SD) shows how much variation there is from the average).

I first did my Apo-B in 1990, but despite this high-grade, ongoing evidence (the above articles are just some of hundreds if not thousands) that ApoB is the best measure of the damaging atherogenic cholesterol particles and, therefore, arguably the most predictive blood test of the risk of a heart attack. It is still not recommended by most doctors or laboratories who only measure LDL.

Recommended Levels

ApoB

- No risk factors: < 130 mg/dL (1.3 g/L)
- Low or intermediate risk: <110 mg/dL (1.1 g/L)
- High-risk (CVD, Diabetes):<90 mg/dL (0.9 g/L)

ApoA1 is the major protein component of HDL.

Apolipoprotein A-I (apo A-I), an indispensable component and a major structural protein of high-density lipoprotein

383 Sever, P., Gouni-Berthold, I., Keech, A. *et al.* 2021, "LDL-cholesterol lowering with evolocumab, and outcomes according to age and sex in patients in the FOURIER Trial", *European Journal of Preventive Cardiology*, Vol. 28, No. 8, pp. 805-812, https://doi.org/10.1177/2047487320902750.

384 Lewis, E. F. & Rhee, J. W. 2020, "IMPROVE-IT: A Final Closure to Carcinogenicity of Ezetimibe?", *JACC: CardioOncology*, Vol. 2, No. 3, pp. 397-399, https://doi.org/10.1016/j.jaccao.2020.08.003.

(HDL), plays a vital role in reverse cholesterol transport and cellular cholesterol homeostasis. Like HDL cholesterol, increased concentrations are associated with reduced risk of cardiovascular disease.

The ApoB/ApoA-1 ratio represents a measure of the balance between particles that promote and protect from atherosclerosis.

- Optimal Result: 0 - 0.77

Table 34: Apolipoprotein B/A1 Ratio.

Risk Category	Male	Female
Optimal	<0.77	<0.63
Moderate	0.77-0.95	0.63-0.78
High	>0.95	>0.78

Other Recommended Cholesterol Tests

Lp(a)

Lipoprotein (a), Lp(a), is a lot like LDL cholesterol, but it's more 'sticky'. If you have high levels in your blood, it can stick to your artery walls and clog them up, leading to heart disease, stroke, aortic valve stenosis, and peripheral arterial disease at a young age.

And there is an inherited trait which can cause overproduction, which an estimated 20% of the population has. It is an independent risk factor, such that levels cannot be controlled by healthy eating and exercising. It is often the cause of a sudden heart attack death in people who were ostensibly fit, eating well, and who had even had their 'cholesterol checked', i.e., LDL and HDL—which were 'normal'.

It is challenging to measure accurately due to the large degree of variation in the molecular weight of Apo(a) isoforms between individuals. I did mine in 1990 and, as it was low, have not repeated it because it is genetically fixed.

If it is high, I would repeat it as it is a difficult test to do, and labs can make errors. But if then it is high, you must seek the advice of a cardiologist. Lipoprotein apheresis, a treatment like dialysis, is the only therapy approved by the Food and Drug Administration although recent drug advances are promising.

Emerging nucleic acid–based therapies have potent Lp(a)-lowering effects and appear safe; phase three trials will establish whether they improve cardiovascular outcomes.[385]

In fact, treatment with zerlasiran produced sustained reductions in lipoprotein(a) [Lp(a)] concentrations out to 1 year in adults with elevated Lp(a), extended data from the APOLLO phase 1 trial showed.[386]

Past (and Present) Dubious Measurements

While most measurements of cholesterol concentrate on LDL-C, as noted, this has a number of contents that simply do not contribute to atheroma. But even further, most previous LDL measurements were not very accurate. Direct LDL cholesterol testing measures the amount of cholesterol found inside low-density lipoproteins (LDL), but in most tests, LDL cholesterol is *estimated* using an equation involving other cholesterol measurements.

A direct LDL cholesterol test is distinct in that it directly *measures* LDL cholesterol in the blood and is, thus, more accurate.

---

385 Lau, F. D. & Giugliano, R. P. 2022, "Lipoprotein(a) and its Significance in Cardiovascular Disease", *JAMA Cardiology*, Vol. 7, No. 7, pp. 760-769, https://doi.org/10.1001/jamacardio.2022.0987.

386 Nissen, S. E., Wolski, K., Watts, G. F. *et al.* 2024, "Single Ascending and Multiple-Dose Trial of Zerlasiran, a Short Interfering RNA Targeting Lipoprotein(a): A Randomized Clinical Trial", *JAMA*, Vol. 331, No. 18, pp. 1534-1543, https://doi.org/10.1001/jama.2024.4504.

Table 35: Usual LDL/HDL & Triglycerides Measurements.
Below 2.6 mmol/L (100 mg/dl) recommended. 1.8 (70) best.

LDL cholesterol (U.S.A)	**LDL cholesterol (Canada / Europe)**	
Below 70 mg/dL	Below 1.8 mmol/L	Ideal for people at very high risk of heart disease
Below 100 mg/dL	Below 2.6 mmol/L	Ideal for people at risk of heart disease
100-129 mg/dL	2.6-3.3 mmol/L	Near ideal
130-159 mg/dL	3.4-4.1 mmol/L	Borderline high
160-189 mg/dL	4.1-4.9 mmol/L	High
190 mg/dL >	Above 4.9 mmol/L	Very high

Table 36: Update – Baseline LDL Cholesterol Has a U-Shaped Association with All-Cause Mortality. All-cause mortality was lowest at an LDL cholesterol level of 140 mg/dL = 3.6 mom/L (*Source: Johannesen, C. D. L., Langsted, A., Mortensen, M. B.* et al. *2020, "Association between low density lipoprotein and all cause and cause specific mortality in Denmark: prospective cohort study"*, BMJ, *Vol. 371, doi: https://doi.org/10.1136/bmj.m4266*).

HDL cholesterol (U.S.A)	**HDL cholesterol (Canada / Europe)**	
Below 40 mg/dL (men) Below 50 mg/dL (women)	Below 1 mmol/L (men) Below 1.3 mmol/L (women)	Poor
40-49 mg/dL (men) 50-59 mg/dL (women)	1-1.3 mmol/L (men) 1.3-1.5 mmol/L (women)	Better
60 mg/dL and above	1.6 mmol/L and above	Best
Triglycerides (U.S.A)	**Triglycerides (Canada / Europe)**	
Below 150 mg/dL	Below 1.7 mmol/L	Desirable <1.3 Recommended
150-199 mg/dL	1.7-2.2 mmol/L	Borderling high
200-499 mg/dL	2.3-5.6 mmol/L	High
500 mg/dL and above	Above 5.6 mmol/L	Very high

How Low Should You Go? Is Very Low LDL-C Safe?

There is an excellent review article an Editorial collaboration of Medscape and the American College of Cardiology, December 01, 2023, for those interested.[387]

Further References/Reading

- Cardiovascular event risk category cut points (optimal, moderate, high) are based on the AMORIS study (Walldius, G. & Jungner, I. 2004, "Apolipoprotein B and apolipoprotein A-I: risk indicators of coronary heart disease and targets for lipid-modifying therapy", *Journal of Internal Medicine*, Vol. 255, No. 2, pp. 188-205, https://doi.org/10.1046/j.1365-2796.2003.01276.x).
- Reiner, Z., Catapano, A. L., De Backer, G. *et al.* 2011, "ESC/EAS Guidelines for the management of dyslipidaemias: The task force for the management of dyslipidaemias of the European Society of Cardiology (ESC) and the European Atherosclerosis Society (EAS)", *European Heart Journal*, Vol. 32, No. 14, pp. 1769-1818, https://doi.org/10.1093/eurheartj/ehr158.
- McQueen, M. J., Hawken, S., Wang, X. *et al.* 2008, "Lipids, lipoproteins, and apolipoproteins as risk markers of myocardial infarction in 52 countries (the INTERHEART study): a case-control study", *Lancet*, Vol. 372, No. 9634, pp. 224-233, https://doi.org/10.1016/S0140-6736(08)61076-4
- Thompson, A. & Danesh, J, 2006, "Associations between apolipoprotein B, apolipoprotein AI, the apolipoprotein B/AI ratio and coronary heart disease: a literature-based meta-analysis of prospective studies", *Journal of Internal*

387 Newman, C. B. & Martin, S. S. 2023, "How Low Should You Go? Is Very Low LDL-C Safe?", *Medscape*, 1 December.

Medicine, Vol. 259, No. 5, pp. 481-492, https://doi.org/10.1111/j.1365-2796.2006.01644.x.

- Jacobson, T. A., Ito, M. K., Maki, K. C. *et al.* 2014, "National Lipid Association recommendations for patient-centered management of dyslipidemia: Part 1-executive summary", *Journal of Clinical Lipidology*, Vol. 8, No. 5, pp. 473-488, https://doi.org/10.1016/j.jacl.2014.07.007.
- Expert Panel on Integrated Guidelines for Cardiovascular Health and Risk Reduction in Children and Adolescents, 2011, "Expert Panel on Integrated Guidelines for Cardiovascular Health and Risk Reduction in Children and Adolescents: Summary Report", *Pediatrics*, Vol. 128, No. Supplemenr 5, pp. S213-S256, https://doi.org/10.1542/peds.2009-2107C.

Further Heart Tests (FYI)

ECG/EKG

Detects any abnormalities of heart rhythm and rate at rest and evidence of any old infarcts.

Unnecessary ECGs/EKGs

Asymptomatic adults at low risk for developing cardiovascular disease do not benefit from cardiac screening with electrocardiography, stress electrocardiography, or myocardial perfusion imaging.

There is, however, an epidemic of atrial fibrillation as we age. It is often asymptomatic. I recommend an ECG/EKG after the age of 60, even if you have no symptoms.

Young Athletes

Athletes have a 2.5 higher risk of sudden death. They should have a full CVS screen (history, exam, & ECG/EKG) every two years from 12 years. This practice could cut heart deaths by 50–70%, especially for HCM (Hypertrophic Cardiomyopathy).[388]

Cardiac Stress Test

This determines any sinister changes with exercise and, if okay, indicates that exercise does not provoke dangerous changes.

Coronary Scoring

Detects any calcium in coronary arteries, which is one indicator of degenerative disease. It is of some 51% help with respect to predicting acute cardiac events (heart attacks); that is, it is not the full answer. However, it further helps provide more information about the most important aspect of our health (our heart).

CT Angiography/CTA (CAT scan)

CT Angiography is a non-invasive way to detect arterial narrowing of blood vessels in the heart, as well as structural abnormalities of the heart, before there are symptoms. It can detect atherogenic plaques (which cause heart attacks), which no other non-invasive tests can. The next test along is Angiography, wherein a catheter is threaded into the coronary arteries. CT Angiography may obviate the need for this. Overall, non-invasive CT angiograms accurately detected or ruled out artery blockages in 91% of patients, compared with 69% for stress testing. Ultra-high-resolution coronary CT Angiography has been developed for special cases.

5. Gynecology check- Pap, Mammogram, DEXA

Different nations have different regimes and recommendations.

388 Elliott, P. M., Poloniecki, J., Dickie, S. *et al.* 2000, "Sudden death in hypertrophic cardiomyopathy: identification of high risk patients", *Journal of the American College of Cardiology*, Vol. 36, No. 7, pp. 2212-2218, https://doi.org/10.1016/s0735-1097(00)01003-2.

Women and people with a cervix aged 25 to 74 years of age are recommended to have a Cervical Screening Test every 5 years through their healthcare provider. This test replaces the Pap test and looks for the human papillomavirus (HPV), which is the main cause of cervical cancer.

The Cervical Screening Test is a new, more accurate way of protecting people with a cervix against cervical cancer. It was introduced in Australia in December 2017 and is expected to protect almost one third more people from cervical cancer than the old Pap test.

The Cervical Screening Test looks and feels the same as the Pap test. However, if your results are normal, it is only done every five years instead of every two years. If you are a person aged 25 to 74 with a cervix, you should have your first cervical screening test two years after your last Pap test.

The Cervical Screening Test is performed by a doctor or nurse. You also have the option to collect your own sample for a Cervical Screening Test. This is called self-collection. This means that you can take your own sample for the test from your vagina, using a swab.

The U.S. Preventive Services Task Force (USPSTF) recommends that women who are at average risk for breast cancer start breast cancer screening at age 40 instead of the previously recommended starting age of 50 and get screening mammograms every other year from ages 40 to 74.

The American Cancer Society (ACS) recommends that women aged 45 to 54 should get mammograms every year, and women 55 and older should switch to mammograms every two years or can continue yearly screening.

Screening should continue as long as a woman is in good health and is expected to live 10 more years or longer.

High Risk Patients

In another editorial accompanying the USPSTF guidelines, it was agreed that "MRI is the supplement of choice at this time" for women meeting high-risk criteria for supplemental breast screening.

The DEXA test is a type of x-ray that is painless, fast, and involves minimal radiation exposure. It measures the density or thinning of your bones that women develop more than men, especially after menopause.

6. Prostate check (MRI)

PSA – Prostate-Specific Antigen and 4K Score

Indicates either prostate enlargement—Benign Prostatic Enlargement (BPH)—or cancer.

PSA presents an ethical problem in that, if it is elevated, it is not diagnostic.

The 4Kscore Test is an in vitro diagnostic test system designed to evaluate a patient's likelihood of aggressive prostate cancer by measuring concentrations of four proteins (total PSA, free PSA, intact PSA, and kallikrein).

However, an MRI picks up 45% more prostate pathology than a PSA. It is an evolving debate.

Latest

Researchers at the University of Michigan have developed a urine test that detects high-grade prostate cancer more accurately than existing tests, including PHI, SelectMDx, 4Kscore, EPI, MPS, and IsoPSA.[389]

---

389 Tosoian, J. J., Zhang, Y., Xiao, L. *et al.* 2024, "Development and Validation of an 18-Gene Urine Test for High-Grade Prostate Cancer", *JAMA Oncology*, Vol. 10, No. 6, pp. 726-736, https://doi.org/doi:10.1001/jamaoncol.2024.0455

7. Colon cancer check—Colonoscopy/Sigmoidoscopy

A camera on the end of a photo-optic cable is inserted via the anus to examine the lower gut. Patients are mostly sedated, and the actual procedure is painless. It can detect Cancer of the Colon (CAC) early enough to effect a cure.

FOBT (Fecal Occult Blood Tests) are blotting paper tests on your feces for minute amounts of blood. They are cheaper, less embarrassing, but not as good. A colonoscopy is "The Gold Standard", providing the best results with regards to survival. A rigid sigmoidoscope, which is about 25cm long, allows examination of up to about 20cm of the rectum and distal sigmoid colon, though it is best suited for rectal assessments only. The flexible sigmoidoscope is made of a flexible fiberoptic tube and can be up to 60cm long.

Endoscopes are passed via the mouth into the stomach to look for ulcers or cancers.

Physicians should perform an individualized risk assessment for CRC in all adults. In this updated guidance, the American College of Physicians (ACP) suggests that clinicians:

- Start screening for colorectal cancer in asymptomatic average-risk adults at age 50 years.
- Consider not screening asymptomatic average-risk adults between the ages of 45 to 49. Clinicians should discuss the uncertainty around benefits and harms of screening in this population.
- Stop screening for colorectal cancer in asymptomatic average-risk adults older than 75 years or in asymptomatic average-risk adults with a life expectancy of 10 years or less.
- Select a screening test for colorectal cancer in consultation with their patient based on a discussion of

benefits, harms, costs, availability, frequency, and patient values and preferences.

- Select among screening tests for colorectal cancer: a fecal immunochemical or high-sensitivity guaiac fecal occult blood test every 2 years, colonoscopy every 10 years, or flexible sigmoidoscopy every 10 years plus a fecal immunochemical test every 2 years.
- Should not use stool DNA, computed tomography colonography, capsule endoscopy, urine, or serum screening tests for colorectal cancer.

The net benefit of colorectal cancer screening is much less favourable in average-risk adults between the ages of 45 to 49 years than in 50 to 75 years. Although there has been a small increase in CRC incidence among individuals aged 45 to 49 years, the incidence is much lower than in individuals aged 50 to 64 years and 65 to 74 years. Harms associated with CRC screenings include cardiovascular and gastrointestinal events (e.g., serious bleeding, perforation, myocardial infarction, angina). Unnecessary follow-ups and costs for findings are deemed clinically unimportant.[390]

Special Note:

Colorectal cancer cases increased a whopping 333% among 15- to 19-year-olds and 185% among 20- to 24-year-olds from 1999 to 2020, according to new research being presented at Digestive Disease Week (DDW) 2024, a major medical conference in Washington, DC. In addition to the increases in the 15- to 19-year-old and 20- to 24-year-old groups, the rates in 2020 compared to 1999 showed a:

- 68% increase for ages 25 to 29
- 71% increase for ages 30 to 34

390 American College of Physicians Statement, 10 August 2023

- 58% increase for ages 35 to 39
- 45% increase for ages 40 to 44

8. Skin check—dermoscopy

These are hand-held or cable-optic microscopes that optically take away the top layer of skin so the examiner can better see the histology of the mole or skin lesion underneath; it enhances the diagnosis of melanoma and skin cancers.

9. Coeliac Disease

IgA TTG and serum IgA [tissue transglutaminase immunoglobulin A], as well as a total IgA level, is the gold-standard test.

Endoscopy and biopsy are sometimes needed.

10. Hormones—not all these tests are needed unless clinically indicated.

TSH/FT3/FT4

These are thyroid function tests. Someone who has a low-functioning thyroid (hypothyroid) appears slow, may be gaining weight, and even lose the outer third of their eyebrows. An auto-immune cause is Hashimoto's Disease.

By contrast, someone who has too much thyroid function is super-fidgety, super-active, and if severe, as in Grave's Disease, bug-eyed. It, too, is an auto-immune disease, and people with any auto-immune disease such as Diabetes 1, Celiac Disease, and such should be screened for others.

Adrenal Axis: Cortisol

Often called the stress hormone, Cortisol peaks mid-morning to face the challengers of the day but is lowest at around 4 a.m., which generals in the Old Testament realised when they attacked their sleepy, un-stimulated enemy.

It is measured to evaluate how well the pituitary and adrenal glands are working, helping to diagnose diseases, such as Cushing's Syndrome and Addison's Disease.

Women

- Estradiol
- Progesterone
- Follicle Stimulating Hormone
- Luteinizing Hormone
- Prolactin

Female hormones are usually done perimenopause to assess the current status.

Men

Testosterone Loss in Older Men: Factors Beyond Age[391]

A range of sociodemographic, lifestyle, and medical factors influence testosterone levels in men and should be considered when assessing levels.

Testosterone levels are, in fact, stable until the age of about 70 years then drop with age.

BMI was inversely associated with testosterone levels. Only men with a BMI over 32 had higher estradiol concentrations.

Similarly, men who did less vigorous physical activity for 75 minutes or less per week saw significantly lower testosterone levels, as did former smokers.

Interestingly, married men—or those otherwise in a relationship—also had significantly lower testosterone levels after age 70.

391 Marriott, R. J., Murray, K., Adams, R. J. *et al.* 2023, "Factors Associated With Circulating Sex Hormones in Men: Individual Participant Data Meta-analyses", *Annals of Internal Medicine,* Vol. 176, No. 9, https://doi.org/10.7326/M23-0342.

In addition, researchers found that having a history of several health factors was associated with significantly lower testosterone levels after surpassing age 70, including:

- Hypertension
- Cardiovascular disease
- Cancer
- Diabetes

Sex hormone-binding globulin (SHBG) was likewise associated with age and inversely associated with BMI. Luteinizing hormone was also directly linked with age in men over 70.

SHBG

Sex hormone-binding globulin (SHBG) transports androgens and estrogens in blood and regulates their access to target tissues. Hepatic (liver) production of SHBG fluctuates throughout the life cycle and is influenced primarily by metabolic and hormonal factors.

DHEA

Dehydroepiandrosterone (DHEA) is a hormone that your body naturally produces in the adrenal gland. DHEA helps produce other hormones, including testosterone and estrogen. Natural DHEA levels peak in early adulthood and then slowly fall as you age.

- Although circulating concentrations of DHEA and DHEAS decline with age, cortisol and 11-keto androgens do not decline or rise slightly.
- Modulation of cortisol signalling could be beneficial in a host of diseases that become more common in older men and women.

- Systemic DHEA supplementation has not shown major benefits in older individuals.[392]

Growth Hormone Axis

- At present, no therapy to increase GH secretion or action is approved as an anti-aging intervention.
- Studies with rhGH and GH secretagogues failed to demonstrate benefits that outweigh risks. However, it is possible that benefit could be maximized with the use of lower doses in study populations with worse physical function and in combination with exercise and adequate nutrition, without the adverse effects seen in previous studies.

11. Low-dose CT Chest

Lung cancer is the deadliest cancer in the US, with over 350 people dying from it every day—more than breast, colorectal, and cervical cancers combined.

Screening for lung cancer, in the USA, is fairly new, starting in 2013. But the lung cancer screening rate has increased by only 2%, mostly because the screening criteria are bureaucratic, burdensome to implement, and accompanied by unprecedented insurance requirements such that the lung cancer screening rate is just 5.7%, compared to 70%-75% for mammograms, colonoscopies, and Pap smears.

The low-dose CT scan is quick and painless. With radiation exposure approaching that of mammograms. and with the other lung diagnostic benefits as for the detection of emphysema, heart disease, and others, it can be a good choice.

392 Cappola, A. R., Auchus, R. J., Fuleihan, G. E. 2023, "Hormones and Aging: An Endocrine Society Scientific Statement," *The Journal of Clinical Endocrinology & Metabolism*, Vol. 108, No. 8, pp. 1835-1874, https://doi.org/10.1210/clinem/dgad225.

12. DEXA

This is a special x-ray to detect osteoporosis. It is also used to measure visceral fat. Get both at the same time.

13. Vision and Hearing

Get both professionally tested.

14. MRI

MRIs are the best tests available to radiologists, and there are no radiation risks, just magnetic alignment pictures that provide the greatest detail. They are relatively expensive and best done in expert centres. There is a vogue for 'whole body MRIs', but this raises questions as to the ethics of doing an unnecessary test and the likelihood of finding a mass, which then requires invasion/surgery only to find it is benign. It is a decision best discussed with your doctor, but I would recommend anyone with a family history of cerebral aneurysms should get a specific MRI.

In an analysis as to 'The use of whole-body MRI for cancer screening and regular health checks', 229 patients underwent whole-body MRIs as part of a routine health examination and cancer screening. Two cases were found to involve malignancy, but mostly, they found disc tears, bulging or protrusion, followed by shoulder bursitis and uterine myoma. But WB MRIs did not evaluate for all malignant diseases, such as breast cancers and small pituitary tumors. Evaluation of lung and bowel lesions was also limited and the inability to detect small (<6 mm) lung nodules.[393]

393 Lee, S. Y., Park, H. J., Kim, M. S. *et al.* 2018, "An initial experience with the use of whole body MRI for cancer screening and regular health checks", *PLOS One*, Vol. 13, No. 11, https://doi.org/10.1371/journal.pone.0206681.

The American College of Preventive Medicine (ACPM) has published formal guidance recommending against full-body scans in asymptomatic patients. The American College of Radiology released a statement in April: "There is no documented evidence that total body screening is cost-efficient or effective in prolonging life."

Radiologists in the Netherlands who conducted a meta-analysis of studies on preventive full-body MRI screenings found scans yielded false positives 16% of the time, on average.[394]

Given this, it would be my recommendation not to get a WB MRI but to get specific tests as per symptoms, signs, or the results of other tests—e.g., a prostate MRI is the best test for prostate cancer.

Further, a review concluded that whole-body MRIs should not be offered for preventive health screening to asymptomatic subjects[395] and medical groups, including the American College of Preventive Medicine, American College of Radiology, and the U.S. Food and Drug Administration, also do not recommend WB MRIs, observing that there is limited evidence they provide significant benefit to ostensibly healthy people. But celebrities like the Kardashians promote it, so if you have a lazy $1,000 for a torso scan, $1,800 for a head-and-torso scan, and $2,500 (USD) for a whole-body scan, you, too, can have one.

As I said in the introduction, I now feel this is an individual decision and, given the current vogue for people to ostensibly take charge of their health, I suspect whole-body MRIs will become de rigueur among these people.

---

394 Kwee, R. M. & Kwee, T. C. 2019, "Whole-body MRI for preventive health screening: A systematic review of the literature", *Journal of Magnetic Resonance Imaging*, Vol. 50, No. 5, pp. 1489-1503, https://doi.org/10.1002/jmri.26736.

395 *Ibid.*

15. STD

Guidelines recommend yearly screening for:

- Sexually active women under age 25
- Women older than 25 and at increased risk of STIs—such as having sex with a new partner or multiple partners.
- Men who have sex with men
- People with HIV
- Transgender women who have sex with men
- People who have been forced to have intercourse or engage in sexual activity against their will.

A study shows that almost one in three men over the age of 15 are infected with at least one genital human papillomavirus (HPV) type, and one in five are infected with one or more of what are known as high risk, or oncogenic, HPV types. The majority of HPV infections in men and women are asymptomatic, but they can lead to long-term sequelae and mortality. Each year, more than 340,000 women die of cervical cancer. HPV prevalence was high in young adults, reaching a maximum between the ages of 25 years and 29 years.[396] At a minimum, the STI screen involves blood tests for HIV, hepatitis B, and syphilis, and swabs or PCR/LCR urine tests for chlamydia and gonorrhoea. Depending on risk assessment, tests for hepatitis A and hepatitis C may also be considered.

At-home test kits for certain STIs, such as HIV, chlamydia, and gonorrhoea have become more common and popular. For home STI testing, you collect a urine sample or an oral or genital swab and then send it to a lab. However, tests done on samples you collect yourself may not always be accurate.

---

396 Bruni, L., Albero, G., Rowley, J. *et al.* 2023, "Global and regional estimates of genital human papillomavirus prevalence among men: a systematic review and meta-analysis", *The Lancet Global Health,* Vol. 11, No. 9, pp. E1345-E1362, https://doi.org/10.1016/S2214-109X(23)00305-4.

In addition, after a baseline complete check, not all need be done again—or at five- to 10-year intervals, if normal.

16. Aortic Aneurysm Ultrasound

Males, especially smokers > 65 years, should have an abdominal ultrasound. Abdominal aneurysms are found in 4 to 8% of men, but a 43% reduction in fatal ruptures is possible.

Einstein died of a ruptured abdominal aortic aneurysm on April 18, 1955. He was 76.

17. VO_2max

It is a free app on a smartphone that comes with the Fitbit and Apple Watch. This is called the "cardio fitness level" and is worth noting, as it is a measure of your fitness and, hence, a motivator, too. A direct measure of your VO_2max requires special equipment.

To measure mitochondrial fitness, the best metric is VO_2max, which represents the maximum rate that your body can use oxygen during exercise. Essentially, it reflects the body's ability to utilize oxygen for energy production.

18. Pulse Wave Velocity

This tests the elasticity of our arteries, and I wouldn't do it except through an app on a smartphone.

19. Troponin

I am not sure if I should include this, but patients were nearly four times as likely to die if their cardiac troponin test result was high (45%) compared to those whose test results fell within the normal range (12%). Further analysis revealed that an abnormally high cardiac troponin level was independently associated with a

76% heightened risk of death, not only from both cardiovascular diseases but also other causes. In fact, the most common cause of death was cancer (46%), followed by cardiovascular disease (13%).[397]

As such, I now include it.

Troponin, especially high-sensitive troponin (cTnI), is used to detect heart muscle damage, i.e., a heart attack, but recently, as pointed out, in a large, unselected hospital population, in 91.4% of whom *there was no clinical indication for testing*, cTnI concentration was independently associated with medium-term cardiovascular and non-cardiovascular mortality in the statistical model tested. The mortality over the course of about 2½ years was 44% in those whose blood test was elevated versus only about 12% in those in whom it wasn't.

The causes of death were not just heart attacks, so it may be a screening test to go look further, and I would get it done.

Addenda FYI

Further Tests as Indicated

This is a relatively random assortment of the latest information and tests you may wonder about or be encouraged to buy. At present, I do not think any are indicated and most just pander to our natural curiosity to see if we are 20 years younger (inaccurate), have longevity genes (there's nothing to be done), and on and on.

Some, of course, are fascinating, but the above tests are known and evidenced at this present time. They are all you need.

I tentatively also append some 'second line' tests I contemplate for this initial baseline according to the patient's

---

397 Hinton, J., Mariathas, M. N., Gabara, L. *et al.* 2023, "Association between troponin level and medium-term mortality in 20,000 hospital patients", *Heart*, Vol. 109, No. 23, pp. 1772-1777, https://doi.org/10.1136/heartjnl-2023-322463.

examination, e.g., if they have high blood glucose and are overweight, I may recommend an HbA1c or a Glucose Tolerance Test (GTT).

Insulin and Insulin Resistance

I have never seen the need to do these tests. If a patient's blood glucose, or HbA1c, was elevated, I may pursue it with a Glucose Tolerance Test, but clinically, the diagnosis of Diabetes was pretty obvious just from the first two. But all the biohackers, who never see a patient, and the labs, who want the money, 'recommend' them, so I looked up the informed, ethical recommendations. I found the following:

"Note that such testing is time and resource-intensive, and there is no universal agreement on its value, especially where there are other (bio) markers of insulin resistance, for example, increased waist circumference, dyslipidemia (low HDL-c, high triglycerides) already give very strong leads."[398]

Iron

Low in blood loss—from piles to cancer

Ferritin

Ferritin is a blood protein that contains iron. A ferritin test helps estimate how much iron your body stores. If a ferritin test reveals that your blood ferritin level is lower than normal, it indicates your body's iron stores are low and you have iron deficiency.

This is not usually done unless your FBC reveals you are anaemic.

---

398 *Sonic Pathology Handbook*

Homocysteine

May be considered if you have been diagnosed with heart or blood vessel disease or if you have conditions that increase your risk for heart and blood vessel disease, such as high blood pressure or high cholesterol. You may also have this test done to check for low levels of vitamin B_{12} or folate.

B_{12}

Vitamin B_{12} deficiency is not common in the Western nations. However, people who follow a vegetarian or vegan diet might be prone to deficiency because plant foods don't contain vitamin B_{12}. Older adults and people with digestive tract conditions that affect absorption of nutrients also are susceptible to vitamin B_{12} deficiency.

The National Institute for Health and Care Excellence has issued its first guidelines for diagnosing and managing vitamin B_{12} deficiency. It said that older people are one of the main groups at risk. One in ten over-75s are estimated to be affected, with lot of elderly people wrongly diagnosed with Alzheimer's or dementia rather than B_{12} deficiency.

Risk factors include age, previous surgery involving the digestive system, and autoimmune conditions. They may also include a diet low in animal-source foods, such as a vegan diet, without the regular use of over-the-counter supplements. However, certain commonly taken drugs interfere with the absorption of B_{12}. This includes some heartburn medicines, including proton pump inhibitors (PPIs), such as esomeprazole (Nexium), lansoprazole (Prevacid), omeprazole (PrilosecOTC), pantoprazole (Protonix), and rabeprazole (Aciphex), H2 blockers such as famotidine (Pepcid AC), and certain Diabetes medicines such as metformin.

Vitamins

The number of vitamin tests ordered in general practice have increased substantially in developed countries in recent years. For example, the regional number of test requests for vitamin B_{12} in Utrecht, the Netherlands, increased almost sixfold between 2004 and 2014. Vitamin D was the fifth most common laboratory test ordered for Medicare patients in the USA in 2016, at a total cost of US$350 million.[399]

The problem is that people are vitamin obsessed and ascribe any feelings from tiredness, poor sleep, anxiety, or what-have-you to a vitamin deficiency. This is encouraged and exploited by the vitamin manufacturers and the DIY laboratories.

Any tests should be assessed by a competent physician and not just a scatter-gun selection for interest only.

The U.S. Preventive Services Task Force (USPSTF) reconsidered the benefits and harms of routine screening. The group's consensus view was that there's still not enough evidence that routine vitamin D blood testing leads to better health outcomes. The task force came to this conclusion during an update of its 2014 recommendation.

There is no need for vitamin tests unless there are clinical symptoms and signs or if the patient does not consume animal proteins. This, however, will not stop the public from taking vitamins or supplements, as 56% of the population does.

Fresh food provides all the vitamins we need—and in the correct and most biologically available form whereas tablets only provide expensive urine.

---

399 Hofstede, H, van der Burg, H. A. M., Mulder, B. C. *et al.* 2019, "Reducing unnecessary vitamin testing in general practice: barriers and facilitators according to general practitioners and patients", *BMJ Open*, Vol. 9, No. 10, https://doi.org/10.1136/bmjopen-2019-029760.

ApoE and Allelles

See Dementia and Alzheimer's disease chapter.

Tests for Chronic Inflammation

Unfortunately, there are no specific tests.

- High levels of hs-CRP indicate inflammation.
- Fibrinogen
- Serum protein electrophoresis (SPE)
- Pro-inflammatory cytokines, like tumor necrosis factor-alpha (TNF-alpha), interleukin-1 beta (IL-1beta), interleukin-6 (IL-6), and interleukin-8 (IL-8) are expensive but may identify specific factors.

Telomeres

Some companies that offer at-home testing promise your DNA will reveal your true biological age and provide insight into your cellular health. But not only is there no standard for what constitutes a "healthy" telomere length by age, there are also multiple methods for evaluating telomere length and, often, significant variations in the results.

"If you are being tested, you might view it as an experiment and not take the result too seriously… It is always possible that a measure has significant error in it… There are no clear hard cut-offs for what telomere length should be at each age. It is also hard to know how companies determine what telomere length should be at any age. Given the wide variance at any age, for an individual, actual comparisons with what may be expected at your age at one time point might not be as meaningful as tracking how you change over time. No one has determined what the right amount of time is to do repeat testing…"[400]

---

400 University of California San Francisco Aging, Metabolism and Emotion Center, Extracts, 3 July 2017

We are now discovering that telomeres are an unreliable aging clock, which raises questions about the validity of aging tests based on them. The links between telomere length and lifestyle choices also aren't as straightforward as we once thought. In fact, long telomeres can even be bad news.[401]

α-Klotho

α-Klotho is a geroprotective protein that can attenuate or alleviate deleterious changes with aging and disease. Levels were decreased in healthy individuals because of the physiological decline from the aging process. Routine assessments using ELISA as a simple and cheap detectable marker of aging may improve quality of life in the elderly.[402] The orally active senolytic, Dasatinib, plus Quercetin (D+Q) can increase α-Klotho in mice and humans.[403] Desatinib is used to treat Chronic Myeloid Leukaemia and has side effects. I would await more trials.

Serum and CSF levels of α-klotho are positively correlated and both predict scores on the Mini-Mental State Examination (MMSE) and Clinical Dementia Rating (CDR), regardless of sex or apoE4 status.[404]

401 *New Scientist*, 17 February 2021

402 Espuch-Oliver, A., Vázquez-Lorente, H., Jurado-Fasoli, L. *et al.* 2022, "References Values of Soluble α-Klotho Serum Levels Using an Enzyme-Linked Immunosorbent Assay in Healthy Adults Aged 18–85 Years", *Journal of Clinical Medicine*, Vol. 11, No. 9, p. 2415, https://doi.org/10.3390/jcm11092415.

403 Zhu, Y., Langhi Prata, L. G. P., Wissler Gerdes, E. O. *et al.* 2022, "Orally-active, clinically-translatable senolytics restore α-Klotho in mice and humans", *eBioMedicine,* Vol. 77, No. 103912, https://doi.org/10.1016/j.ebiom.2022.103912.

404 Kundu, P., Zimmerman, B., Quinn, J. F. *et al.* 2022, "Serum Levels of α-Klotho Are Correlated with Cerebrospinal Fluid Levels and Predict Measures of Cognitive Function," *Journal of Alzheimer's Disease*, Vol. 86, No. 3, pp. 1471-1481, https://doi.org/10.3233/JAD-215719.

FOXO3

This is **"The"** anti-aging gene, according to Craig Willcox co-author of *The Okinawa Way.*

It inhibits inflammation of CVS. Everybody has FOXO3, but only one in three have the protective version, which triples the chance of reaching 100. But exercise and diet activate the normal FOXO3 to be somewhat protective.

Biomarkers

The basic definition of a biomarker is deceptively simple: "A defined characteristic that is measured as an indicator of normal biological processes, pathogenic processes, or responses to an exposure or intervention." This broad definition encompasses therapeutic interventions and can be derived from molecular, histologic, radiographic, or physiologic characteristics. For the sake of clarity, biomarkers should be distinct from direct measures of how a person feels, functions, or survives.[405]

Confusion reigns! Experts disagree. Different experts recommend different biomarkers or tests.

To put it simply, a biomarker or marker is *any* measurement that can assess changes.

When I studied physics, 'measurement' was defined as 'the comparison of a similar object against a known standard'. Thus, once a standard has been established, it is possible, as say with cholesterol, to say it is high or low.

While the standard pathological tests, such as our haemoglobin or sodium have been sorted out long ago, the new laboratory markers for aging have not.

---

405 Califf, R. M. 2018, "Biomarker definitions and their applications", *Experimental Biology and Medicine*, Vol. 243, No. 3, pp. 213-221, https://doi.org/10.1177/1535370217750088.

Be that as it may, I do have my own aging clinical biomarkers:

1. Do they look their age?
2. Are they unkempt (undress the patient: look at their feet, heels and nails)?
3. Are they overweight?
4. Do they have missing teeth?
5. Are they vague or confused?
6. Does the person look ill?

These may not sound satisfactory to the biohackers, scientists, and researchers measuring their biological clock or telomeres, but they sure have served me (and my patients) well. Whereas the human genome research was begun in 1990, and 33 years later, there's no improvement in our longevity.

Longevity is the new fad and has taken off because you don't have to be a medical graduate, let alone a clinician, to sell it… anyone can do it!

For scientists, new laboratories, and researchers, longevity means extending, pausing, reversing, or even stopping aging. Whereas the clinical definition I agree with is, as stated, *the prevention of premature death.*

The only recommendations to prevent you from dying before you should, at this moment in time, are what the *Live Longer* program provides.

Here, clinical medicine and longevity research, to a degree, part company. The researchers have come up with 'biomarkers' of aging… but there are no agreed upon biomarkers.

Biological Age

The concept is that the health of your cells and, thus, organs may be older or younger than your actual chronological age.

These tests measure or assess DNA methylation to create epigenetic age clocks. Initially, they were research projects but now have been snapped up by the labs and home-kits. They are widely inaccurate, up to 15% or so. Some offer advice based on your results, but such advice is generalised, such as adopting a plant-based diet, exercising more, sleeping better… oh really!

And then, the clincher: Take our 'Special Supplement' and get re-tested every six months (or so)! While they may be more accurate in the future, they are not to be recommended at present, with results varying widely from lab to lab. Any advice received may well be dubious.

Some informed longevity doctors no longer use the epigenetic clock.

What Is Aging?

Aging means different things to different people, and there is no consensus as to what ging is or what causes it; is aging a disease, and what is rejuvenation? Some people think of aging as increased mortality rate. Others think of it as age-related changes, decreased fitness, functional decline, damage accumulation, increased biological age, or a continuation of development.

These different concepts are obviously inter-related but would require their own biomarkers. But the various longevity programs cannot even agree which are the best biomarkers.

To complicate matters more, different organs and tissues in the same person age at a different rate, and then, even different cells in the same tissue age at a different rate.

At least some 25 of the major labs have formed a consortium to try and fix these issues, but the work involved is simply enormous: Not only the human body, not only each tissue, not only each organ, not only each cell, not only each constituent of the cells, but the constituents of the constituents of each cell and their metabolic pathways and…well, you get the picture. And this research has to be done mostly on mice.

Or you can plug into a longevity clinic and get 200 arguably useless tests, get your blood taken every day (or at least every two months), and measure the calories in your food and their micronutrient content and join a gym and…

The tests and investigations I recommend have been evidenced to measure the most important markers to keep us healthy (such as ApoB). The intention is to then treat any abnormalities and/or diagnose illnesses that are mostly preventable.

Largest study of centenarian blood biomarkers[406]

"Despite the claim that chance plays an important role in the achievement of exceptional longevity, it has repeatedly been shown that already earlier in life, centenarians are a selected group with fewer disabilities, comorbidities, hospitalizations, and better cognitive function compared to non-centenarians. While the cited studies focus on specific health outcomes, blood-based biomarkers can provide additional information about health status already before other observable outcomes occur. A Japanese cohort study found that low inflammation defined by cytomegalovirus titre, interleukin-6, tumor necrosis factor-alpha, and C-reactive protein (CRP) was an important predictor for exceptional survival. Improved survival in old age has also been linked to lower creatinine, higher albumin, and several circulating biomarkers (N-terminal pro-B-type natriuretic peptide, interleukin-6, cystatin C, and cholinesterase). Cross-sectional studies have found centenarians to have lower total cholesterol and insulin tolerance than younger elderly. However, since

406 Murata, S., Ebeling, M., Meyer, A. C. *et al.* 2024, "Blood biomarker profiles and exceptional longevity: comparison of centenarians and non-centenarians in a 35-year follow-up of the Swedish AMORIS cohort", *Geroscience*, Vol. 46, pp. 1693-1702, https://doi.org/10.1007/s11357-023-00936-w.

biomarkers change with age, it is difficult to draw conclusions from cross-sectional studies that compare samples drawn at different ages".

For those able to access such tests, they may well be added to these below.

Table 37: Further tests. These, while not in common use, may prove useful in the future.

Insulin	blood/serum	Diabetic state
IL6 [IA]	blood/plasma	Inflammation
Tumor necrosis factor alpha (TNFα) [IA]	blood/serum	Inflammation, cancer
Insulin-like growth factor 1 (IGF-1)	blood/serum	Metabolic disease
Creatinine [PA]	blood/plasma	Kidney dysfunction
Glycated hemoglobin (Hba1c)	blood/EDTA	Diabetic state
Cystatin C	blood/plasma	Kidney dysfunction
N-terminal prohormone of brain natriuretic peptide (NT-proBNP)	blood/EDTA	Heart failure
D-dimer	blood/citrate monovette	Hypercoagulable state
IL8 [IA]	blood/plasma	Inflammation
Plasminogen activator inhibitor-1 (PAI1)	blood/EDTA	Prothrombotic state in cancer and other acute phases
IL15	blood/plasma	Inflammation
CD4/CD8 ratio	blood/EDTA	Immune deficiency, autoimmunity
C-peptide (preferable to insulin)	blood/serum	Diabetic state
IL1-β [IA]	blood/plasma	

Table 38: Frequently mentioned potential "routine laboratory" biomarkers.

Potential biomarkers	**Material**	**Age linked processes**	**e-score**	**rc-score**	**c-score**
Lymphocytes/ WBC [CDC] [PA]	blood/ EDTA	Inflammation autoimmune disorders	–	202	2240
Insulin	blood/serum	Diabetic state	–	148	1143
Glucose/ glucose fastened [PA]	blood/ glucose monovette	Diabetic state	–	111	1175
C-reactive protein (CRP/ hsCRP) [IA] [PA]	blood/ plasma	Inflammation, cancer, cardiovascular disease	–	71	1146
Cholesterol	blood/ plasma	Cardiovascular disease	–	67	896
Albumin [PA]	blood/ plasma	Kidney and liver dysfunction	–	65	1062
IL6 [IA]	blood/ plasma	Inflammation	–	58	979
Tumor necrosis factor alpha (TNFα) [IA]	blood/serum	Inflammation, cancer	–	51	751
Hemoglobin [CDC]	blood/ EDTA	Anemia, other hematopoietic disorders	–	39	471
Insulin-like growth factor 1 (IGF-1)	blood/serum	Metabolic disease	–	29	263
LDL-cholesterol	blood/ plasma	Cardiovascular disease	–	24	280
Triglycerides	blood/ plasma	Cardiovascular disease	–	23	498
HDL-cholesterol	blood/ plasma	Cardiovascular disease	–	23	349
Creatinine [PA]	blood/ plasma	Kidney dysfunction	–	19	479
Monocytes	blood/ EDTA	Inflammation	–	16	378

Glycated hemoglobin (Hba1c)	blood/ EDTA	Diabetic state	–	13	220
Cystatin C	blood/ plasma	Kidney dysfunction	–	12	142
N-terminal prohormone of brain natriuretic peptide (NT-proBNP)	blood/ EDTA	Heart failure	–	10	119
Alkaline phosphatase [PA]	blood/ plasma	Liver damage, bone disorder	–	9	252
Hematocrit/ RBC [CDC]	blood/ EDTA	Anemia	–	8	159
D-dimer	blood/citrate monovette	Hypercoagulable state	–	8	91
IL8 [IA]	blood/ plasma	Inflammation	–	7	164
Plasminogen activator inhibitor-1 (PAI1)	blood/ EDTA	Prothrombotic state in cancer and other acute phases	–	6	72
Bilirubin	blood/ plasma	Liver dysfunction	–	5	46
Urea	blood/ plasma	Renal dysfunction	–	3	137
IL15	blood/ plasma	Inflammation	–	3	55
Mean corpuscular volume/MCV [CDC] [PA]	blood/ EDTA	Anemia, other hematopoietic disorders	–	2	42
Mean corpuscular hemoglobin concentration/ MCHC [CDC]	blood/ EDTA	Anemia, other hematopoietic disorders	–	2	32

CD4/CD8 ratio	blood/ EDTA	Immune deficiency, autoimmunity	–	1	103
C-peptide (preferable to insulin)	blood/serum	Diabetic state	–	1	32
IL1-β [IA]	blood/ plasma				

Natriuretic Peptide Tests (BNP, NT-proBNP)

Natriuretic peptides are substances made by the heart. Two main types of these substances are brain natriuretic peptide (BNP) and N-terminal pro b-type natriuretic peptide (NT-proBNP). Normally, only small levels of BNP and NT-proBNP are found in the bloodstream. High levels can mean your heart isn't pumping as much blood as your body needs. When this happens, it's known as heart failure (HF), sometimes called congestive heart failure. BNP is very helpful in diagnosing HF.

A normal BNP level makes HF less likely, freeing doctors to hunt for other conditions that may be causing shortness of breath or fluid retention. Slightly high BNP levels are less conclusive; but patients with suspected HF and very high BNP levels can get started on therapy with less delay.

MRIs

I would recommend you read, in full, a lovely article: "They Can See Right Through You: Why all the cool kids are getting full-body MRIs".[407]

I feel she captures and reflects the marketplace and current trends:

407 Long, A. 2023, "They Can See Right Through You: Why all the cool kids are getting full-body MRIs", *Town & Country*, Vol. 177, No. 5495, November.

"I confess, I had a moment of weakness. Just after I slipped into the surprisingly tailored scrub set provided in the private dressing room at the new Prenuvo clinic in Manhattan, I thought, These are cute. There's a mirror. Should I take a selfie? Remembering that I was about to slide into the maw of a very serious MRI machine, I resisted. But still, what madness was this? I've never had an impulse to Instagram a mammogram.

In my defense, everybody else is doing it. Among those who have stepped into Prenuvo's full-body MRI and posted about it: celebrity Harvard longevity scientist David Sinclair, self-proclaimed "father of biohacking" Dave Asprey, TV host Maria Menounos (who credited the scan with detecting her stage 2 pancreatic cancer), Paris Hilton, Miranda Kerr, and Kyle MacLachlan. (Cindy Crawford and iPhone co-creator Tony Fadell are investors.) Prenuvo's viral ubiquity can be credited partly to the company's decision to offer free scans to influencers and partly to the indisputable power of Kim Kardashian, who shared a photo of herself on Instagram, dressed in those fetching scrubs, perched on the edge of what she captioned "this life-saving machine." She was promptly lambasted for being tone-deaf, and her critics weren't entirely wrong. Who among Kardashian's followers can afford to get a $2,500 medical scan, not covered by insurance, just for the heck of it?

But such are the times in which we live. We are fixated on fixing everything—fast—and money is no object. There is no wrinkle that a vial of neurotoxin can't erase, no pocket of flab that CoolSculpting can't freeze away, no bikini body that Ozempic can't rapidly manifest. A pricey MRI is the latest Silicon Valley–driven dream: that we can buy our way out of anything, even death. Or, if not the grand finale itself, at least out of infirmity, disease, old age. It is the pinnacle (so far) of the quantified health movement—the obsession with tracking everything from REM sleep to body temperature to changes in the cellular genome.

You can biohack all you want, but at some point you'll want to lift the hood, as it were, and see if by optimizing all those data points you've kept the engine pristine".

MRI + AI heart studies

Artificial Intelligence (AI) can compare your study with hundreds of others, which radiologists can't do, and can work out the relative age of your heart. The earliest signs of premature aging can be so subtle that even expert cardiologists are unable to detect them—but the AI tool can because it has also been fed the images of 40,000 people of varying heart health, along with their health outcomes. The system analyses hundreds of tiny details in the 3D motion of the patient's MRI scan and compares them with those of 5,000 people of varying ages who had led healthy lifestyles. It is not known whether premature heart aging comes down to your genes or down to your lifestyle.

Cancer

There was a headline-catching study in a recent medical journal how 'Screening for Cancer Doesn't Save Lives' which, having saved innumerable lives from screening, I found more than curious. But then I read Dr. Perry Wilson's analysis on Medscape's Impact Factor to wit, a brief extract:

"In other words, the screening tests are unlikely to help most people because most people will not die of the particular type of cancer being screened for. But it will help some small number of those people being screened a lot, potentially saving their lives. If we knew who those people were in advance, it would be great, but then I suppose we wouldn't need the screening test in the first place."[408]

408 Wilson, F. P. 2023, "Really? Cancer Screening Doesn't Save Lives?", *Medscape Impact Factor*, 29 August.

To take up Dr. Wilson's point, *Live Longer* does list the risk factors and who should screen for what.

Tumor Markers in Common Use

A tumour marker is anything present in or produced by cancer cells or other cells of the body in response to cancer or certain benign (noncancerous) conditions that provides information about a cancer, such as how aggressive it is, whether it can be treated with a targeted therapy, or whether it is responding to treatment. The presence of tumor markers alone is not enough to diagnose cancer. You will probably need other tests. Tumour marker tests are not perfect and are often not specific for cancer. They may not be sensitive enough to pick up a cancer recurrence.

The NIH National Cancer Institute lists over 70 such tests, and you are directed to their very good website.

Some markers are pretty useless, such as Prostatic Specific Antigen which, if elevated, is not diagnostic and causes confusion and distress, yet my blood collectors (phlebotomists) tell me it's what men request most. An MRI is better.

Liquid Biopsies

More than 100 years ago, it was found that tumours shed molecules and cells into bodily fluids. Recently, it has been found that these molecules and cells, by taking a sample of blood or urine, cerebrospinal fluid, or saliva, called a liquid biopsy, can reveal some of the same information that tissue biopsies provide.

Multi-cancer early detection tests (MCEDs), sometimes called liquid biopsy tests, are a new method of detecting cancer early. While the *concept* is promising, these untested tests currently pose significant problems.

So far, none of the multiple tests in development have been approved by the Food and Drug Administration. Yet because of a loophole in how diagnostic tests are regulated in the U.S., one of these tests is available for $949.

If desired or offered, you must check just what the laboratory can do and how reliable the test is. At present, liquid biopsies lack the required accuracy in predicting tumour origin in patients who test positive, but this may well change soon.

Tests for Suspected Liver Disease

Alpha-fetoprotein and ultrasound for hepatocellular cancer.

AFP testing, in conjunction with ultrasonography, is used to screen high-risk patients for hepatocellular carcinoma. AFP testing alone isn't used for diagnostic purposes. Instead, it's combined with other tests to get a fuller picture of the patient's condition. The testing may also be done as a baseline measurement once a diagnosis has been made.

AFP blood testing may also be performed during pregnancy to determine a baby's risk for a congenital disability or genetic disorder.

Genetic Testing

These types of testing may be indicated when there is a family history of an inherited disease. They are performed by a blood, saliva, or tissue sample. This is best supervised by a genetic counsellor, who can review your family history and provide advice. Common conditions and diseases that benefit from genetic testing include:

- Colon cancer (Lynch syndrome)
- Breast cancer (BRCA gene)
- Down syndrome
- Cystic fibrosis
- Tay-Sachs disease

- Sickle cell disease
- Spina bifida
- Turner syndrome
- Von Willebrand Disease
- Albinism
- Duchenne muscular dystrophy

Caution: At-Home Medical Tests

An Australian-first study[409] has identified that only 10% of these direct-to-consumer (DTC) tests – a few of which cost almost $2000 – offer any potential clinical utility.

The team found that healthy people made up most of the consumers targeted in this market and that most of the products would not provide useful, actionable information.

Some of the commercial "health check" tests that were found to have no evidence behind them included tests to determine biological age, bone health, fertility status, microbiome analysis, and sleep quality. Other tests targeted conditions that are not recognised by the medical community, including hair metal and mineral analysis to test environmental toxin exposure, as well as tests for cancer, autism, adrenal fatigue, leaky gut, and mental health checks analysing neurotransmitters in urine.

The small percentage of online tests that were regarded as having potential clinical use included bowel cancer test kits, STI home tests and cardiovascular disease risk factor tests.

DIY or at-home medical tests allow you to test for, screen, or monitor certain diseases and conditions in the privacy of your

---

409 Shih, P., Ding, P., Carter, S. M. *et al.* 2023, "Direct-to-consumer tests advertised online in Australia and their implications for medical overuse: systematic online review and a typology of clinical utility", *BMJ Open*, Vol. 13, No. 12, https://doi.org/10.1136/bmjopen-2023-074205.

own home. But their unreliability has been questioned both in the UK and USA.[410,411]

Common at-home tests include:

- Pregnancy tests
- Glucose (blood sugar) tests, which may be used on a regular basis to help manage Diabetes
- Fecal occult blood tests, which screen for colon cancer
- Tests that check for signs of infectious diseases, such as hepatitis, HIV, and COVID-19
- Genetic tests that may show if you are at higher risk for certain diseases.

Most test kits involve taking a sample of a body fluid, such as blood, urine, or saliva, and applying it to the kit as directed. Some tests provide immediate results, while others need to be packaged and mailed to a lab.

- **Only use FDA-approved or FDA-authorized tests.** The FDA has strict requirements for quality and accuracy in home test kits.
- **Follow test instructions exactly.** Even minor changes can affect your results.
- **Don't buy or use expired tests.** Chemicals in the test may lose their effectiveness over time.

There has been a boom in private blood tests being sold online, with one piece of market research predicting that the global blood testing market will rise by 60% from around $80.5 billion in 2021 to $128 billion in 2028.[412]

---

410 Wilkinson, E. 2023, "Unreliable private online hormone tests sold for months despite accuracy concerns", *BMJ*, https://doi.org/10.1136/bmj.p1898.

411 Greene, D., Pannu, J. & Berke, A. 2023, "The Danger of 'Invisible' Biolabs Across the U.S.", *Time Magazine*, 31 August.

412 Wilkinson, E. 2023, "Unreliable private online hormone tests sold for months despite accuracy concerns", *BMJ*, https://doi.org/10.1136/bmj.p1898.

An array of online companies offer blood tests for a range of conditions and deficiencies. These online retailers send the tests to private laboratories and, often, an online retailer will use multiple labs for the same or different tests. The results are then sent back to consumers by the online retailer, often without the consumer ever knowing which laboratory processed their test.

There is no regulator of any laboratories in the UK and it would seem the same elsewhere, as the Theranos fiasco revealed in the USA.

You must ascertain the quality assurance of your tests and if they actually reveal anything of use.

Theranos Inc was founded in 2003 by the then 19-year-old Elizabeth Holmes, and raised more than US$700 million from resulting in a $10 billion valuation at its peak in 2013 and 2014. The company claimed that it had devised blood tests that required very small amounts of blood and that could be performed rapidly and accurately, all using compact automated devices which the company had developed. These claims were later proven to be false, and Elizabeth Holmes is in jail.

The bottom line is: *for your own sake, you should not trust mail-order, DIY tests.* Even then, find out what laboratory your tests are going to and what their quality control standards are.

Omics

The "omics" started in the 1980s with genomics, the study of the genome, an organism's entire complement of DNA. After that came proteomics, the study of proteins, lipidomics, which focus on fats, then microbiomics, which deals with the bacteria, viruses, and fungi that reside in and on our body.

These, and more, provided lines of investigation into health issues, known as 'Deep Phenotyping', to try and find the causes of cancer, heart disease, allergies, Parkinson's Disease, addiction, and more.

Ageotypes

But then, the omics have been applied to aging, as all of our parts are susceptible to the ravages of time. However, some of our 'parts' age more quickly than others. Which parts fail first differ from individual to individual.

Studies by Michael Snyder, a geneticist at Stanford University in California, has identified 608 molecules, genes, and microbial species that changed significantly as the studied people aged. Many were already known biomarkers of aging, but many weren't and revealed that people aged in one of four distinct organs or systems—the kidneys, liver, immune system, and general metabolism.

But not everybody showed the same pattern of change. Most aged along all four trajectories at once, but with one or two predominating.

Snyder dubbed these four broad categories ageotypes.

The principal way in which an individual is aging is their "ageotype". The oldest part of your body may be dragging the rest of it down, but by working out your ageotype, you might be able to target it to live healthier for longer.

Gene Studies[413]

A study shows that screening every single 30-year-old in the United States for three particular genetic conditions may not only save lives but be reasonably cost-effective.

413 Guzauskas, G. F., Garbett, S., Zhou, Z. *et al.* 2023, "Population Genomic Screening for Three Common Hereditary Conditions A Cost-Effectiveness Analysis", *Annals of Internal Medicine*, Vol. 176, No. 5, https://doi.org/10.7326/M22-0846

Getting your genome sequenced is a double-edged sword. Of course, there is the potential for substantial benefit; finding certain mutations allows for definitive therapy before it's too late. That said, there are genetic diseases without a cure and without a treatment. Knowing about that destiny may do more harm than good.

Three conditions are described by the CDC as "Tier 1" conditions, genetic syndromes with a significant impact on life expectancy that also have definitive, effective therapies.

These include mutations like BRCA1/2, associated with a high risk for breast and *ovarian cancer*, mutations associated with *Lynch syndrome,* which confer an elevated risk for colon cancer, and mutations associated with *familial hypercholesterolemia*, which confer elevated risk for cardiovascular events.

In each of these cases, there is clear evidence that early intervention can save lives. Individuals at high risk for breast and ovarian cancer can get a prophylactic mastectomy and (maybe) salpingo-oophorectomy. Those with Lynch syndrome can get more frequent screening for colon cancer and a polypectomy, and those with familial hypercholesterolemia can get aggressive lipid-lowering therapy.

SECTION K

RÉSUMÉ: TO LIVE LONGER

1. Choose your parents.
2. Be female.
3. Be facially attractive.
4. BLEDS: Blood Pressure, Lipids, Exercise, Diet, Smoking
5. Avoid life-shortening factors:
    a. High-risk behaviours
        i. Smoking
        ii. Fast food—anything packaged.
        iii. Sunburn
        iv. Pollution
        v. Driving
        vi. Drugs
        vii. Alcohol
        viii. >60, avoid heat, no solo activities, heights
        ix. carry a phone/smart-watch, hold the rails
        x. Get a wrist/portable Blood Pressure machine
    b. Constant stress
6. Get basic pathology/medical screen (F/CBC, MBA, Lipids, Pap, Mammogram, ?PSA)
7. Know the priority order of fatal illness for your age and screen for them i.e Predictive Analysis

8. Be happy:
    a. 'Yin-yang' partner
    b. Regular support network—family/friends
    c. Move on. Avoid nasty people.
    d. Laugh. Get a dog/meditate/relax/take breaks.
    e. Don't retire if you enjoy your job or, if you retire, ensure social activity
    f. Have an Artistic Activity
9. 3Ps (Projects, Purpose, Participate)
10. Financial Security-Planning: Save and invest 10% of your salary
11. Keep fit
    a. Exercise daily: Stretch; walk, fast, use green spaces, garden, take stairs, play tennis
    b. Don't sit: Vigorous bouts of activity lasting three to five minutes >22 minutes in total
    c. Lift heavy objects like weights and groceries
    d. Stay lean. 'The lean live longest'.
12. Diet
    a. Fresh food (Newtrition-Longevity Diet)
    b. No processed foods
    c. Reduce calories by 12% or more
    d. Drink coffee – no more than 3 cups a day
13. Education. Use your brain.
14. Any illness or injury
    a. "Get it seen; get it diagnosed; get it fixed."
    b. Minimise medications.
    c. Blood tests/dentist/vaccinate/hygiene.
15. "Moderation in all things".
16. Resilience
17. Medicines
    a. Statins
    b. GLP-1 agonists
    c. Metformin
    d. ?Rapamycin

SECTION L

CONCLUSION

We are at the gate or start of potential major changes to our health and lifespans, with the identification of growth genes and pathways common to many life-forms.

These growth pathways, however, have evolved over billions of years and are incredibly complex. It is a very attractive suggestion that there is one master regulator, mTOR, which senses our intake of amino acids and helps us grow, anabolism, or clears the degradation products of catabolism.

Time will tell.

The advocates point out that such an approach is primary or basic, whereas treating illnesses or abnormalities, like high cholesterol, secondary.

This may well be so, but our modern lifestyles have helped create these illnesses, and it would be reasonable to address these, too—and, of course, any resultant abnormalities or illnesses, while we wait.

Nutrition is a new science created in WW2 then abandoned by Oxford University, as it was thought to have been completed, and those scientists were snapped up by the new fast-food industry, who now effectively control what we eat. In the

USA, however, Ancel Keys, who pioneered the K-Rations, the minimum food needed for troop survival, promoted the Mediterranean diet. At the same time, John Yudkin, in London, thought sugar was the culprit for what was, and still is, our greatest killer—heart disease. Both were right.

To me, it is no coincidence that the pandemic of obesity and Type 2 Diabetes (T2D) shadows this introduction of fast and ultra-processed delicious, synthetic foods, which are cheaper than fresh foods and available 24/7. But, of course, our increasingly sedentary lifestyles and labour-saving devices contribute.

What *Live Longer* contends is that humans evolved to be opportunistic omnivores. To survive, we had to eat anything and everything, unlike most other animals, but our choices were restricted by seasons, famines, paucity of game and so on. They were also varied, such that this variety supplied the essential 13 vitamins we need but also the 5,000(+) micronutrients required. We also had to walk, run, and live in a tight-knit tribe that offered mutual support.

We are living longer, but this is mainly due to improved public health measures such as pure water, better sewerage, and hygiene—especially at birth.

Fast food is cheap(er), available 24 hours a day, seven days a week (as are heart attacks), while the cleanest coronary arteries in the world belong to meat-eating Bolivian hunter-gatherers the Tsmaine.

Obviously, we are not about to mimic their running through the jungle to spear the occasional lean monkey while eating berries, fruits, roots, and the odd fish… but at least we should be made aware of these facts.

While rapamycin may well promote longevity, our present lifestyle of excess fast-foods, sedentary behaviour, and increasing loneliness will still see the onslaught of obesity, Type 2 Diabetes, heart attacks, and cancers continue to increase.

And, while we wait, I don't think rapamycin is going to lower your cholesterol or provide the roughage/fiber that seems to help prevent colon cancer.

Live Longer's approach results from actually seeing patients and logically prioritising what kills or disables them to avoid, prevent, or treat illnesses.

Obviously, prevention is the desired objective, but the forces against us are incredible—and very, very well-funded.

However, it would seem that AI will have a profound beneficial effect, helping to diagnose illnesses incredibly early and making them preventable or curable.

It is, or will be, so much easier to just take a pill, even to mimic exercise. In the meantime…

Then again: "The doctor of the future will give no medicine but will interest his patients in the care of the human frame, in diet and in the cause and prevention of disease." Thomas Edison 1903.

STOP PRESS

The following extracts were able to be tagged on after *Live Longer* went to the publisher. Only those that are helpful and practical are included.

Healthy Lifestyle and the Likelihood of Becoming a Centenarian

Individuals aged 80 years or older were evaluated, those with the highest healthy lifestyle score (constructed from smoking, exercise, and dietary diversity) had a significantly higher likelihood of becoming a centenarian, compared with those with the least healthy lifestyle behaviors. Adhering to a healthy lifestyle appears to be important even at late ages.[414]

Heart disease and stroke

Heart disease and stroke claimed more lives in the U.S. in 2021 than all forms of cancer and chronic lower respiratory disease combined. No matter what your actual age is, better heart-healthy behaviors and managing heart disease risk factors were associated

414 Li Y, Wang K, Jigeer G, *et al.* 2024, "Healthy Lifestyle and the Likelihood of Becoming a Centenarian", JAMA Network Open, Vol. 7, No. 6, https://doi.org/10.1001/jamanetworkopen.2024.17931.

with a younger biological age and a lower risk of heart disease and stroke, death from heart disease and stroke and death from any cause.

The American Heart Association's Life's Essential 8 heart disease and stroke health factors:

1. eat healthy foods;
2. be more active;
3. quit tobacco;
4. get healthy sleep;
5. manage weight;
6. maintain healthy cholesterol, blood sugar and blood pressure levels;
7. using a composite of four behavioral measures (dietary intake, physical activity, hours slept per night and smoking status); and
8. four clinical measurements (body mass index, cholesterol, blood sugar and blood pressure).

Increases in an individual's Life's Essential 8 score, the risk of developing cardiovascular disease for the first time could be reduced by about 35%, death from cardiovascular disease, by 36% and death from any cause was reduced by 29%. In people with a genetic risk profile making them more likely to have an accelerated biological age, the Life's Essential 8 score had a larger impact on outcomes potentially via DNA methylation, i.e., DNA methylation accounted for 39%, 39%, and 78% reduction in the risk of cardiovascular disease, cardiovascular death and all-cause death, respectively.[415]

415 Carbonneau, M., Li, Y., Prescott, B. *et al.* 2024, "Epigenetic Age Mediates the Association of Life's Essential 8 With Cardiovascular Disease and Mortality", *Journal of the American Heart Association*, Vol. 13, No. 11, https://doi.org/10.1161/JAHA.123.032743.

Home test reveals the risk of heart attack in five minutes

A self-report tool has been developed with a good-to-excellent discriminative ability that identifies individuals with moderate to severe coronary atherosclerosis. It can be executed from home and has a similar performance to a clinical tool requiring a clinical visit involving blood tests and physical examination and could serve as an initial step toward a cost-effective screening program to identify high-risk individuals or used to identify individuals who would benefit from further risk refinement by cardiac imaging.[416]

Blood Pressure

For 8 decades, cardiovascular disease (CVD) has been the leading cause of death in the US and most other economically developed countries. More than 7 decades ago, hypertension was recognized as the leading risk factor for heart disease and stroke. For 5 decades, it has been clear that reducing blood pressure (BP) in patients with hypertension reduces the risk of CVD in individuals and in whole populations. However, despite the availability of inexpensive, well-tolerated antihypertensive medications and the overwhelming evidence that lowering of BP levels reduces CVD risk, BP control rates among people in the US have decreased in the past decade rather than shown improvement.[417]

---

416 Bergström, G., Hagberg, E., Björnson, E. *et al.* 2024, "Self-Report Tool for Identification of Individuals With Coronary Atherosclerosis: The Swedish CardioPulmonary BioImage Study", *Journal of the American Heart Association*, online prepublication, https://doi.org/10.1161/JAHA.124.034603.

417 Jones, D. W. 2024, "A Pathway to Better Blood Pressure Control", *JAMA Cardiology*, 18 June, https://doi.org/10.1001/jamacardio.2024.1463.

Child Heart Risks

It has been found that a third of heart attacks, which kills most of us, start in childhood. It may be a good measure to do a kid's Blood and Biochemical screen and ApoB aged 11 and again at 17 if it was normal.

Studies beginning in childhood have shown that children exposed to cardiovascular risk factors are prone to develop preclinical atherosclerosis and cardiovascular events in adulthood. The development of atherosclerosis would probably be prevented by maintaining the concentration of apolipoprotein B-containing lipoproteins in the plasma towards their physiological range from an early age.[418]

Physical performance

Physical performance significantly correlates with increased longevity in individuals aged over 80 years. Participants were aged < 85 years at the time of enrollment (mean age, 82 years). Short Physical Performance Battery (SPPB) tested balance, gait speed, and leg strength based on the ability to stand from a seated position in a chair. Participants were classified as having severe, moderate, mild, or no functional impairment. Higher scores on the SPPB and faster gait speed were linked to a lower risk for mortality before that age. The average gait speed was 0.88 m/s among participants who lived to 95 years of age and 0.78 m/s for those who died at younger ages. About 21% of the participants lived to 95 years of age.[419]

---

418 Raitakari, O., Pahkala, K. & Magnussen, C. G. 2022, "Prevention of atherosclerosis from childhood", *Nature Reviews Cardiology*, Vol. 19, No. 8, pp. 543-554, https://doi.org/10.1038/s41569-021-00647-9.

419 Remaly, J. 2024, "Three Keys to Longevity in Older Adults?", *Medscape,* 21 May.

Jogging

In 2015, researchers in Copenhagen made a surprising discovery when they studied the long-term mortality of light, moderate and strenuous joggers, as well as non-runners. The light and moderate joggers had a lower mortality rate than either the non-runners or the strenuous runners. The strenuous joggers had a mortality rate that wasn't statistically different to the non-runners.[420]

Physical Activity

Higher daily duration of physical activity was consistently associated with lower risk of death, regardless of total sedentary time. For example, the team reported an additional ten minutes of moderate to vigorous physical activity each day could lower mortality risk by up to 15 percent for people who were sedentary less than 10.5 hours a day. For those considered highly sedentary (10.5 hours a day or more), an additional ten minutes lowered mortality risk by up to 35 percent. Even short bouts of exercise can have these positive effects. In this study, the 22 minutes wasn't necessarily done all at once.[421]

TV and Exercise

Researchers defined healthy aging as living to at least 70 years and being healthy across at least four categories, including having no major chronic disease, and no issues with subjective memory, physical health, and mental health. For every two hours of sitting

420 *BBC Science Focus Magazine*, 16 April 2024

421 Sagelv, E. H., Hopstock, L. A., Morseth, B. *et al.* 2023, "Device-measured physical activity, sedentary time, and risk of all-cause mortality: an individual participant data analysis of four prospective cohort studies", *British Journal of Sports Medicine*, Vol. 57, No. 22, pp. 1457-1463, https://doi.org/10.1136/bjsports-2022-106568.

to watch TV, study participants had a 12% drop in the odds that they would age in a healthy way. However, the study also found that having two additional hours of light physical activity at work increased the chances of healthy aging by 6%. People who swapped one hour of sitting and watching TV with light physical activity also were more likely to age in a healthy way.[422]

Evenings Best

Moderate to vigorous aerobic physical activity performed in the evening is associated with the lowest risk for mortality, cardiovascular disease (CVD), and microvascular disease (MVD) in adults with obesity, including those with type 2 diabetes (T2D).[423]

Education and Longevity

Each 4.20 years of additional educational attainment were causally associated with a 3.23-year-longer parental lifespan independently of income and occupation and were causally associated with 30-59% higher odds of self-longevity, suggesting that education was the primary determinant. By contrast, each one-standard-deviation-higher income and one-point-higher occupation was causally associated with 3.06-year-longer and 1.29-year-longer parental lifespans, respectively, but not independently of the other socio-economic indicators. Cigarettes per day, body mass index, waist-to-hip ratio, hypertension, coronary heart disease, myocardial infarction, stroke, Alzheimer's

422 Shi, H., Hu, F. B., Huang, T. *et al.* 2024, "Sedentary Behaviors, Light-Intensity Physical Activity, and Healthy Aging", *JAMA Network Open*, Vol. 7, No. 6, https://doi.org/10.1001/jamanetworkopen.2024.16300.

423 Talwadekar, M. 2024, "Is Nighttime the Best Time for Exercise?" *Medscape*, 25 April.

disease, type 2 diabetes, heart failure and lung cancer individually played substantial mediating roles (proportion mediated, >10%) in the effect of education on specific longevity outcomes.[424]

Vitamins

With as many as 1 in 3 US adults using multivitamin supplements, the question as to whether these supplements reduce mortality is an important public health issue. Drawing on 3 large cohorts including 390,124 participants and more than 20 years of follow-up data, the study by Loftfield and colleagues investigated the association between multivitamin use and mortality, while carefully controlling for potential confounders. Confirming the mostly negative results of prior studies, multivitamin supplementation was not associated with a mortality benefit. On the contrary, mortality risk was 4% higher among multivitamin users, compared with nonusers, in the initial years of follow-up.[425]

But in older individuals, multivitamin supplementation is associated with improved memory and slowed cognitive decline.[426]

---

424 Ye, C. J., Kong, L. J., Wang, Y. Y. 2023, "Mendelian randomization evidence for the causal effects of socio-economic inequality on human longevity among Europeans", *Nature Human Behaviour*, Vol. 7, No. 8, pp. 1357-1370, https://doi.org/10.1038/s41562-023-01646-1.

425 Loftfield, E., O'Connell, C. P., Abnet, C. C. *et al.* 2024, "Multivitamin Use and Mortality Risk in 3 Prospective US Cohorts", *JAMA Network Open*, Vol. 7, No. 6, https://doi.org/10.1001/jamanetworkopen.2024.18729.

426 Vyas, C. M., Manson, J. E., Sesso, H. D. *et al.* 2023, "Effect of multivitamin-mineral supplementation versus placebo on cognitive function: results from the clinic subcohort of the COcoa Supplement and Multivitamin Outcomes Study (COSMOS) randomized clinical trial and meta-analysis of 3 cognitive studies within COSMOS", *The American Journal of Clinical Nutrition*, Vol. 119, No. 3, pp. 692-701, https://doi.org/10.1016/j.ajcnut.2023.12.011.

Recommended daily allowance of vitamin D

Healthy adults under the age of 75 are unlikely to benefit from taking more than the daily intake of vitamin D recommended by the Institutes of Medicine (IOM) and do not require testing for vitamin D levels. For children, pregnant people, adults older than 75 years and adults with high-risk prediabetes, the guideline recommends vitamin D higher than the IOM recommended daily allowance.[427]

New Endocrine Society guidelines call for limiting vitamin D supplementation beyond the daily recommended intake to specific risk groups and advises against routine 25-hydroxyvitamin D [25(OH)D] testing in healthy individuals.[428]

Calorie Restriction

The Comprehensive Assessment of Long-term Effects of Reducing Intake of Energy (CALERIE) study of caloric restriction suggests that 2 years of mild caloric restriction significantly reduces biological age.[429]

There are many reasons why caloric restriction may extend human lifespans. One primary mechanism through which life is extended relates to metabolism in a cell. When energy is consumed within a cell, waste products from that process cause oxidative stress that can damage DNA and otherwise break down

427 Demay, M. B., Pitta, A. G., Bikle, D. D. *et al.* 2024, "Vitamin D for the Prevention of Disease: An Endocrine Society Clinical Practice Guideline", *The Journal of Clinical Endocrinology & Metabolism*, https://doi.org/10.1210/clinem/dgae290.

428 Tucker, M. E. 2024, "'Don't Screen' for Vitamin D: New Endo Society Guideline", *Medscape*, 3 June.

429 Fong, S., Pabis, K., Latumalea, D. *et al.* 2024, "Principal component-based clinical aging clocks identify signatures of healthy aging and targets for clinical intervention", *Nature Aging*, Vol. 243, https://doi.org/10.1038/s43587-024-00646-8.

the cell. When a person's cells consume less energy due to caloric restriction, however, there are fewer waste products, and the cell does not break down as quickly.[430]

Coffee

Non-coffee drinkers who sat six hours or more per day were 1.58 times more likely to die of all causes than coffee drinkers sitting for less than six hours per day, indicating that the association of sedentary with increased mortality from all-cause and CVD was only observed among adults with no coffee consumption but not among those who had coffee intake.[431]

Teeth Cleaning

The assumption has been that scaling and polishing can prevent gingivitis and periodontitis, thus potentially preventing tooth loss, pain, and mobility. However, to our knowledge there are no published clinical trials assessing these outcomes.[432]

Dementia: Alzheimer's

Alzheimer's pathology, which we consider represents Alzheimer's disease, begins to appear in the brain at least 15 to 20 years prior to the onset of symptoms. To be scientifically accurate, we

430 Hastings, W. J., Ye, Q., Wolf, S. E. *et al.* 2024, "Effect of long-term caloric restriction on telomere length in healthy adults: CALERIE™ 2 trial analysis", *Aging Cell,* Vol. 23, No. 6, https://doi.org/10.1111/acel.14149.

431 Zhou, H., Nie, J., Cao, Y. *et al.* 2024, "Association of daily sitting time and coffee consumption with the risk of all-cause and cardiovascular disease mortality among US adults", *BMC Public Health,* Vol. 24, p. 1069, https://doi.org/10.1186/s12889-024-18515-9.

432 Hujoel, P. P. 2024, "Endpoints in periodontal trials: the need for an evidence-based research approach", *Periodontol 2000,* Vol. 36, No. 1, pp. 196-204, https://doi.org/10.1111/j.1600-0757.2004.03681.x.

therefore define high-quality biomarker evidence of Alzheimer's pathology to represent Alzheimer's disease, including in people who are presently asymptomatic.[433]

Dementia test can predict illness nine years before symptoms

A brain scan can predict whether people are likely to develop dementia as much as nine years before they receive a conventional diagnosis, new research has found. The test, which is 80 per cent effective, was developed by looking at MRI scans of 81 people who were later diagnosed with dementia, as well as 21 with a diagnosis. By comparing them with people of a similar age who didn't develop dementia, researchers were able to pinpoint a telltale alteration in their brain function.[434]

Predicting Dementia

In this study, tau-PET showed the best performance as a stand-alone marker to predict progression to dementia among individuals with MCI. This suggests that, for prognostic purposes in MCI, a tau PET scan may be the best currently available neuroimaging marker.[435]

433 Jack, C. R., Andrews, J. S., Beach, T. G. *et al.* 2024, "Revised criteria for diagnosis and staging of Alzheimer's disease: Alzheimer's Association Workgroup", *Alzheimer's & Dementia*, online prepublication, https://doi.org/10.1002/alz.13859.

434 Whipple, T. 2024, "Dementia test can predict illness nine years before symptoms", *The Times of London*, 6 June.

435 Groot, C., Smith, R., Collij, L. E. *et al.* 2024, "Tau Positron Emission Tomography for Predicting Dementia in Individuals With Mild Cognitive Impairment", *JAMA Neurology*, online prepublication, https://doi.org/10.1001/jamaneurol.2024.1612.

Alzheimer's and Vaccinations

Accumulating evidence suggests that several vaccinations, including Tdap/Td, HZ, and pneumococcal, are associated with a reduced risk for developing AD and Alzheimer's disease related dementias.[436]

People who have had a recent vaccine against tetanus appear to be less likely to develop Parkinson's disease, suggesting that the bacterial infection is involved in the condition.[437]

Parkinson's

The risk of developing Parkinson's increased two-fold in people >50 with anxiety.[438]

Loneliness

Chronic loneliness was associated with higher stroke risk independent of depressive symptoms or social isolation in a nationally representative cohort of older U.S. adults independent of social isolation but not depressive symptoms. Only individuals with consistently high loneliness over time (vs consistently low)

---

436 Harris, K., Ling, Y., Bukhbinder, A. S. *et al.* 2023, "The Impact of Routine Vaccinations on Alzheimer's Disease Risk in Persons 65 Years and Older: A Claims-Based Cohort Study using Propensity Score Matching", *Journal of Alzheimer's Disease,* Vol. 95, No. 2, pp. 703-718, https://doi.org/org/10.3233/JAD-221231.

437 Israel, A., Magen, E., Merzon, E. *et al.* 2024, "Anti-tetanus vaccination is associated with reduced occurrence and slower progression of Parkinson's disease", *MedRxiv,* online prepublication, https://doi.org/10.1101/2024.05.03.24306800.

438 Bazo-Alvarez, J. C., Nimmons D., Walters, K. *et al.* 2024, "Risk of Parkinson's disease in people aged ≥50 years with new-onset anxiety: a retrospective cohort study in UK primary care", *British Journal of General Practice,* Vol. 74, No. 744, https://doi.org/10.3399/BJGP.2023.0423.

had 56% significantly higher risk of incident stroke, independent of social isolation and depressive symptoms.[439]

Weight Loss

Endoscopic sleeve gastroplasty sustained greater weight loss over 5 years vs semaglutide (BMI of 31.7 vs 33.0). To achieve nondominance, the annual price of semaglutide, currently $13,618, would need to be $3591. This study suggests that ESG is cost saving compared with semaglutide in the treatment of class II obesity. On price threshold analyses, a 3-fold decrease in the price of semaglutide is needed to achieve nondominance.[440]

Cancer

Breast cancer blood test '100% accurate' at spotting whether disease willreturn. A revolutionary blood test is able to detect if breast cancer will return years before it shows up on a scan, meaning women could start treatment before the disease becomes incurable. The test looks for tiny fragments of tumour DNA in the bloodstream and was found to be 100 per cent accurate at predicting which patients would relapse after surgery.

Prostate cancer screening is currently based on prostate-specific antigen (PSA) testing followed by a detailed multiparametric magnetic resonance imaging (mpMRI) if the PSA is raised. But we know that PSA testing misses some cancers and throws up lots of false alarms, so is it time to ditch it? This decision model analysis used lifetime data from US men aged

---

439 Soh, Y., Kawachi, I., Kubzansky, L. D. *et al.* 2024, "Chronic loneliness and the risk of incident stroke in middle and late adulthood: a longitudinal cohort study of U.S. older adults", *eClinicalMedicine*, online prepublication, https://doi.org/10.1016/j.eclinm.2024.102639.

440 Haseeb, M., Chhatwal, J., Xiao, J. *et al.* 2024, "Semaglutide vs Endoscopic Sleeve Gastroplasty for Weight Loss", *JAMA Network Open*, Vol. 7, No. 4, https://doi.org/10.1001/jamanetworkopen.2024.6221.

over 55 years with no prior screening or diagnosis of prostate cancer to compare biennial PSA testing (with or without second-line mpMRI if PSA >4 µg/L) with biparametric MRI (bpMRI) as a screening test (with MRI guided biopsy or ultrasound as a secondary test). Biparametric MRI is quicker than mpMRI and doesn't involve an injection of dye which some people react badly to. Compared with PSA testing, bpMRI prevented 2-3 deaths from prostate cancer and added 4-11 days of life. The disadvantage of bpMRI was a marked increase in the number of biopsies (1506 to 4174) and overdiagnosis (38 to 124). The current practice of first-line PSA testing therefore remains the more cost effective option. [441]

Urine Test Accurately Detected High-Grade Prostate Cancer

Researchers say use of the test could substantially reduce biopsies.

Noise

Airplane noise exposure may increase risk of chronic disease. A new study indicates that airplane noise may increase one's risk of developing cardiometabolic diseases, a cluster of conditions such as heart attack, stroke, diabetes, and hypertension. The study found that people who were exposed to airplane noise levels at 45 dB or more were more likely to have higher self-reported body mass index (BMI), with the highest BMI measures linked to aircraft noise levels at 55 dB or above.[442]

---

441 Gulati, R., Jiao, B., Al-Faouri, R. *et al.* 2024, "Lifetime Health and Economic Outcomes of Biparametric Magnetic Resonance Imaging as First-Line Screening for Prostate Cancer: A Decision Model Analysis", *Annals of Internal Medicine*, https://doi.org/10.7326/M23-1504.

442 Bozigar, M., Laden, F., Hart, J. E. *et al.* 2024, "Aircraft noise exposure and body mass index among female participants in two Nurses' Health Study prospective cohorts living around 90 airports in the United States", *Environment International*, Vol. 187, p. 108660, https://doi.org/10.1016/j.envint.2024.108660.

Ventilation and viruses

When a disease is airborne, there's no sensor that can track how many infectious aerosols are floating around us in real time but the amount of carbon dioxide in the air can act as a proxy. We exhale it when we breathe, so in spaces that aren't well-ventilated, it accumulates. The more CO_2 in the air, the more virus-friendly that air becomes.[443]

Statins

A meta-analysis by the Cholesterol Treatment Trialists' Collaboration using individual level data from 23 trials confirms that statin therapy increases the risk of diabetes. The explanation is that statins cause a small dose dependent upward shift in blood glucose levels. In people with baseline glycaemic markers that are close to the diagnostic threshold for diabetes, this is enough to tip them over the edge. However, any adverse effects from this small rise in glucose have already been accounted for in the estimates of reduced cardiovascular risk seen in these statin trials. So it's almost certainly nothing to worry about.[444]

What is Old Age

Middle-aged and older adults believe that old age begins later in life than their peers did decades ago. At age 64, the average

---

443 Haddrell, A., Oswin, H., Otero-Fernandez, M. *et al.* 2024, "Ambient carbon dioxide concentration correlates with SARS-CoV-2 aerostability and infection risk", *Nature Communications*, Vol. 15, https://doi.org/10.1038/s41467-024-47777-5.

444 Cholesterol Treatment Trialists' (CTT) Collaboration, 2024, "Effects of statin therapy on diagnoses of new-onset diabetes and worsening glycaemia in large-scale randomised blinded statin trials: an individual participant data meta-analysis", *Lancet Diabetes & Endocrinology*, Vol. 12, No. 5, pp. 306-319, https://doi.org/10.1016/S2213-8587(24)00040-8.

participant said old age started at 74.7. At age 74, they said old age started at 76.8. On average, the perceived onset of old age increased by about one year for every four to five years of actual aging.[445]

Master Control

The process of how genes change from birth to adulthood and into old age has been largely unknown It was previously thought to be a random process but the researchers have shown it is predictable and is the same in all cell types, regulated by a master controller AP-1. Master controller genes regulate which genes are turned on or off in each of our cells, making sure that each cell does its specific job, just as a conductor directs musicians to produce different sounds. The activity of the master regulator Activator Protein 1 or AP-1 was studied and it was found that it progressively activated adult genes, while the activity of 'early-life' genes involved in development were dialled down, and this process was shared across cell types.[446]

Alzheimer's APOE4 Benefit

In a 3-year randomized clinical trial, ω-3 polyunsaturated fatty acid treatment was safe and well-tolerated but failed to reach significant reductions in WML accumulation or neuronal integrity breakdown among all participants. However, neuronal

445 Wettstein, M., Park, R., Kornadt, A. E., Wurm, S., Ram, N., & Gerstorf, D. 2024, "Postponing old age: Evidence for historical change toward a later perceived onset of old age", *Psychology and Aging*, online prepublication, https://doi.org/10.1037/pag0000812.

446 Patrick, R., Naval-Sanchez M., Deshpande N. *et al.* 2024, "The activity of early-life gene regulatory elements is hijacked in aging through pervasive AP-1-linked chromatin opening", *Cell Metabolism*, online prepublication, https://doi.org/10.1016/j.cmet.2024.06.006.

integrity breakdown was reduced by ω-3 treatment in *APOE*E4* carriers, suggesting that this treatment may be beneficial for this specific group.[447]

Genes 5%

In most cases, your genes have less than five per cent to do with your risk of developing a particular disease.[448]

Coffee limit

Drinking more than three cups of coffee a day is linked to more rapid cognitive decline over time, results from a large study suggest.[449]

Multivitamins No Use

Among 390124 participants multivitamin use was not associated with a mortality benefit. Still, many US adults report using MV to maintain or improve health.[450]

---

447 Shinto, L. H., Murchison, C. F., Silbert, L. C. *et al.* 2024, "ω-3 PUFA for Secondary Prevention of White Matter Lesions and Neuronal Integrity Breakdown in Older Adults", *JAMA Network Open*, Vol. 7, No. 8, https://doi.org/10.1001/jamanetworkopen.2024.26872.

448 Patron, J., Serra-Cayuela, A., Han, B. *et al.* 2019, "Assessing the performance of genome-wide association studies for predicting disease risk", *PLOS ONE*, Vol. 14, No. 12, https://doi.org/10.1371/journal.pone.0220215.

449 Anderson, P. 2024, "Too Much Coffee Linked to Accelerated Cognitive Decline", *Medscape*, 1 August.

450 Loftfield, E., O'Connell, C. P., Abnet, C. C. *et al.* 2024, "Multivitamin Use and Mortality Risk in 3 Prospective US Cohorts", *JAMA Network Open*, Vol. 7, No. 6, https://doi.org/10.1001/jamanetworkopen.2024.18729.

Abdominal Pain Blood Tests

Common blood tests could improve cancer diagnosis for people with stomach pain or bloating

In the UK study sample, the researchers found that, among people aged 30 to 59 years with abdominal pain or bloating, anaemia, low albumin, raised platelets, abnormal ferritin, and increased inflammatory markers strongly predicted a risk of undiagnosed cancer.[451]

Newtrition and Biological Age

Researchers have found a link between following a diet that is rich in vitamins and minerals, especially one without much added sugar, and having a younger biological age at the cellular level.[452]

Malnourishment for those in Care

In the largest study of its kind ever carried out in Australia, researchers from Monash and Griffith universities revealed 40% of care residents are malnourished, and 6% of those are severely malnourished. [453]

---

451 Rafiq, M., Renzi, C., White, B. *et al.* 2024, "Predictive value of abnormal blood tests for detecting cancer in primary care patients with nonspecific abdominal symptoms: A population-based cohort study of 477,870 patients in England", *PLOS Medicine*, Vol. 21, No. 7, https://doi.org/10.1371/journal.pmed.1004426.

452 Chiu, D. T., Hamlat, E. J., Zhang, J. *et al.* 2024, "Essential Nutrients, Added Sugar Intake, and Epigenetic Age in Midlife Black and White Women", *JAMA Network Open*, Vol. 7, No. 7, https://doi.org/10.1001/jamanetworkopen.2024.22749.

453 O'Shea, M.-C., Bauer, J., Barrett, C. *et al.* 2024, "Malnutrition Prevalence in Australian Residential Aged Care Facilities: A Cross-Sectional Study" *Healthcare*, Vol. 12, No. 13, p. 1296, https://doi.org/10.3390/healthcare12131296.

Longevity and Artistic Endeavour

Arts activities combine multiple psychological, physical, social, and behavioural factors with an intrinsic aesthetic motivation to engage and could have a protective association with longevity in older adults. This association might be partly explained by differences in cognition, mental health, and physical activity among those who do and do not engage in the arts but remains even when the model is adjusted for these factors.[454]

Facial Attractiveness and Longevity

Attractiveness, based on independent ratings of high-school yearbook face photographs, may convey underlying health, and it systematically structures critical social stratification processes. At age 20, women in the least attractive sextile had a life expectancy nearly two years less than others'; among men in the least attractive sextile, it was nearly one year less. This finding remained robust to the inclusion of covariates describing high-school achievement, intelligence, family background, earnings as adults, as well as mental and physical health in middle adulthood.[455]

Green Spaces, Rivers and Less Coronary Artery Calcification

Proximity to green and blue spaces directly correlates to an indicator of better cardiovascular health, especially among certain races and socioeconomic groups. The researchers observed the

454 Fancourt, D. & Steptoe A. 2019, "The art of life and death: 14 year follow-up analyses of associations between arts engagement and mortality in the English Longitudinal Study of Ageing", *British Medial Journal*, Vol. 367, https://doi.org/10.1136/bmj.l6377.

455 Sheehan, C. M. & Hamermesh, D. S. 2024, "Looks and longevity: Do prettier people live longer?", *Social Science & Medicine*, Vol. 354, https://doi.org/10.1016/j.socscimed.2024.117076.

most significant impacts among Black individuals and people living in low-income areas. Long-term exposures to urban blue and green spaces from early to middle adulthood were associated with lower odds of having coronary artery calcification in middle adulthood.[456]

Lancet Commission on dementia

The 2024 update of the Lancet Commission on dementia provides new hopeful evidence about dementia prevention, intervention, and care, how reducing vascular damage (eg, by reducing smoking and treating high blood pressure) is likely to have contributed to a reduction in age-related dementia incidence. Evidence is increasing wrt less education, hearing loss, hypertension, smoking, obesity, depression, physical inactivity, diabetes, excessive alcohol consumption, traumatic brain injury [TBI], air pollution, and social isolation, untreated vision loss and high LDL cholesterol. The full article may be access\ed free of charge.[457]

---

456 Carnethon, M. R., Palaniappan, L. & Watson, K. 2024, "Working to Promote Health Equity: The Fourth Annual Disparities Issue", *Circulation*, Vol. 150, No. 3, pp. 169-170, https://doi.org/10.1161/CIRCULATIONAHA.124.070825.

457 Livingston, G., Huntley, J., Liu, K. Y. *et al.* 2024, "Dementia prevention, intervention, and care: 2024 report of the *Lancet* standing Commission", *The Lancet*, https://doi.org/10.1016/S0140-6736(24)01296-0.

SECTION M

ABBREVIATIONS/ INDEX

Abbreviations

APO	Apoprotein
BMJ	British Medical Journal
JAMA	Journal of the American Medical Association
NEJM	New England Journal of Medicine
BG	Blood Glucose
BMD	bone-mineral density
BMI	Body Mass Index
BMJ	British Medical Journal
BP	Blood Pressure
CA, Ca	Cancer
CAC	Cancer of the Colon
CAD	Coronary Artery Disease
CBC	Complete Blood Count
CDC	Centers for Disease Control and Prevention
cf	compared to / with
CHD	Coronary Heart Disease
CVD	Cardiovascular Disease
COPD	Chronic Obstructive Pulmonary Disease
DHA	Docosahexaenoic acid
EAR	Estiamted Average Requirement

EPA	Eicosapentaenoic acid
EPIC	European Prospective Investigation into Cancer and Nutrition
EVOO	Extra Virgin Olive Oil
ECG/EKG	Electrocardiogram
FBC	Full Blood Count
FDA	Federal Drug Administration
FV	Fruit and Vegetables
GI(T)	Gastro Intestinal (Tract)
HEI	Healthy Eating Index
HFCS	High Fructose Corn Syrup
H/L DL	High- or Low-Density Cholesterol
HT	Hypertension – raised BP
IHD	Ischemic Heart Disease – essentially the same as CAD
IARC	International Agency for Research on Cancer
IF	Intermittent fasting
JAMA	Journal of the American Medical Association
MD	Mediterranean Diet
MIND	Mediterranean-DASH Intervention for Neurodegenerative Delay.
MUFA	Monounsaturated Fatty Acid
MVA/RTA	Motor Vehicle/Road Traffic Accidents
n-3 LCPUFAs	Long Chain Polyunsaturated Fatty Acids
NHANES	National Health and Nutrition Examination Survey
NHS	National Health Scheme – the UK Government Health system

OO	Olive Oil
PAH	Polycyclic aromatic hydrocarbons
PCB	Polychlorinated biphenyls
PFA	Perfluoroalkylated substances
POPs	Persistent organic pollutants
PUFA	Polyunsaturated Fatty Acid
QOL	Quality of Life
RDA	Recommended daily Allowance
RCT	Random Controlled Trial/Test
RTA	Road Traffic Accident
SCS	Seven Countries Study
SFA	Saturated Fatty Acids
SSB	sugar-sweetened beverages
TF(A)	Trans fats (Acid)
TMD	Traditional Mediterranean Diet
WHO	World Health Organization

Index

D

E

F

G

H

N

Made in the USA
Monee, IL
04 November 2026

67385327R00351